# Management of the Patient at High Risk for Breast Cancer

Nora M. Hansen
Editor

# Management of the Patient at High Risk for Breast Cancer

Springer

*Editor*
Nora M. Hansen
Feinberg School of Medicine
Division of Breast Surgery
Northwestern University
Chicago, IL, USA

ISBN 978-1-4614-5890-6 ISBN 978-1-4614-5891-3(eBook)
DOI 10.1007/978-1-4614-5891-3
Springer New York Heidelberg Dordrecht London

Library of Congress Control Number: 2012954563



Printed on acid-free paper

Springer is part of Springer Science+Business Media (www.springer.com)

# Preface and Acknowledgements

This book *Management of the Patient at High Risk for Breast Cancer* is designed to meet the needs of physicians involved in the care of patients who are at increased risk for developing breast cancer. The goal is to provide up-to-date and evidence-based information on all aspects of care for those who are at an increased risk for developing breast cancer. I am extremely grateful to all of the contributing authors for their time and their expertise, and I thank them for their contributions. I would also like to thank my assistant Burton Korman for all the hard work he put into making this book become a reality. I would especially like to thank Maria Smilios, my developmental editor, who worked tirelessly on this project and kept the project moving forward.

I believe as physicians we cannot underestimate the psychological stress that patients experience when they realize that they are at an increased risk for developing breast cancer. Our goal is to provide our patients with the necessary information which will allow them to make informed decisions about either surveillance of their breasts or interventions to reduce their risk from either a medical or a surgical approach. I hope that the information in this book will serve as a strong foundation of knowledge in order to better care for this group of patients.

I would like to dedicate this book to my parents who have always supported me in everything I do. My late father, Dr. Gerard Hansen, who was a practicing obstetrician and gynecologist would have been thrilled to see this book become a reality. My mother, Peggy Hansen, has been a true inspiration to me and her strength, courage, and support have helped shape me into the person I have become.

Chicago, IL, USA　　　　Nora M. Hansen MD

# Contents

# Contributors

**Jennifer E. Cheesborough, MD** Division of Plastic and Reconstructive Surgery, Northwestern Memorial Hospital, Chicago, IL, USA

**Brian Drohan, PhD** Department of Surgical Oncology, Avon Comprehensive Breast Evaluation Center, Massachusetts General Hospital, Boston, MA, USA

**Paula Grabler, MD** Department of Radiology, Northwestern Memorial Hospital, Chicago, IL, USA

**Christine M. Gresik, MD** Lynn Sage Comprehensive Breast Center, Feinberg School of Medicine of Northwestern University, IL, USA

**Nora M. Hansen, MD** Feinberg School of Medicine, Northwestern University, Chicago, IL, USA

**Ashley N. Hardy, MD** Department of Surgery, Northwestern Memorial Hospital, Chicago, IL, USA

**Kevin S. Hughes, MD, FACS** Department of Surgical Oncology, Avon Comprehensive Breast Evaluation Center, Massachusetts General Hospital, Boston, MA, USA

**Jacqueline S. Jeruss, MD, PhD** Department of Surgery, Northwestern Memorial Hospital, Chicago, IL, USA

**Virginia Kaklamani, MD, DSc** Division Hematology/Oncology, Northwestern University, Chicago, IL, USA

**Seema A. Khan, MD** Robert H. Lurie Comprehensive Cancer Center, Feinberg School of Medicine of Northwestern University, Chicago, IL, USA

**John Y.S. Kim, MD** Division of Plastic and Reconstructive Surgery, Northwestern Memorial Hospital, Chicago, IL, USA

**Swati A. Kulkarni, MD** Department of Surgery, The University of Chicago Medical Center, Chicago, IL, USA

**Thomas J. Lawton, MD** Pacific Breast Pathology Medical Corporation, Novato, CA, USA

**Susan M. Love, MD, MBA, FACS** Dr. Susan Love Research Foundation, Santa Monica, CA, USA

**Megan E. Miller, MD** Department of Surgery, University of Chicago Medical Center, Chicago, IL, USA

**Sarah M. Nielsen, MS, CGC** Department of Hematology/Oncology, The University of Chicago Medical Center, Chicago, IL, USA

**Erin Neuschler, MD** Department of Breast Imaging, Northwestern Memorial Hospital, Chicago, IL, USA

**Timothy Pearman, PhD** Supportive Oncology, Robert H. Lurie Comprehensive Cancer Center of Northwestern University, Chicago, IL, USA

Department of Medical Social Sciences, Department of Psychiatry & Behavioral Sciences, Northwestern University Feinberg School of Medicine, Chicago, IL, USA

**Vinay Rawlani, MD** Division of Plastic and Reconstructive Surgery, Northwestern Memorial Hospital, Chicago, IL, USA

**Constance Roche, BSN, MSN, ANP-BC, ONC, APNG** Department of Surgical Oncology, Avon Comprehensive Breast Evaluation Center, Massachusetts General Hospital, Boston, MA, USA

**Lee P. Shulman, MD** Division of Clinical Genetics, Feinberg School of Medicine of Northwestern University, Chicago, IL, USA

Northwestern Ovarian Cancer Early Detection and Prevention Program, Feinberg School of Medicine of Northwestern University, Chicago, IL, USA

Cancer Genetics Program, Robert S. Lurie Comprehensive Cancer Center, Feinberg School of Medicine of Northwestern University, Chicago, IL, USA

Department of Obstetrics and Gynecology, Prentice Women's Hospital, Northwestern Memorial Hospital, Chicago, IL, USA

**Lisa Renee-Palko Spiguel, MD** McGaw Medical Center, Feinberg School of Medicine, Northwestern University, Chicago, IL, USA

**Elizabeth Tarasewicz, BS** Department of Surgery, Northwestern Memorial Hospital, Chicago, IL, USA

**Scott M. Weissman, MS, CGC** NorthShore University HealthSystem, Center for Medical Genetics, Evanston, IL, USA

# 1 Identifying Women at High Risk of Breast Cancer: Understanding the Risk Models

Scott M. Weissman

## Introduction

Breast cancer risk assessment is increasingly becoming part of routine medical care. For women who have not been affected with breast cancer, identifying those that have personal and/or family history risk factors increasing their risk can benefit from increased screening with breast MRI, chemoprevention with tamoxifen, and/or prophylactic bilateral mastectomy, especially in women found to have a hereditary susceptibility to breast cancer [1–5]. Similarly, women who have already been affected with breast cancer can benefit in the same fashion for the same reasons with respect to developing an ipsi- or contralateral tumor, in addition to the potential of recognizing other sites in the body that may be at increased risk for tumor development (e.g., ovarian, gastric, endometrium). One integral tool in assessing breast cancer risk is the incorporation of one or more breast cancer risk models.

There are two main types of breast cancer risk models that can be employed for assessing risk: models that quantify a woman's breast cancer risk (either as a 5-year, 10-year, or lifetime risk) and models that provide a probability that a woman harbors a mutation in a gene known to cause a hereditary cancer predisposition syndrome; models have been created for hereditary breast and ovarian cancer syndrome (i.e., the *BRCA1* and *BRCA2* genes) and Cowden syndrome (*PTEN* gene). These different model types can be further subdivided into two broad categories: empirical and genetic models [6, 7]. Empirical breast cancer risk models use a number of variables, typically a combination of personal and/or family history factors, and the effect of each variable is then combined using a statistical analysis, commonly logistic regression, to produce risk estimates. Empirical models do not take into account genetic factors like mode of inheritance, mutation prevalence, or penetrance (i.e., the chance of developing cancer if someone carries a gene mutation). Further, empirical models cannot take into account exact family structure or unaffected individuals to adjust risks. Genetic models, as discussed by Amir and colleagues, make explicit assumptions about the number of susceptibility genes involved, the mutation frequencies in the general population, and the cancer risks conferred by mutations in the genes [7]. Genetic models use pedigree analysis in the form of Bayesian and segregation analysis which are based on exact family relationships and ages (current, age at cancer diagnosis, or age at death); this is the main advantage of a genetic model over an empiric model. However, genetic

S.M. Weissman, M.S., C.G.C. (✉)
NorthShore University HealthSystem, Center for Medical Genetics, 1000 Central Street—Suite 620, Evanston, IL 60201, USA
e-mail: sweissman@northshore.org

N.M. Hansen (ed.), *Management of the Patient at High Risk for Breast Cancer*,
DOI 10.1007/978-1-4614-5891-3_1, © Springer Science+Business Media New York 2013

models can be limited if an individual is unaware of their family's medical history with respect to cancer or if someone has a particularly small family size or, in the case of breast cancer, a limited number of female relatives.

Regardless of model type, the most important feature of a risk model is its performance with respect to calibration, discrimination, and accuracy [8]. Calibration evaluates the model's ability to predict the number of events in a specific group of a population and is usually measured by using goodness-of-fit or chi-square statistics which compare the number of expected to observed events. Models that have good calibration will adequately predict disease burden in a population. Discrimination assesses the ability of a model to distinguish who will and will not develop a disease at the individual level and is measured by calculating the concordance statistic (c-statistic); the c-statistic is typically presented as the area under a receiver operating curve (i.e., AUC). An AUC of 0.50 would be representative of a chance occurrence, so a model that has good discrimination generally as an AUC of 0.70 or higher [7]. Lastly, a model's accuracy is represented by values of sensitivity, specificity, positive predictive value (PPV), and negative predictive value (NPV). Accuracy and discrimination are of importance when trying to make clinical decisions at the level of the individual [8].

This chapter describes the most commonly used empiric and genetic breast cancer risk models and summarizes the pros and cons of each model. Tables 1.1 and 1.2 provide quick overviews of the characteristics of each model reviewed. While some of the models included are out-of-date and are not used as frequently as some of the other models, they were included because they are incorporated in CancerGene© (copyright), a software package that includes nine different breast cancer and family history models as well as colon and pancreatic cancer models [9, 10]. Many healthcare professionals use this software as it incorporates many risk models into one program. Risk models not included in this chapter have been reviewed elsewhere [6].

## Empiric Models: Breast Cancer Risk

### Gail Model

The Gail model is one of the most recognized and widely used breast cancer risk assessment models. The model provides 5-year and lifetime breast cancer risks based on a woman's current age and risk factors compared to a woman of the same age with average risk factors [11]. The original Gail model was developed from a population of Caucasian women participating in the Breast Cancer Detection Demonstration Project (BCDDP), a mammography screening program conducted between 1973 and 1980 [12, 13]. After examining a number of potential risk factors between 2,852 incident cases of breast cancer (which included both in situ and invasive disease) and 3,146 unaffected controls, in addition to a woman's current age, four major risk factors were identified; these included: family history of breast cancer in first-degree relatives (either 0, 1, or ≥2 affected relatives), age at first live birth (<20, 20–24, 25–29 or ≥30) or nulliparity, age at menarche (<12, 12–13, or ≥14), and previous breast biopsy (0, 1, or ≥2) relative to age at the biopsy (<50 or ≥50). Using unconditional logistic regression, Gail and colleagues calculated relative risk coefficients for each risk factor, concurrently adjusting for the other risk factors. The relative risk for each individual risk factor is multiplied to create a single relative risk which is then combined with background breast cancer incidence rates to generate an absolute age-specific risk through a baseline proportional hazards estimation. The model will predict breast cancer between the ages of 20–80.

Three different studies evaluated and validated the original Gail model [14–16]. While all three studies had slightly different populations of various sizes, all found that the Gail model significantly overestimated breast cancer risk, especially in younger women. Spiegelman et al. found that it overestimated risk in women with two or more first-degree relatives affected with breast cancer and in women who had their first live birth < age 20 [15]. Additionally, Bondy et al.

**Table 1.1** Input variables and features of the empiric risk models[a]

| Variable | Gail | PENN I | PENN II | Myriad I | Myriad II | NCI CART[b] | LAMBDA[b] |
|---|---|---|---|---|---|---|---|
| *Model characteristics* | | | | | | | |
| Requires a computer | • | | • | | | | |
| Requires a pedigree | | | | | | | |
| Available in CancerGene© (copyright) | • | • | | • | •[c] | • | |
| *Model input* | | | | | | | |
| Exact family structure | | | | | | | |
| Age of unaffected proband | • | | | | | • | • |
| Age of unaffected relatives | | | | | | | |
| Reproductive and personal risk factors | • | | | | | | |
| Ashkenazi Jewish ancestry | | • | • | • | | • | • |
| Non-Caucasian ethnicity | • | | | | | | |
| Breast cancer status, proband | | • | • | • | • | • | • |
| Breast cancer status, relatives | • | • | • | • | • | • | • |
| Breast cancer age of onset, proband | | • | • | • | • | • | • |
| Breast cancer age of onset, relatives | | • | • | | • | | • |
| Ovarian cancer status, proband | | • | • | • | • | • | • |
| Ovarian cancer status, relatives | | • | • | • | • | • | • |
| Ovarian cancer age of onset, proband | | | | • | | • | |
| Ovarian cancer age of onset, relatives | | | | | | | |
| Male breast cancer status, proband | | | • | | | | |
| Male breast cancer status, relatives | | | • | | | | |
| Male breast cancer age of onset, proband | | | | | | | |
| Male breast cancer age of onset, relatives | | | | | | | |
| Both breast and ovarian cancer in proband | | • | • | • | • | | • |
| Both breast and ovarian cancer in relatives | | • | • | • | | • | • |
| Bilateral breast cancer status, proband | | | • | • | • | | • |
| Bilateral breast cancer status, relatives | | | • | | | | |
| Bilateral breast cancer, both ages of onset, proband | | | | | | | |
| Bilateral breast cancer, both ages of onset, relatives | | | | | | | |
| Prostate cancer in family | | | • | | | | |
| Pancreatic cancer in family | | | • | | | | |
| *Model output* | | | | | | | |
| Breast cancer risk | • | | | | | | |
| Ovarian cancer risk | | | | | | | |
| Predictions for *BRCA1* and *BRCA2* separately | | | • | | • | | |
| Predictions for *BRCA1* and *BRCA2* together | | | • | | • | • | • |
| Predictions for *BRCA1* only | | • | | • | | | |
| Probability of carrying a mutation | | | | | | | |
| Probability of finding a mutation if tested | | • | • | • | • | • | • |

Adapted and modified from [29]

[a] Does not include the *PTEN* mutation risk calculator

[b] These models are for people of Ashkenazi Jewish ancestry only

[c] This model was included in CancerGene© (copyright) up until version 3.3

**Table 1.2** Input variables and features of the genetic risk models

| Variable | Claus | BRCAPRO | BOADICEA | IBIS |
|---|---|---|---|---|
| *Model characteristics* | | | | |
| Requires a computer | | • | • | • |
| Requires a pedigree | | • | • | • |
| Available in CancerGene© (copyright) | • | • | | |
| *Model input* | | | | |
| Exact family structure | | • | • | • |
| Age of unaffected proband | | • | • | • |
| Age of unaffected relatives | | • | • | • |
| Reproductive and personal risk factors | | | | • |
| Ashkenazi Jewish ancestry | | • | • | • |
| Non-Caucasian ethnicity | | • | | |
| Breast cancer status, proband | | • | • | |
| Breast cancer status, relatives | • | • | • | • |
| Breast cancer age of onset, proband | | • | • | |
| Breast cancer age of onset, relatives | • | • | • | • |
| Ovarian cancer status, proband | | • | • | • |
| Ovarian cancer status, relatives | | • | • | • |
| Ovarian cancer age of onset, proband | | • | • | • |
| Ovarian cancer age of onset, relatives | | • | • | • |
| Male breast cancer status, proband | | • | • | |
| Male breast cancer status, relatives | | • | • | |
| Male breast cancer age of onset, proband | | • | • | |
| Male breast cancer age of onset, relatives | | • | • | |
| Both breast and ovarian cancer in proband | | • | • | |
| Both breast and ovarian cancer in relatives | | • | • | • |
| Bilateral breast cancer status, proband | | • | • | |
| Bilateral breast cancer status, relatives | | • | • | • |
| Bilateral breast cancer, both ages of onset, proband | | • | • | |
| Bilateral breast cancer, both ages of onset, relatives | | • | • | • |
| Prostate cancer in relatives | | | • | |
| Pancreatic cancer in relatives | | | • | |
| *BRCA1/2* genetic test results from the proband | | • | • | • |
| *BRCA1/2* genetic test results from relatives | | • | • | • |
| *BRCA1/2* genetic test sensitivity and specificity | | • | • | |
| *Model output* | | | | |
| Breast cancer risk | • | • | • | • |
| Ovarian cancer risk | | • | • | |
| Predictions for *BRCA1* and *BRCA2* separately | | • | • | • |
| Predictions for *BRCA1* and *BRCA2* together | | • | • | • |
| Probability of carrying a mutation | | • | • | • |
| Probability of finding a mutation if tested | | | | |

Adapted and modified from [29]

found that the model underestimated risk in older women [16]. Interestingly, none of women in the validation studies were undergoing routine annual mammography as was done in the BCDDP study which led all of the studies to suggest that the Gail model may be most accurate for populations of women undergoing routine annual mammography.

The Gail model was subsequently modified (a.k.a., Gail 2, or the Breast Cancer Risk Assessment Tool (BCRAT)) for the National Surgical Adjuvant Breast and Bowel Project (NSABP) Breast Cancer Prevention Trial (BCPT) [17, 18]. The model was changed so that it projected the absolute risk of invasive breast cancer only for women 35 years or older; age-specific invasive breast cancer rates, and attributable risk estimates to obtain baseline hazard rates were taken from Surveillance Epidemiology and End Results (SEER) data instead of the BCDDP and the model formally incorporated atypical hyperplasia, although adding atypical hyperplasia was first discussed in the discussion section of the original Gail model publication [12, 19]. Costantino and colleagues sought to validate the original (model 1) and modified (model 2 or Gail 2) Gail models from the women enrolled in the placebo arm of the BCPT P-1 Trial [19]. Model 1 provided "reasonable" absolute risk estimates for women under the age of 60 and overestimated risk in women older than 60. Model 2, overall, had good calibration with an expected to observed ratio of 1.03 (158.99 expected vs. 155 observed), but it overestimated risk for women in the highest risk quintiles and underestimated risk for women in the lowest risk quintiles. Further, when evaluating the individual risk factors, both models overestimated risk in women with more than two biopsies under the age of 50 and in women who had their first live birth under the age of 20 (as seen in Spiegelman study) and underestimated risk for women with one biopsy under the age of 50 and for most categories of women without a family history of breast cancer. With respect to the models' calibration, measures of goodness of fit were assessed; model 1 showed a lack of fit whereas model 2 had no evidence for lack of fit.

Rockhill and colleagues validated the modified Gail model in the Nurses' Health Study population, as they did for the original Gail model and had the exact same findings as Costantino et al. [20]. Interestingly, they also looked at the discriminatory accuracy of the modified Gail model (none of the previous studies evaluated this) and found the c-statistic to be very low at 0.58. However, as they discussed, this finding was not unexpected due to the low relative risks associated with many of the risk factors used for the Gail model and described how incorporating other risk factors (e.g., mammographic density) could help improve its discriminatory accuracy (which, to date, has not been done).

The Breast Cancer Risk Assessment Tool website is the version of the model that is used today [11]. Figure 1.1a and b demonstrates what the current input looks like as well as an example of how the results are displayed. The Gail model has been updated as SEER data has changed and now includes race-specific risks for African-American, Asian, and Pacific Islander women [21, 22]. Validation in a Hispanic population is still needed. With the development of more complex breast cancer risk assessment models over the years, the Gail model is primarily used for chemoprevention discussions. In fact, Gail et al. created a benefit-to-risk index that assesses the benefits of taking tamoxifen for breast cancer risk reduction against the risks of adverse events associated with tamoxifen use [23]. It needs to be noted that the Gail model should not be used to determine breast MRI eligibility as was specifically noted in the Appendix of the American Cancer Society breast MRI screening guidelines [1]. Part of the reason for this is that the Gail model is not a family history-based risk model. The Gail model does not factor in second-degree relatives, age of onset, or any genetic factors; although a few papers have looked at increasing the discriminatory accuracy by incorporating single nucleotide polymorphisms (SNPs) that have been linked to increased breast cancer risk [24–26]. Therefore, the Gail model is not a model that should be used to assess breast cancer risk in women with a paternal family history of breast cancer (any affected relatives would have to be second-degree or more distant) or women with a strong family history of breast cancer (e.g., three or more or multiple early onset breast cancer cases).

a b

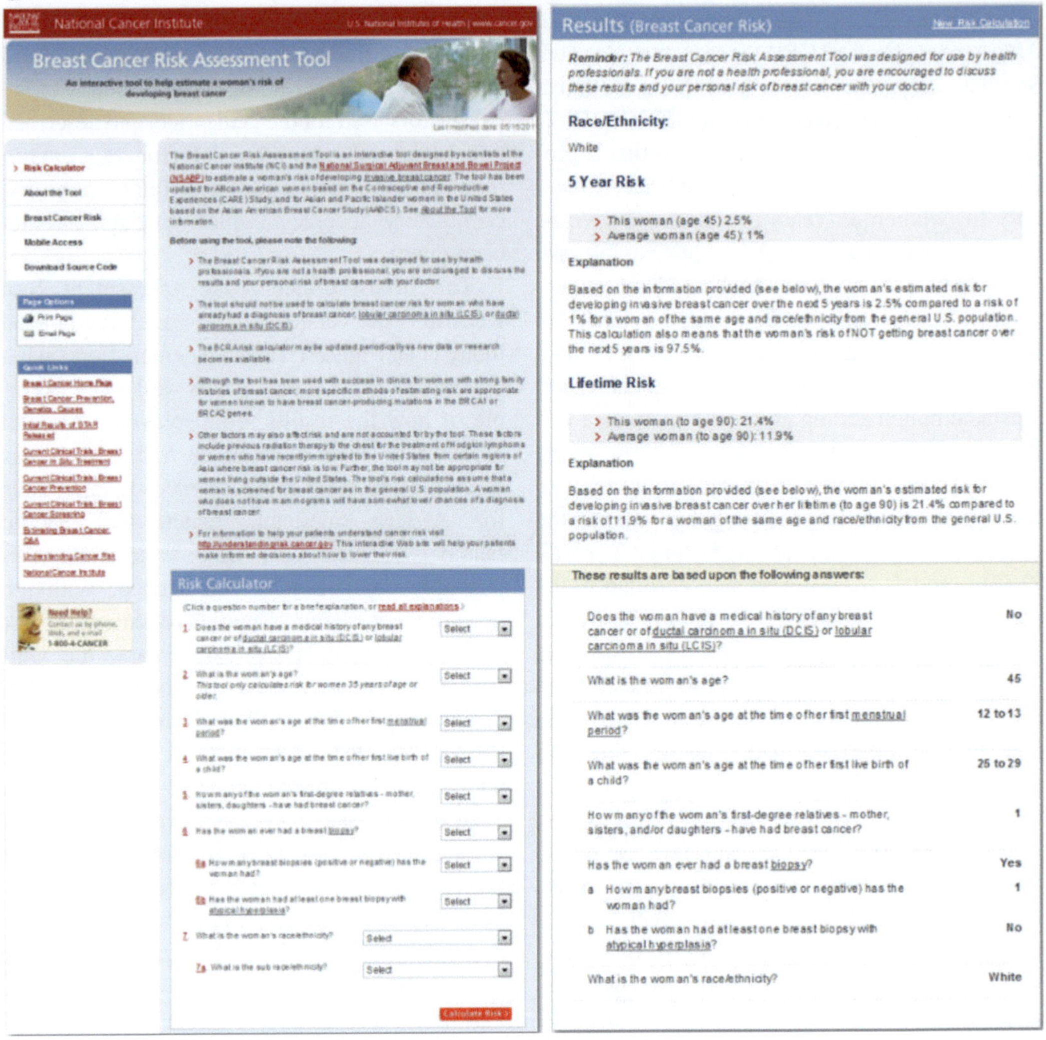
National Cancer Institute
Breast Cancer Risk Assessment Tool
An interactive tool to help estimate a woman's risk of developing breast cancer
Risk Calculator
About the Tool
Breast Cancer Risk
Mobile Access
Download Source Code
Risk Calculator
Need Help?
1-800-4-CANCER
Results (Breast Cancer Risk)
Reminder: The Breast Cancer Risk Assessment Tool was designed for use by health professionals. If you are not a health professional, you are encouraged to discuss these results and your personal risk of breast cancer with your doctor.
Race/Ethnicity:
White
5 Year Risk
This woman (age 45) 2.5%
Average woman (age 45) 1%
Explanation
Based on the information provided (see below), the woman's estimated risk for developing invasive breast cancer over the next 5 years is 2.5% compared to a risk of 1% for a woman of the same age and race/ethnicity from the general U.S. population. This calculation also means that the woman's risk of NOT getting breast cancer over the next 5 years is 97.5%.
Lifetime Risk
This woman (to age 90): 21.4%
Average woman (to age 90): 11.9%
Explanation
Based on the information provided (see below), the woman's estimated risk for developing invasive breast cancer over her lifetime (to age 90) is 21.4% compared to a risk of 11.9% for a woman of the same age and race/ethnicity from the general U.S. population.
These results are based upon the following answers:
Does the woman have a medical history of any breast cancer or of ductal carcinoma in situ (DCIS) or lobular carcinoma in situ (LCIS)?
No
What is the woman's age?
45
What was the woman's age at the time of her first menstrual period?
12 to 13
What was the woman's age at the time of her first live birth of a child?
25 to 29
How many of the woman's first-degree relatives - mother, sisters, and/or daughters - have had breast cancer?
1
Has the woman ever had a breast biopsy?
Yes
a How many breast biopsies (positive or negative) has the woman had?
1
b Has the woman had at least one breast biopsy with atypical hyperplasia?
No
What is the woman's race/ethnicity?
White

**Fig. 1.1** (**a** and **b**) Example of the Gail model

## Empiric Models: *BRCA1/2* Mutation Probabilities

### PENN Models

In 1997, Couch et al. published a model for assessing the likelihood of identifying *BRCA1* mutations in women with or without a personal history of breast cancer [27]. They created their model using 263 unrelated women with breast cancer from families (both Ashkenazi and non-Ashkenazi Jewish) with a history of breast with or without ovarian cancer. Using both univariate and multivariate analyses, they examined possible associations between the presence of a *BRCA1* mutation in a family and the following family characteristics: unilateral breast cancer, bilateral breast cancer, ovarian cancer, combined breast and ovarian cancer in the same individual, the number of women at risk in a family (>20 years of age), the average age of diagnosis for breast and ovarian cancer, and Ashkenazi Jewish ancestry. A predicted probability of harboring a *BRCA1* mutation in the family was calculated using logistic regression analysis; from this, they created two sets of tables (one each for Ashkenazi and non-Ashkenazi Jewish individuals) that take the average age of onset of breast cancer only in the family in combination with one of four family features: families with breast cancer only, families with breast and ovarian cancer, families with a single individual with breast and ovarian cancer, and families with both breast and ovarian cancer who have one individual in the family who had both breast and ovarian cancer.

For example, take a non-Ashkenazi woman who had breast cancer at age 42, who has a mother, maternal aunt, and maternal first cousin with breast cancer at ages 52, 48, and 38, respectively, the PENN model would predict a 5% chance of identifying a *BRCA1* mutation in this family since this is a breast cancer only family with an average age of onset of 45 years. If the same family had a grandmother with ovarian cancer, the PENN model predicts a 23.4% chance of finding a *BRCA1* mutation and if you switch the ovarian cancer diagnosis to the maternal aunt with breast cancer, the likelihood of identifying a *BRCA1* mutation now increases to 82.9%. Once the likelihood of identifying a mutation is determined, you can then use basic Mendelian principles of autosomal dominant inheritance to calculate the chance of other people in the family also having a *BRCA1* mutation (e.g., any of the maternal aunt's children would have an ~41.5% chance of harboring a *BRCA1* mutation, 50% of the aunt's risk).

The PENN model is easy to use and has been built into CancerGene©. The PENN model performs similarly to other *BRCA* mutation prediction models with an AUC between 0.62 and 0.80 depending on the population studied [28–30]. The PENN model requires knowledge of all breast and ovarian cancer diagnoses in the family; only takes into account one side of the family so if there is breast and/or ovarian cancer in both lineages of a proband, the model would need to be run separately for each side of the family; and is based on *BRCA1* genetic testing that occurred when genetic testing first became available which means it: (1) identified variants of uncertain significance (i.e., inconclusive test results) at much higher rate (30–40% vs. 3–5% today); and (2) did not evaluate for large deletions or duplications. Therefore, the PENN model underestimates the likelihood of finding a *BRCA1* mutation. However, the biggest limitation of the PENN model is that it does not evaluate for *BRCA2* mutations. Genetic testing for the *BRCA1* and *BRCA2* genes almost uniformly includes both genes; *BRCA* genetic may be limited to one gene in situations where there is a known *BRCA* mutation in the family or the family is of a specific ethnic background that has founder mutations in only one gene (e.g., *BRCA1* founder mutations in Poles). Another limitation is that the group does not report on whether the breast cancers included are invasive, in situ, or both or whether the ovarian cancers are epithelial only or a combination of epithelial and non-epithelial tumors. Non-epithelial ovarian cancers are generally not associated with *BRCA* mutations [31, 32].

The PENN model has been updated (PENN II) and expanded to include the *BRCA2* gene. The new model factors in additional cancers including prostate and male breast cancer (the number of cases in the family) as well as pancreatic cancer (present or absent in the family) and mother-daughter concordance. At the time of writing this chapter, a full description of the PENN II model has not yet been published in a peer-reviewed journal, although some information about the model has been published and the model performs equally to other *BRCA* risk models in the high-risk clinic setting [30]. The model is available online for free at http://www.afcri.upenn.edu/itacc/penn2/ (Fig. 1.2) and at least one major insurance carrier (Aetna) recognizes the PENN II model in determining coverage for *BRCA1* and *BRCA2* genetic testing.

## Myriad Models: Shattuck-Eidens and Myriad II

### Shattuck-Eidens Model (Myriad I)

Shortly after clinical *BRCA1* and *BRCA2* genetic testing became available, Myriad Genetic

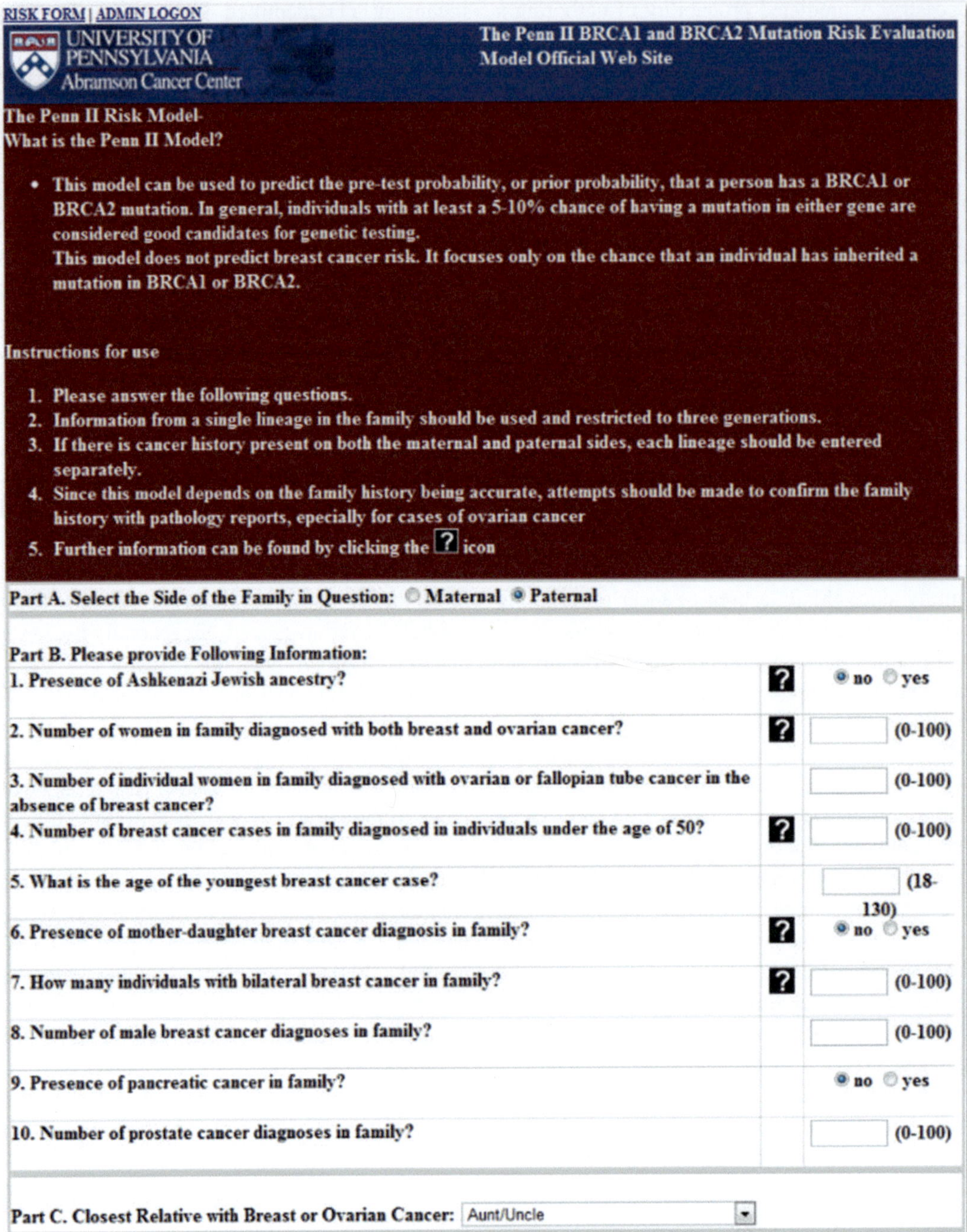

RISK FORM | ADMIN LOGON

UNIVERSITY OF PENNSYLVANIA Abramson Cancer Center

The Penn II BRCA1 and BRCA2 Mutation Risk Evaluation Model Official Web Site

The Penn II Risk Model-
What is the Penn II Model?

- This model can be used to predict the pre-test probability, or prior probability, that a person has a BRCA1 or BRCA2 mutation. In general, individuals with at least a 5-10% chance of having a mutation in either gene are considered good candidates for genetic testing.
  This model does not predict breast cancer risk. It focuses only on the chance that an individual has inherited a mutation in BRCA1 or BRCA2.

Instructions for use

1. Please answer the following questions.
2. Information from a single lineage in the family should be used and restricted to three generations.
3. If there is cancer history present on both the maternal and paternal sides, each lineage should be entered separately.
4. Since this model depends on the family history being accurate, attempts should be made to confirm the family history with pathology reports, epecially for cases of ovarian cancer
5. Further information can be found by clicking the ? icon

Part A. Select the Side of the Family in Question: Maternal Paternal

Part B. Please provide Following Information:

| | | |
|---|---|---|
| 1. Presence of Ashkenazi Jewish ancestry? | ? | no yes |
| 2. Number of women in family diagnosed with both breast and ovarian cancer? | ? | (0-100) |
| 3. Number of individual women in family diagnosed with ovarian or fallopian tube cancer in the absence of breast cancer? | | (0-100) |
| 4. Number of breast cancer cases in family diagnosed in individuals under the age of 50? | ? | (0-100) |
| 5. What is the age of the youngest breast cancer case? | | (18-130) |
| 6. Presence of mother-daughter breast cancer diagnosis in family? | ? | no yes |
| 7. How many individuals with bilateral breast cancer in family? | ? | (0-100) |
| 8. Number of male breast cancer diagnoses in family? | | (0-100) |
| 9. Presence of pancreatic cancer in family? | | no yes |
| 10. Number of prostate cancer diagnoses in family? | | (0-100) |

Part C. Closest Relative with Breast or Ovarian Cancer: Aunt/Uncle

**Fig. 1.2** Example of the PENNII model (© Copyright 2012 The Trustees of the University of Pennsylvania, owner and operator of the University of Pennsylvania Health System. ALL RIGHTS RESERVED.)

Laboratories, in collaboration with the USA and European groups, published data intended to identify predictive characteristics of harboring a *BRCA1* mutation [33]. They collected *BRCA1* genetic testing data from 798 unrelated individuals from 20 high-risk clinics selected for testing based on features suggestive of a *BRCA1* mutation (e.g., early age of onset of breast cancer, multiple breast cancer diagnoses, ovarian cancer). Most of the individuals had family history information available from first-degree relatives, but some individuals included information on second-degree relatives as well. There is no mention of including third-degree relatives or male relatives affected with breast cancer.

Complete information was available on 621 affected individuals and their families and, from this data set, they examined the relationship between phenotype and the presence of a deleterious *BRCA1* mutation (all uncertain *BRCA1* variants of uncertain significance were excluded) for 593 individuals by logistic regression. Six factors were considered in their modeling algorithm: (1) patient disease status using five different classifications—unilateral breast cancer/no ovarian cancer, bilateral breast cancer/no ovarian cancer, unilateral breast cancer with ovarian cancer, bilateral breast cancer with ovarian cancer, ovarian cancer/no breast cancer; (2) patient age at first diagnosis; (3) Ashkenazi or non-Ashkenazi Jewish ancestry; (4) number of relatives affected with breast cancer but not ovarian cancer; (5) number of relatives affected with ovarian cancer, but not breast cancer; and (6) number of relatives affected with both breast and ovarian cancer. No distinction was made between degree of relatedness of family members in the model. When fitting the model, an individual with unilateral breast cancer and ovarian cancer who also had a family history of ovarian cancer ended up as a negative risk factor because only a few individuals met this criteria, so this variable was removed from the modeling. The overall number of women positive for a *BRCA1* mutation was 102.

The data generated from the model is presented in graphical format in the paper. There are two sets of graphs, one each for patients of Ashkenazi and non-Ashkenazi Jewish descent. Unfortunately, this model is not particularly user-friendly in this format, but it has been built into the CancerGene© (copyright) for easier use. The Shattuck-Eidens model has the same limitations as the original PENN model.

## Myriad II Model (The Frank Model)

About a year after the Shattuck-Eidens model was published, Myriad Genetic Laboratories and collaborators (12 sites from the USA were included) published a report of an update to their initial model that included the *BRCA2* gene and a uniform selection criteria [34]. The Myriad II model is based on a cohort of 238 women who either had invasive breast cancer before age 50 or ovarian cancer at any age and had at least one first- or second-degree female relative with either diagnosis at any age (most of the cancer diagnoses in the proband and family members were verified with a medical records review); 105 women met this minimal criteria; and 123 women had more significant histories. Family histories collected included primarily first-, second-, and third-degree relatives. Four eligible women reported a family history of male breast cancer, but there were not enough cases to factor male breast cancer into the model.

All but 27 women had genetic testing for both *BRCA1* and *BRCA2*; 27 women declined *BRCA2* genetic testing after they were found to have a *BRCA1* mutation. The final number of women positive for either a *BRCA1* or *BRCA2* mutation was 94 (63 *BRCA1* and 31 *BRCA2*); of these, 70 were women with breast cancer before the age of 50 only ($n=200$), 10 were women with ovarian cancer only ($n=22$), and 14 were in women with a history of breast and ovarian cancer ($n=16$).

After applying a model-fitting procedure to their polychotomous logistic regression analysis of their selected risk factors, they developed a mathematical fit for the probability of detecting either a *BRCA1* or *BRCA2* mutation in women diagnosed with breast cancer under the age of 50 only plus additional personal or family history. No significant factors appeared when the analyses were applied to women ascertained based on a diagnosis of ovarian cancer. Therefore in order to use the Myriad II model, to start, the patient must be a woman with breast cancer under the age of 50 and has to have at least one relative with breast cancer under the age of 50. If both of these criteria are not met, the Myriad II model cannot be used. For patients who meet these criteria, the Myriad II model will then adjust the likelihood of testing positive for a *BRCA1/2* mutation on whether: (1) there is any relative with ovarian cancer; (2) the patient had bilateral breast cancer (with one under the age of 50) or ovarian cancer (in addition to breast cancer under age 50); and (3) if the patient had breast cancer under the age of 40 or any combination of the above factors. For example, if a woman had breast cancer at 39, has a relative with breast cancer under age 50, and a relative with ovarian cancer, her chance of testing positive for a *BRCA1* mutation is 50.9%, 7.9% for *BRCA2*, and 59% for either *BRCA* or *BRCA2*. Unlike with the Myriad I model, Ashkenazi Jewish ancestry was not associated with an increased likelihood of finding a *BRCA* mutation and was not factored into their analysis.

The Myriad II model was a major improvement over the Myriad I model since it took into account the *BRCA2* gene, had uniform selection criteria, and verified histological diagnoses in most cases and in its simplicity to use (look-up table). However, there are two major weaknesses of this model; first, is that it is based on a highly selective patient population as evidenced by their nearly 40% detection rate of *BRCA1* or *BRCA2* mutations which is not representative of most cancer genetics clinics. Secondly, the Myriad II model is highly restrictive in respect to who the model can be applied to which limits its application. As discussed above, if the patient does not have a diagnosis of breast cancer in themselves and at least one family both under the age of 50, the model cannot be used. Other issues with the model include some of the same issues as in the Myriad I and PENN I models with respect to the genetic testing technology and high variant of uncertain significance rate, the lack of incorporation of male breast cancer, and the potential for inclusion of low malignant potential/borderline or mucinous ovarian tumors and non-epithelial ovarian cancers.

The Myriad II model used to be included in CancerGene© (copyright) but has since been removed (starting in version 3.3) in favor of the Myriad prevalence table data which is also available as a *BRCA* risk calculator [35]. The Myriad prevalence data is not a model, but reflects the likelihood of finding a mutation based on certain personal and family history features from Myriad's internal database for both Ashkenazi and non-Ashkenazi Jewish individuals. This data is purely based on the personal and family history and ancestral information recorded on Myriad's test requisition forms by healthcare professionals who order clinical *BRCA* genetic testing; individuals tested under research protocols are not included. Whether or not the diagnoses recorded are confirmed or if the ages are accurate are unknown and are the major limitations of this data set. The risk calculator can be found at https://www.myriadpro.com/brca-risk-calculator?page_id=165 and the prevalence tables can be found at https://www.myriadpro.com/bracanalysis-prevalence-tables. At the time of writing this, the prevalence tables were last updated in February of 2010. Various studies have validated the Myriad I, II and the prevalence tables and these models are comparable with respect to its discrimination and accuracy with other empiric and genetic models [28–30, 36, 37].

## NCI CART Model

The NCI CART model provides *BRCA1* and *BRCA2* mutation frequencies for individuals of Ashkenazi Jewish ancestry [38]. The model is based on data collected from a population survey of 5,318 Ashkenazi Jewish men and women from the Washington, DC area. Information on cancers and ages of onset in the study participant, first- and second-degree relatives was collected and all individuals were tested for the three Ashkenazi Jewish founder *BRCA* mutations (*BRCA1* 187delAG, *BRCA1* 5385insC, and *BRCA2* 6174delT). They applied the classification and regression tree (CART) procedure to evaluate prediction algorithms on the following factors: the decade of age the individual was tested in (i.e., <40, 40–49, 50–59, ≥60), the decade of age at diagnosis for affected individuals, breast or ovarian cancer in the participant, first-degree relative with breast or ovarian cancer, and a history of breast and ovarian cancer in the same woman. They opted not to include second-degree family history information.

Personal and family history combinations and mutation frequencies are presented in tabular format which makes the NCI CART model very easy to use; it is also in CancerGene©(copyright). However, based on the categories, there are certain histories that cannot be accounted for, which is a limitation of this model. For instance, if a woman has a family history of breast and/or ovarian cancer and also has a personal history of breast cancer under the age of 40, the family history information will not be factored in to adjust her likelihood of having a mutation. The reason for this is that the authors concluded family history had less influence on the chance of having a *BRCA* mutation for women with cancer compared to unaffected individuals with a family history. This conclusion was challenged by two separate groups who reanalyzed the data using different statistical methods and found that family history was a significant factor for women with a personal history of cancer [39–41].

While the model can be used for men or women, it is only applicable to Ashkenazi Jewish individuals, only includes affected first-degree relatives, does not factor in male breast or bilateral breast cancer, and does not differentiate maternal and paternal lineages (i.e., to effectively use the model, risk should be calculated independently for each side of the family). Additionally, the genetic testing done on individuals in this study included the three Ashkenazi Jewish founder mutations and likely missed some families that have a non-Ashkenazi Jewish founder mutation [35]; this would lead to the model likely underestimating risk, albeit slightly. In a study comparing seven different *BRCA* risk prediction models, the NCI CART model had the lowest c-statistic of all the models (0.63) for risk predictions for Ashkenazi Jewish families [29]. This in part may be due to the original purpose of the study which is to calculate population-based penetrance estimates for mutation carriers and the majority of their participants were unaffected individuals [42, 43].

Further, using the NCI CART (or the LAMBDA model discussed below) has limited value for determining when *BRCA* genetic testing should be offered to an Ashkenazi Jewish individual since guidelines in the USA recommended genetic counseling and *BRCA* testing for all Ashkenazi Jewish women with a personal and/or family history of breast and/or ovarian cancer in first- and second-degree relatives [4, 5, 44]. The model could be used to help patients better understand their chances of testing positive during pretest genetic counseling.

## LAMBDA Model

A second *BRCA* prediction model developed specifically for Ashkenazi Jewish individuals is the *L*og odds of an *A*ncestral *M*utation in ***BRCA1*** or *BRCA2* for a *D*efined personal and family in an *A*shkenazi Jewish woman (LAMBDA) [43]. The LAMBDA model was primarily developed out of the response the authors published to the NCI CART model [39]. The LAMBDA model was developed from data sets from two different Ashkenazi Jewish populations: (1) Australian women who had a diagnosis of breast or ovarian cancer or had a family history of breast or ovarian cancer in first- or second-degree relatives ($n=240$); and (2) women from the UK who had a previous diagnosis of breast or ovarian cancer ($n=184$) [45]. All probands were screened for the three Ashkenazi Jewish founder *BRCA* mutations, and then through logistic regression analysis, they modeled the probability that the proband carries one of the three mutations. To be consistent with the NCI CART study, they used many of the same predictive factors including the same age breakdowns (decade of age of onset of cancer and decade of age at genetic testing), personal history of breast or ovarian cancer, and the number of first- and second-degree relatives affected with breast or ovarian cancer in the modeling. They also included a history bilateral breast cancer in the proband or a first- or second-degree relative. After they analyzed the combined Australian and the UK populations, they again used logistic regression to combine this data set with the data generated from their analysis of the NCI CART data to generate the LAMBDA model.

The final factors that ended up having significance and being included in the model are shown in Fig. 1.3. Breast cancer diagnosed 60 or older, second-degree relatives with breast cancer

**Probability that an Ashkenazi Jewish Woman Carries an Ancestral Mutation in BRCA1 or BRCA2**

For <u>each</u> personal feature listed below, identify those relevant to the consultand and then write the corresponding coefficient in the shaded box alongside.
For <u>each</u> family history feature listed below, identify those relevant to the consultand. First multiply the corresponding coefficient by the number of affected relatives with that feature, and then write this in the shaded box alongside.
<u>Add</u> all the scores to obtain LAMBDA, then use the LAMBDA CONVERSION TABLE to give the estimated PROBABILITY that an Ashkenazi Jewish woman carries an ancestral mutation in BRCA1 or BRCA2.

| | coefficient | | SCORE |
|---|---|---|---|
| BASELINE | -3.75 | | -3.75 |

**Personal history features**

| CONSULTAND HAS HAD BREAST OR OVARIAN CANCER | coefficient | | SCORE |
|---|---|---|---|
| diagnosed with a primary breast cancer before age 40 | +3 | one of | |
| age 40 - 49 | +2 | | |
| age 50 - 59 | +1 | | |
| diagnosed with bilateral breast cancer at any age | +1 | | |
| diagnosed with a primary ovarian cancer at any age | +3 | | |
| CONSULTAND HAS <u>NOT</u> HAD BREAST OR OVARIAN CANCER | | | |
| age 40 - 49 | -0.5 | one of | |
| age 50 - 59 | -1.0 | | |
| age 60 or older | -1.5 | | |

**Family history features**

| FIRST DEGREE RELATIVES | no. affected relatives | | coefficient | SCORE |
|---|---|---|---|---|
| diagnosed with breast cancer before age 40 | [ ] | multiplied by | +1.5 | |
| age 40 - 49 | [ ] | multiplied by | +1 | |
| age 50 - 59 | [ ] | multiplied by | +0.5 | |
| diagnosed with ovarian cancer at any age | [ ] | multiplied by | +1.5 | |
| SECOND DEGREE RELATIVES (on either side of the family) | | | | |
| diagnosed with breast cancer before age 40 | [ ] | multiplied by | +0.5 | |
| diagnosed with ovarian cancer at any age | [ ] | multiplied by | +1.0 | |

LAMBDA CONVERSION TABLE

| LAMBDA | probability | LAMBDA | probability |
|---|---|---|---|
| 2.5 or more | >90% | -0.5 | 36% |
| 1.5 | 82% | -0.75 | 32% |
| 1.25 | 78% | -1.0 | 27% |
| 1.0 | 73% | -1.25 | 22% |
| 0.75 | 68% | -1.5 | 18% |
| 0.5 | 62% | -2.0 | 12% |
| 0.25 | 56% | -2.5 | 8% |
| 0 | 50% | -3.0 | 5% |
| -0.25 | 44% | -3.75 | 2% |

LAMBDA [ ]

↓

PROBABILITY [ ]

**Fig. 1.3** (**a–c**) Example of the LAMBDA risk assessment tool

after the age of 40 or with bilateral breast cancer and age of onset of ovarian cancer were not included in the model as the authors found no evidence these factors influenced risk. The authors tested the internal consistency of the LAMBDA model and there was no evidence of systematic bias. The LAMBDA model is simple to use and requires adding up all of the risk factors to get the LAMBDA score which in turn is compared to the conversion table which provides a pretest probability of having one of the three Ashkenazi Jewish *BRCA* mutations.

Apicella and colleagues validated the LAMBDA model on a population of over 1,200 Ashkenazi Jewish women from North America that were pooled from clinic-, community-, and population-based cohorts [46]. Overall, the AUC was 0.79 but the model seemed to have better prediction for *BRCA1* mutations over *BRCA2*. The model was overdispersed, predicting 18% more carriers than observed. When compared to BRCAPRO (discussed below) risk estimates on the same population, the LAMBDA model was comparable with respect to AUC (0.78 for BRCAPRO) and did better with dispersion as BRCAPRO was markedly overdispersed predicting 86% more carriers than observed. A second study was published in 2007 that compared the LAMBDA model to the Myriad II, BRCAPRO, and Couch models in 200 women presenting to a high-risk clinic at the Mayo Medical Center in Rochester [28]. Interestingly, Lindor and her colleagues only had 30 Ashkenazi Jewish women in their cohort (15% of the total), but they ran the LAMDA model on all 200 women and performed complete DNA sequencing for both *BRCA1* and *BRCA2* as well as a deletion and duplication panel for 5 *BRCA1* mutations. Like Apicella et al. reported [46], the LAMBDA was overdispersed, but was less likely to miss mutation carriers than the three other models. Further, they found the LAMBDA model outperformed or at least matched most of the models in a high-risk clinic setting in which 85% of the patients were not of Ashkenazi Jewish ancestry suggesting the LAMBDA model may have utility in non-Ashkenazi Jewish women. However, further studies are needed to confirm their findings.

Limitations of the LAMBDA model include the lack of inclusion of relatives beyond second-degree, male breast cancer, age of onset in relation to bilateral breast cancer, and other *BRCA*-related cancers. Like some of the other models, the model does not differentiate the maternal from the paternal lineage and, at this time, it can only be used in individuals of Ashkenazi Jewish ancestry, although Apicella notes her group is working on modifying the model for individuals not of Ashkenazi Jewish descent [46]. While the LAMBDA is not computerized which would speed up the time it takes to use the model, the math involved is straightforward and simple.

## Genetic Models: Breast Cancer Risk

### Claus Model

The Claus model, sometimes referred to as the Claus tables, is another well-known model for breast cancer risk assessment. The Claus model provides age-specific breast cancer risk estimates for women with family history of breast cancer [47]. The actual model was developed from data obtained from the Cancer and Steroid Hormone (CASH) Study, a multicenter, population-based, case–control study conducted by the Centers for Disease Control [48]. The study included 4,730 women with a confirmed diagnosis of breast cancer, "most" of which were invasive, between the ages of 20–54 and 4,688 control subjects matched according to 5-year age intervals and geographic region. Family history information was collected on specific female relatives, but for the development of the model, only mothers and sisters of Caucasian cases and controls were used. Second-degree relatives and non-Whites were excluded due to underreporting of diagnoses for these groups. Daughters were also excluded due to the relatively few cases of affected daughters in both the case and control arms; this was likely a byproduct of the age eligibility for the study.

Through goodness-of-fit tests, they compared the observed age-specific risk patterns with those predicted under a variety of genetic models and determined a rare allele inherited in autosomal dominant manner with an allele frequency of 0.0033 best explained the risk in these families; it is important to remember that the *BRCA* genes had not yet been fully elucidated at the time the Claus model was published. Assuming an autosomal dominant rare allele was responsible for breast cancer, complex segregation analysis was used to calculate age-specific risks for women with either one or two first- or second-degree relatives affected with breast cancer by the age of onset of the affected relative. The results of this analysis are presented in lookup tables that provide cumulative probabilities of developing breast cancer between ages 29 and 79 in 10-year increments for different family history combinations of affected relatives by age of onset including: 1 first-degree relative; 1 second-degree relative; 2 first-degree relatives; a mother and maternal aunt; a mother and paternal aunt; 1 maternal and 1 paternal second-degree relative; and 2 second degree relatives.

There are several limitations to the Claus model, most important of which is that there is no independent validation of the Claus model. Numerous studies have compared the Claus model to other models. In a study comparing the estimated risks for the Gail and Claus models for 111 women attending a high-risk clinic at the University of California in Los Angeles, McGuigan et al. showed that there was poor concordance between the two models with Claus model estimate falling within the 95% confidence interval of the Gail risk only 22% of the time [49]. However, the models were more concordant for women who had more than one affected first-degree relative, so the authors postulated that some of these differences in agreement could be due to the personal risk factors factored into the Gail model that are not included in the Claus model. A second group comparing the Claus and Gail models had similar findings to McGuigan et al. [50]. Amir and colleagues found the Claus model underestimated absolute breast cancer when comparing expected to observed cases as well as breast cancer risk among women with a single affected first-degree relative in a cohort of 3,170 women from the UK undergoing comprehensive risk assessment [51]. Since the Claus model only takes into account two affected relatives, the Claus model will also underestimate risk for women who have very strong family histories of breast cancer (four or more cases) who are negative for a *BRCA* mutation. The model also is limited by the fact that certain combinations of affected first- and second-degree relatives are not accounted for by the tables (e.g., sister and aunt or mother and paternal grandmother), so this requires some manipulation of the models to get risk numbers for patients. For instance, in a sister/aunt combination, the sister may need to be reflected as an affected mother to accurately capture her first-degree relationship. Other issues to be aware of are that model's accuracy in non-Caucasian populations is unknown, the model likely underestimates risk for women who have relatives diagnosed in the twenties because there were few women in the CASH study diagnosed with breast cancer in this age range, bilateral breast cancer is not taken into account, and non-familial risks are not factored in [47, 52].

The Claus model was created from a large data set and is useful for women who have 2–3 affected relatives who have not undergone *BRCA* genetic testing or when a *BRCA* mutation has not been identified as the cause of the breast cancer in the family. This last point was assessed by Claus and the creators of the BRCAPRO model and they concluded the Claus model may be better than BRCAPRO for estimating breast cancer risk in *BRCA* negative families [53]. The model has been incorporated into the CancerGene© (copyright) for easy use. Additionally, when using the Claus model in CancerGene© (copyright), the program will provide risk estimates for the most genetic looking combination of affected individuals. For example, if a woman has a mother affected at 49, a sister affected at 42, and a paternal aunt diagnosed at 35, CancerGene© (copyright) will automatically provide the risk for having two affected first-degree relatives (35.4%) over the mother/paternal aunt risk (19.7%). The Claus model is one of the models recognized by the American Cancer Society for calculating breast cancer risk to determine breast MRI screening eligibility [1].

A couple of variations of the Claus model exist although they are not commonly used. Prior to the publication of the Claus model, Claus and

syndromes (PTHS) [103, 104]. Briefly, Cowden syndrome is a multisystem disorder that has features including macrocephaly, dermatologic, neurologic, and gastrointestinal manifestations as well as an increased risk for various cancers including breast, thyroid, endometrial, and renal. Specifically, the lifetime risk of developing breast cancer for a woman who carries a *PTEN* mutation is 25–50% [105]. The International Cowden Consortium (ICC) created operational diagnostic criteria in 1996 to help identify individuals that should be offered genetic testing for *PTEN* mutations which has subsequently been revised on two occasions [105–107]; Table 1.5 lists the current diagnostic criteria.

The rationale for generating the *PTEN* risk calculator is that current Cowden syndrome guidelines do not differentiate features found in adult and pediatric populations, the number of major and minor criteria combinations makes the guidelines difficult to use, the guidelines do not allow a clinician to quantitate the likelihood of finding a *PTEN* mutation, and chiefly none of the existing guidelines are based on data generated from a prospectively collected population of *PTEN* mutation carriers.

The *PTEN* risk calculator was developed using an international cohort of 3,042 prospectively collected individuals recruited into a protocol at the Ohio State University initially and then at the Cleveland Clinic. Individuals were eligible for the protocol if they met relaxed ICC operational criteria for Cowden syndrome; this includes pathognomonic criteria or at least two criteria, either major or minor. All individuals underwent extensive molecular analysis for *PTEN* mutations that included testing for large deletions and duplications as well as DNA sequencing of the *PTEN* promoter region. The cohorts were a mix of children and adults, so the risk calculator can be used for pediatric or adult patients suspected of having a PTHS. The rest of the discussion will focus on the factors used in the creation of the risk calculator for an adult population.

To start, Tan and colleagues compared the prevalence of the different benign and malignant manifestations of Cowden syndrome in the general population (primarily North American reports) to their cohort of individuals who met relaxed ICC criteria as well as those who had identifiable *PTEN* mutations. One of the limitations with their adult cohort is that many individuals were referred to the study due to a personal and/or family history of one or more cancers that in turn may have led to a referral bias; this prevented the use of conventional regression modeling, so they used a clinically driven modeling approach. For each manifestation, they generated a relative risk from the Cleveland Clinic cohort (by using the one cohort, they could then use the Ohio State cohort to validate the risk calculator) relative to

**Table 1.5** ICC criteria for an operational diagnosis of Cowden syndrome

| *Pathognomonic criteria* |
|---|
| Adult Lhermitte-Duclos disease, defined as the presence of a cerebellar dysplastic gangliocytoma |
| Mucocutaneous lesions—trichilemmomas, acral keratoses papillomatous lesions +/– mucosal lesions |
| *Major criteria* |
| Breast cancer |
| Epithelial thyroid cancer (non-medullary), especially follicular thyroid cancer |
| Macrocephaly |
| Endometrial cancer |
| *Minor criteria* |
| Other thyroid lesions (e.g., adenoma, multinodular goiter) |
| Intellectual disability (IQ ≤ 75) |
| Hamartomatous intestinal polyps |
| Fibrocystic breast disease |
| Lipomas or fibromas |
| Genitourinary tumors (especially renal cell carcinoma) or malformations |
| Uterine fibroids |
| *An operational diagnosis of Cowden syndrome is made if an individual meets any one of the following criteria:* |
| Pathognomonic mucocutaneous lesions combined with one of the following: |
| Six or more facial papules, of which three or more must be trichilemmoma |
| Cutaneous facial papules and oral mucosal papillomatosis |
| Oral mucosal papillomatosis and acral keratoses |
| Six or more palmo-plantar keratoses |
| Two or more major criteria |
| One major and three or more minor criteria |
| Four or more minor criteria |

Adapted from [108]

colleagues developed two tables that provide age-specific breast cancer risks for women with either: (1) one or two first-degree relatives affected with ovarian cancer by age of onset or (2) two affected first-degree relatives, one with breast cancer and one with ovarian cancer, by age of onset [54]. The same CASH data set was used with all the same parameters as discussed above including an additional 493 women who had epithelial ovarian cancer. The utility of this model has never been evaluated.

The other Claus model variation is an extension of the original Claus model called the Claus extended method [55]. Using newer information about risk factors for hereditary breast cancer, van Asperen and colleagues used linear regression analysis and incorporated three additional factors into the Claus model: (1) family history of ovarian cancer; (2) family history of bilateral breast cancer; and (3) whether there are more than two affected relatives with breast cancer in the family. This last factor can also, in theory, include male breast cancer but the model did not specifically take this into account. They created a regression formula factoring in these three risk factors plus the original Claus model score for the family. In their analyses, the Claus extended method had lower agreement with the Claus model than the Claus tables, but the extended method correlated better with risk estimates from BRCAPRO and another lesser used model called the Jonker model (a.k.a., BRCA1/2/u model) [56]. The main issue with the Claus extended method is that the formula has never been made available in any computerized format, so using the Claus extended method requires inputting data into their formula and doing the math to calculate the risks which is not the most practical approach in a busy clinic setting.

## Genetic Models: Breast Cancer Risk and *BRCA1/2* Mutation Probabilities

### BRCAPRO

BRCAPRO is by far the most studied and widely used model for assessing *BRCA1/2* mutation carrier probabilities. It is a mathematical model that uses Mendel's laws of inheritance, in this case autosomal dominant inheritance, and Bayes theorem to combine information about a person's personal and family history with published *BRCA* mutation prevalence data and age-specific cancer rates [57–61]. Unlike the BOADICEA or Tyrer-Cuzick model (discussed below), the BRCAPRO model works on the assumption that the cancer in the family is either due to a *BRCA*1/2 mutation or is sporadic in nature, so no other genes (real or theoretical) are including in its statistical equations. The BRCAPRO model will produce a *BRCA* carrier probability for men or women based on: a person's current age; history of invasive breast (unilateral or bilateral, as well as male breast cancer) and/or ovarian cancer and age of onset; all maternal and paternal first- and second-degree relatives including their current age or age at death, their history of invasive breast (unilateral or bilateral, as well as male breast cancer) and/or ovarian cancer and if affected, the age of onset; Ashkenazi Jewish ancestry (BRCAPRO uses different mutation prevalences for Ashkenazi and non-Ashkenazi Jewish individuals); and results of *BRCA1/2* testing for anyone in the family who has undergone testing. The sensitivity and specificity of *BRCA* genetic testing is modifiable in the model. Background cancer rates come from SEER data. Technically, BRCAPRO does not factor in DCIS since age-specific DCIS risks for BRCA carriers are not known. However, some genetics providers will include DCIS when using BRCAPRO in one of two ways: (1) the provider will perform two separate calculations, one including and one excluding the relative with DCIS, and then provide both probabilities to the consultand and explain that the actual carrier probability is somewhere in between the two risks or (2) some providers will include the relative but add 10 years to the age of onset given the potential that in 10 years, if left in the breast, DCIS would transform into invasive disease [62]. Neither of these methods for using BRCAPRO has ever been validated.

Over the years, the BRCAPRO model has undergone a variety of updates. The age-specific penetrance estimates for breast and ovarian cancer have gone from the original higher estimates to more conservative levels [63–68]. BRCAPRO will now factor in both the ovarian and breast cancer risk reduction afforded to women who have undergone prophylactic bilateral salpingo-oophorectomy, for whatever reason, in the family based on the age at surgery; the protective effect on breast cancer risk only benefits women who have the surgery under the age of 60 [69, 70]. Estrogen and progesterone receptor, HER2-neu, CK14, and CK5/6 status can also be inputted to adjust risk predictions [36, 71, 72]. Further, BRCAPRO will consider different races and ethnicities for both penetrance and mutation prevalence estimates and pedigrees of any size can now be included (e.g., third- and fourth-degree relatives can be added).

Multiple studies have looked at the ability of BRCAPRO to discriminate between *BRCA* mutation carriers and noncarriers. Antoniou and Easton provide a summary of some of the studies which show a range of concordance between 60 and 83% [6]. Bellcross compiled data showing the sensitivity, specificity, and PPV of BRCAPRO range between 73–79%, 24–79%, and 24–46%, respectively [73]. BRCAPRO generally overestimates risk for individuals with high carrier probabilities and underestimates risk for individuals with low carrier probabilities [6]. The BRCAPRO model generally poorly discriminates between mutations in *BRCA1* and *BRCA2*, but it seems as though the addition of breast cancer tumor markers into the model has increased the model's discriminatory power [36, 71, 72]. BRCAPRO has been found to overestimate risk for women with bilateral breast cancer [74, 75] and appears to have high discriminatory capacity for men with breast cancer [76]. The BRCAPRO model has been evaluated for individuals of African-American, Hispanic, Asian-American, and Native American background [77–82]. In general, BRCAPRO seems to have the same discriminatory ability and calibration for minority populations compared to Caucasian populations. Some of the studies found slight differences but none of the differences were statistically significant.

In addition to *BRCA* mutation carrier probabilities, the BRCAPRO model provides lifetime breast and ovarian cancer risks for unaffected individuals or contralateral breast cancer risk for an affected individual based on the weighted average of the penetrance for mutation and non-mutation carriers, with the estimated carrier probabilities as weights. The risk is presented in 5-year increments and will calculate risk out until the eighth decade of life. Interestingly, if the patient is in the eighth decade of life, BRCAPRO will provide risks for a minimum of 20 years (i.e., tenth decade). This function of the BRCAPRO model is not as well studied or fully validated. The BRCAPRO model may be underestimating risk since it is not factoring in any personal history and/or other genetic factors. At least one study found that the BRCAPRO model significantly underestimated breast cancer risk and performed the worst compared to the Gail, Claus, and Tyrer-Cuzick models [51].

BRCAPRO requires a computer to use the program and may take 10–15 min to input the history to generate carrier probabilities. BRCAPRO also requires a complete family history to get the most accurate prediction; any family history that is omitted will cause the model to overestimate risk. As with most of the other *BRCA* mutations prediction models, BRCAPRO does not factor other *BRCA*-related cancers (e.g., prostate, pancreas) and as mentioned above, does not include DCIS. It is important to note that not all of the additions discussed above have been incorporated into the BRCAPRO model in the CancerGene© (copyright) software [18] (most recent version is 5.1), but they will soon be added (D. Euhus, personal communication). The most up-to-date version can be downloaded from the BayesMendel website [61].

## BOADICEA Model (Breast and Ovarian Cancer Analysis of Disease Incidence and Carrier Estimation Algorithm)

The BOADICEA model uses complex segregation analysis and Bayes theorem to compute *BRCA1* and *BRCA2* mutation carrier probabilities as well as age-specific invasive breast and ovarian cancer risks [83–86]. The BOADICEA model accounts for the allele frequencies and age-specific breast and ovarian cancer risks for

*BRCA1* and *BRCA2* mutations as well as a polygenic component (i.e., an unknown number of genes that confer a low risk of cancer and act multiplicatively with one another) that represents the familial aggregation of breast cancer not due the *BRCA* genes, but that can also influence breast cancer penetrance in *BRCA* mutation carriers; the polygenic component has no influence on ovarian cancer risk in this model.

The original model version of the BOADICEA model was fit from a combined data set of 1,484 population-based cases of breast cancer diagnosed under the age of 55 and "multiple case" breast cancer families that included ≥2 affected individuals, at least one of whom was diagnosed under the age of 50 [84, 85]. Family history information was included for first-degree relatives only. All of the index cases underwent *BRCA1* and *BRCA2* genetic testing, albeit with an inferior testing technique (conformation sensitive gel electrophoresis (CSGE)) that has an ~70% detection rate; this means they missed some mutations which in turn would have affected the calibration of the model. The baseline breast and ovarian cancer risks are from an English and Welsh population from 1983 to 1987. These rates (5% for breast and 1% for ovarian cancer) are lower than typical rates from the USA. The incidences were assumed to change in 5-year intervals as opposed to an even and gradual change in risk. Further, the model assumed a fixed set of calendar incidences over all groups instead of accounting for the change in risks with advancing age. The *BRCA* penetrance estimates for breast and ovarian cancer selected were on the lower end of the spectrum as well (breast and ovarian cancer by age 70: 35% and 26%, respectively, for *BRCA1* and 50% and 9.1%, respectively, for *BRCA2*). The lower penetrance estimates, in turn, led the BOADICEA model to provide lower carrier probabilities when compared to an early version of BRCAPRO. Finally, only breast and ovarian cancer were included in the model and only one cancer was factored in (e.g., bilateral breast cancer was not counted).

BOADICEA was subsequently expanded to include a much larger data set of population-based breast (which included some male breast cancers) and ovarian cancer diagnoses from three additional studies, one of which was from a meta-analysis of 22 separate population-based studies which totaled 2,785 families and 537 *BRCA1* or *BRCA2* mutation carriers [86, 87]. Family history was again reported for all first-degree relatives and some studies went beyond first-degree relationships. All of the index cases had *BRCA1* and *BRCA2* genetic testing, but given the variety of techniques used across all studies, a 70 and 80% mutation detection rate for *BRCA1* and *BRCA2*, respectively, was assumed (however, when using BOADICEA online, the model allows the user to set the genetic testing sensitivity to provide more accurate risks). Baseline breast and ovarian cancer rates were again taken from English and Welsh populations, but calendar period and cohort-specific incidences were used and the authors employed a method of "smoothing" to account for the gradual changes in risk over time. They used the same techniques for determining penetrance estimates for *BRCA* mutation carriers which were substantially higher and closer to the believed penetrance estimates. Further, family history of male breast, prostate, and pancreatic cancer was added into the model for determining *BRCA* carrier probabilities and male breast cancer was included for adjusting age-specific breast cancer risks, but the model will not provide breast cancer risks for men. History of more than one cancer for women has been included in BOADICEA. This allows the model to factor in bilateral breast cancer diagnoses for *BRCA* mutation carrier probabilities as well as contralateral breast cancer risk for women with and without *BRCA* mutations who have already been affected. Also added were *BRCA* genetic test results and Ashkenazi Jewish ancestry for each individual versus the entire family; this is helpful for individuals who are Ashkenazi Jewish through only one lineage. Breast cancer tumor pathology is an additional factor that will be added soon [88].

The BOADICEA model is available in a Web-based program and will generate a PDF report with a pedigree, *BRCA* carrier probabilities, and breast and ovarian cancer risks [89] (Fig. 1.4a–c). Pedigrees can be created online or uploaded from a pedigree drawing program. A complete family history is needed for the most accurate risk estimates. BOADICEA can include half sibling and relatives beyond second-degree. However, the online model is rather labor-intensive and not very user-friendly. For example, in order to add aunts, uncles, and cousins, grandparents need to be entered first, but this information is not found on the website. Additionally, since the BOADICEA model is calendar- and cohort-specific, it requires year of birth or death for each person in the family which is information most people do not have, so it takes additional time to try and calculate years of birth/death based on the ages provided by patients. While there is an "unknown" option if this information is not available, selecting "unknown" will cause that relative to be ignored by the model which in turn will lead BOADICEA to underestimate risks highlighting the need for specific ages. BOADICEA will not calculate cancer risks beyond the age of 80. BOADICEA does not factor in any reproductive or hormonal risk factors or preventative surgeries. To include preventative surgeries, a woman's age should be censored at the age she had the surgery [89]. In situ disease and non-epithelial ovarian cancers were not used to develop the model, so including this information may lead to overestimation of risks. Another limitation of the model relates to age-specific ovarian cancer risks in women who have tested negative for a *BRCA* mutation. Since the polygenic component was not applied to ovarian cancer risks, the BOADICEA model will assume low ovarian cancer risks if negative *BRCA* results are entered into the model. Further, BOADICEA also underestimates risk for families with a strong history of ovarian cancer [89]. Other than Ashkenazi Jewish ancestry, the model cannot be adjusted for any other races or ethnicities, though the original BOADICEA has been shown to provide comparable risk estimates for African-Americans, but may underperform in Hispanics [82].

Despite all of these limitations, BOADICEA predicts *BRCA* carrier probabilities just as well as some of the other models. At least three separate studies have validated both the original [37, 82, 90] and current version [91–93]. Areas under the ROC curves, sensitivities, specificities, and PPVs are shown in Table 1.3. The breast and ovarian cancer risks produced by BOADICEA have not been well studied or validated. The initial publications for the original and updated version show that the model predicts breast cancer risks well compared to a large combined analysis of familial risk [94], though it may underestimate the risk for very early onset cases (< age 30) in the family and may overpredict risk at older ages [85, 86]. Jacobi and colleagues compared BOADICEA

**a**

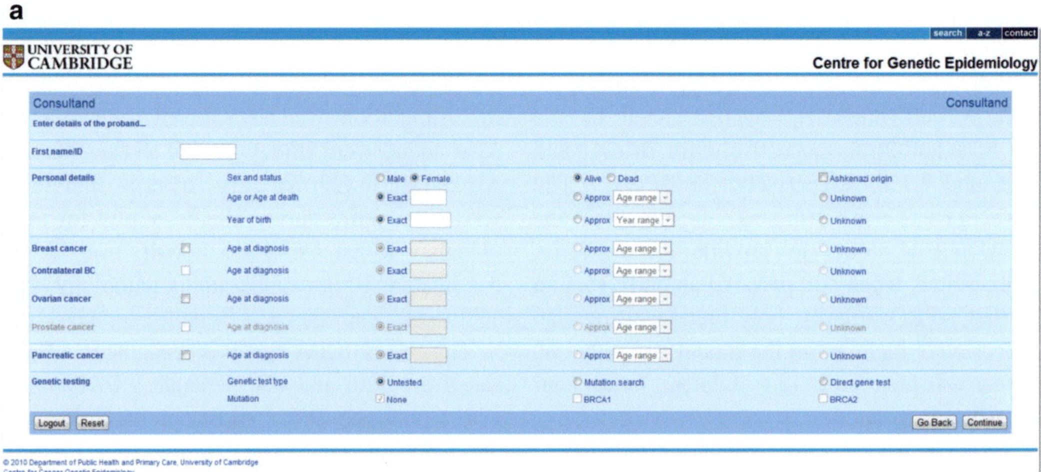


**Fig. 1.4** (a–c) Example of the BOADICEA model including the typical data input page and results output

b

## 2.0 BOADICEA risk calculation results

### Index or subject of the BOADICEA calculation

Firstname/identifier of index: Scott
Unique identifier of index: 1

The BOADICEA model predicts the following BRCA1/BRCA2 mutation carrier probabilities and breast/ovarian cancer risks for this individual:

| Genetic status | Mutation carrier probabilities |
|---|---|
| No mutation | 0.8841 |
| BRCA1 | 0.0609 |
| BRCA2 | 0.0550 |

| Model parameters | |
|---|---|
| Family member | Scott (1) |
| Mutation frequencies | Ashkenazi<br>BRCA1: 0.008<br>BRCA2: 0.006 |
| Mutation search sensitivities | Custom<br>BRCA1: 0.9<br>BRCA2: 0.9 |

| Age | Breast cancer risks | Ovarian cancer risks |
|---|---|---|
| 36 | 0.0023 | 0.0001 |
| 37 | 0.0049 | 0.0003 |
| 38 | 0.0077 | 0.0006 |
| 39 | 0.0109 | 0.0009 |
| 40 | 0.0143 | 0.0013 |
| 45 | 0.0362 | 0.0045 |
| 50 | 0.0656 | 0.0087 |
| 55 | 0.0986 | 0.0149 |
| 60 | 0.1304 | 0.0229 |
| 65 | 0.1589 | 0.0299 |
| 70 | 0.1841 | 0.0362 |
| 75 | 0.2073 | 0.0422 |
| 80 | 0.2279 | 0.0478 |

c

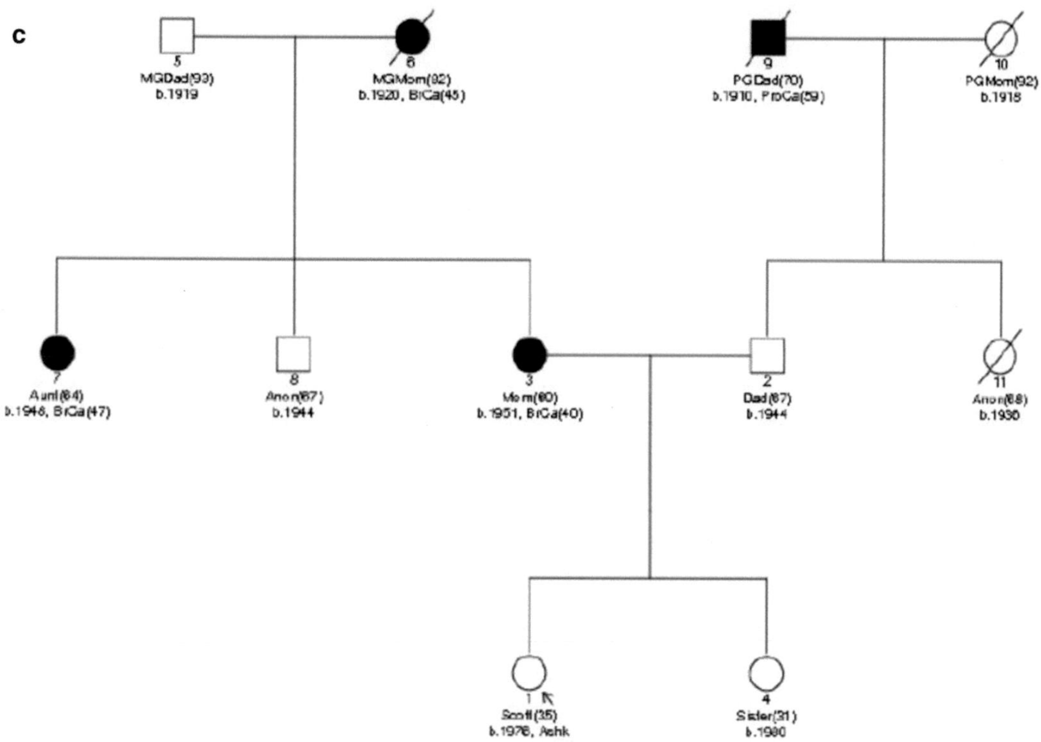


**Fig. 1.4** (continued)

**Table 1.3** Performance characteristics of the BOADICEA model

| | BRCA1 | | | | BRCA2 | | | | BRCA1/2 | | | |
|---|---|---|---|---|---|---|---|---|---|---|---|---|
| Original model | AUC | Sens | Spec | PPV | AUC | Sens | Spec | PPV | AUC | Sens | Spec | PPV |
| Barcenas et al. [8][ab]—F/SDR only | 0.772 | 0.500 | 0.877 | 0.339 | 0.758 | 0.483 | 0.864 | 0.229 | 0.781 | 0.671 | 0.774 | 0.405 |
| Barcenas et al. [8][ab]—extended | 0.773 | 0.571 | 0.856 | 0.333 | 0.763 | 0.552 | 0.803 | 0.189 | 0.775 | 0.729 | 0.711 | 0.367 |
| Roudgardi et al. [9][c] | 0.700 | 0.460 | 0.840 | – | 0.590 | 0.180 | 0.930 | – | 0.680 | 0.530 | 0.780 | – |
| Kurian et al. [10][d] | – | – | – | – | – | – | – | – | 0.826 | – | – | |
| *Updated model* | | | | | | | | | | | | |
| Panchal et al. [11][b] | 0.800 | – | – | – | 0.630 | – | – | – | 0.740 | 0.700 | 0.650 | – |
| Antoniou et al. [12]—extended | – | – | – | – | – | – | – | – | 0.810 | – | – | – |
| Antoniou et al. [13][b] | 0.820 | 0.829 | 0.638 | 0.219 | 0.680 | 0.675 | 0.591 | 0.125 | 0.770 | 0.904 | 0.395 | 0.258 |

*AUC* area under the curve, *Sens* sensitivity, *Spec* specificity, *PPV* positive predictive value, *F/SDR only* first- and second-degree family members only, *extended* entire family structure
[a]Non-Ashkenazi Jewish families only
[b]Sensitivity, specificity, and PPV using a 10% cutoff for offering genetic testing
[c]Sensitivity, specificity, and PPV using a 20% cutoff for offering genetic testing
[d]Data in table for Caucasian pts only

breast cancer risk estimates with other breast cancer models for different fictitious personal and family history scenarios and found that BOADICEA tended to produce lower risk estimates than many of the other models [95]. Studies assessing age-specific ovarian cancer risk estimates have not been performed. Finally, one study evaluated the breast and ovarian cancer risks provided by BOADICEA for unaffected *BRCA* mutation carriers and it seemed to be comparable to what would be expected for the study population, but further studies are needed to confirm their findings [93].

## IBIS Model (*Tyrer-Cuzick Model*)

The IBIS model is a complex model that provides both lifetime breast cancer risk estimates as well as *BRCA1* or *BRCA2* mutation probabilities [96]. The model uses a two locus genetic model with one of the genes being either *BRCA1* or *BRCA2* and the other being a hypothetical low penetrant, highly prevalent gene that causes breast cancer only; the theoretical prevalence of this gene is 11% in the general population with a lifetime risk of 24% to age 70. The purpose of the hypothetical gene is to account for all other unknown genes modifying familial breast cancer risk which can help account for effects of the family history of cancer if a *BRCA* gene mutation is not present in the family. The same approach was not applied to ovarian cancer, so the IBIS model does not provide ovarian cancer risks. The IBIS model uses a proportional hazards modeling to combine both genetic and nongenetic factors to calculate breast cancer risks. It does this by combining the absolute risk based purely on family history and the relative risk for an individual based on her personal factors. For *BRCA* probabilities, the model uses segregation analysis based on Bayes theorem to predict the risk of having a *BRCA1* or *BRCA2* mutation from family history information.

The data used to generate the model comes from a variety of populations. Baseline breast and ovarian cancer risks were taken from the UK national statistics whereas the *BRCA* breast and ovarian cancer penetrance estimates (i.e., lifetime risks) were from the Breast Cancer Linkage Consortium (BCLC) which is a population of European and North American *BRCA* families [66].

*BRCA1* and *BRCA2* mutation prevalence data come from a population of the UK women with early onset breast cancer. Lastly, family history risk estimates were comprised from a Swedish registry that reported breast and ovarian cancer risks for women whose mothers and/or sisters had breast (unilateral or bilateral) and/or ovarian cancer [97].

The IBIS model is one of the most comprehensive models as it factors in a variety of personal risk factors including current age, age at menarche, parity and, if parous, age at first live birth, height and weight for body mass index, menopausal status and age at menopause, atypical hyperplasia, and lobular carcinoma in situ. Since the model was first published, additional personal risk factors have been added including hyperplasia without atypia [98], personal history of ovarian cancer, hormone replacement therapy use and length of use, and Ashkenazi Jewish ancestry for the whole family (i.e., a person who is half Ashkenazi Jewish has to be entered as either non-Ashkenazi or 100% Ashkenazi) [42]. For an individual's family history, the IBIS model allows for the incorporation of both maternal and paternal lineage and initially included both affected and unaffected first- and second-degree female relatives and has been updated to include cousins and half sisters. A diagnosis and age of onset for breast cancer can be added for any relative, but bilateral breast cancer can only be inputted for mothers and sisters. Diagnoses and age of onset for ovarian cancer can be added for most relatives except nieces, cousins, and half sisters and the model will account for up to two aunts with ovarian cancer on each side of the family. Other *BRCA*-related cancers (e.g., pancreatic) and male breast cancer are not included in the IBIS model.

The IBIS model has a number of benefits. The model itself is easy to use with regard to data entry (although it does require a complete family history to be most accurate) and can be found online at www.ems-trials.org/riskevaluator/. The model output is very nice as it represents age-adjusted risks in both numerical and graphical form and provides a small pedigree (Fig. 1.5a–c). IBIS incorporates personal and reproductive risk factors in addition to pretty complete family history information and will adjust risk based on the number of affected and unaffected female relatives. *BRCA* genetic test results can be added into the model and it will calculate residual breast cancer risks. The original model's breast cancer predictive value was compared to both the Gail and Claus models in a cohort of women from the UK who was seen for risk assessment and undergoing regular mammography [51]. Overall, the IBIS model outperformed both models, predicting breast cancer risk more accurately as shown by its goodness of fit and discriminatory value (Table 1.4), though the same type of study has not been performed on a population of women with different baseline breast cancer risks than the UK women to see if this finding would be consistent in a different population of Caucasian women than was used to create the model. This is relevant as one of the main uses of the IBIS model is to aid genetics professionals in determining breast MRI eligibility [1, 52].

Many downsides have been raised by multiple authors as well. To start, the model will not factor in a diagnosis of breast cancer in a proband; so IBIS model cannot be used to calculate *BRCA* carrier probabilities for women affected with breast cancer. Concerns about the IBIS model include the possibility that the penetrance may be underestimated and the mutation frequency could be overestimated for the hypothetical gene which would lead to an underestimation of breast cancer risk for women with a strong family history of breast cancer and overestimation of risk for women with weaker family histories [99]. The IBIS model was developed by modeling recurrence risks in mother–daughter pairs only so it may not predict risks for other affected relative groupings as accurately and it is not based on a real sample of women [6, 100]; instead it is an amalgamation of different populations and data sets. The model assumes that the nongenetic risk factors are multiplicative on risk and has the same degree of effect on both *BRCA* mutation carriers and non-*BRCA* mutation carriers [6]. The risk of breast and ovarian cancer for *BRCA* mutation carriers used from the BCLC is based on high-risk families [6] and may lead to overestimates of *BRCA* probabilities. The IBIS model seems to

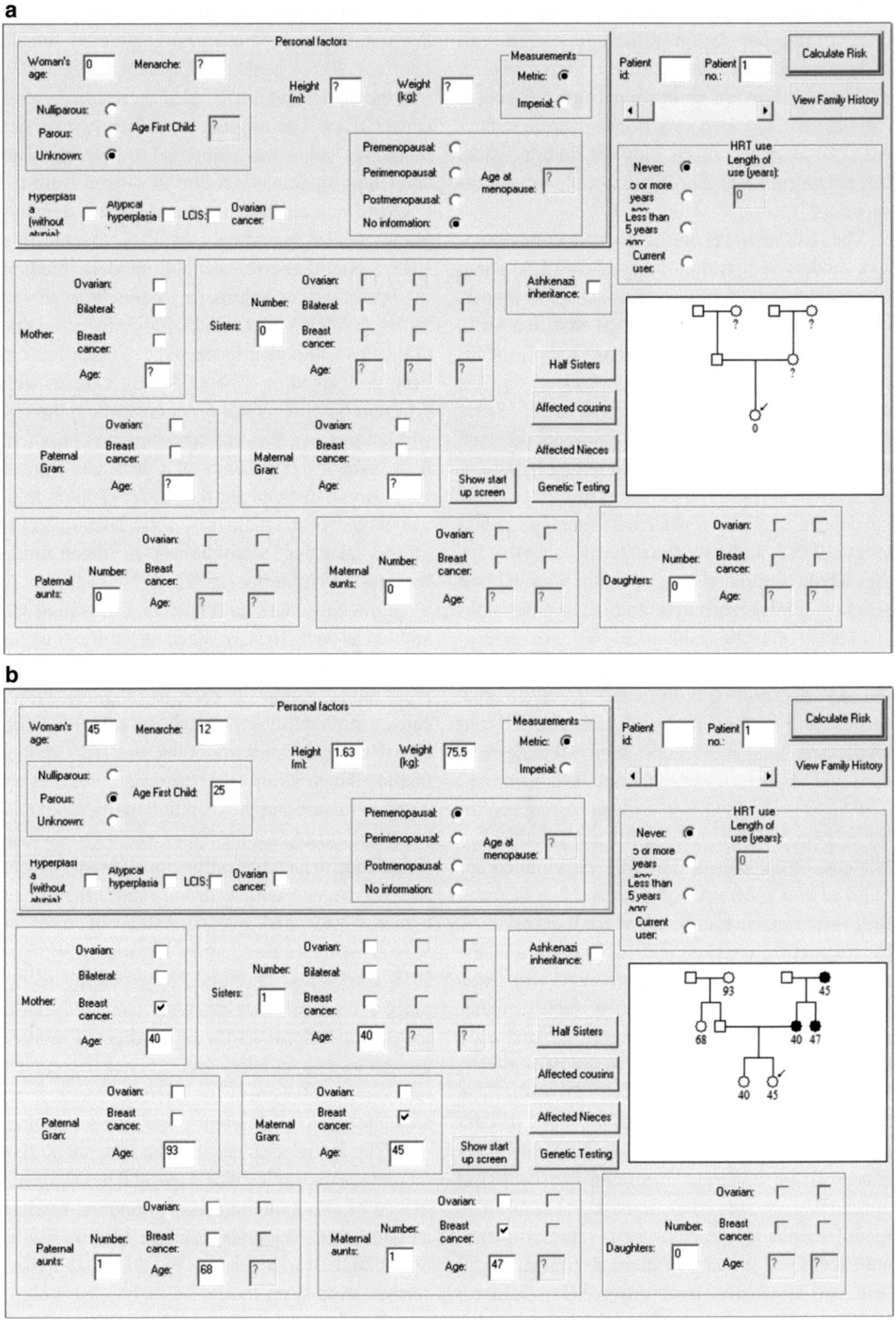

**Fig. 1.5** (**a–c**) Example of the IBIS model including the data input page and the results output

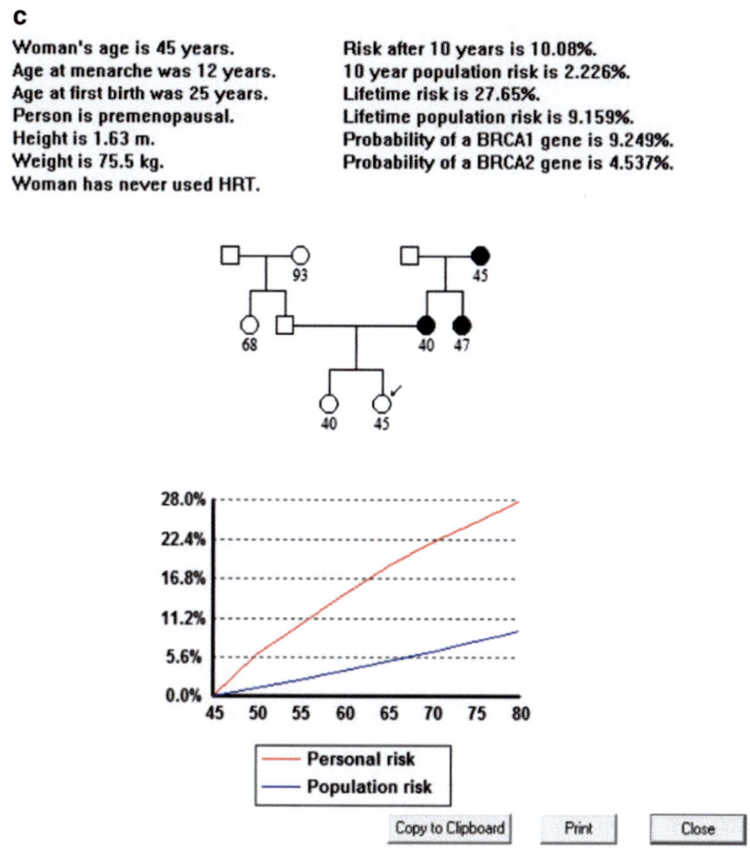


**Fig. 1.5** (continued)

**Table 1.4** Comparison of calibration and discrimination between IBIS, Claus, and Gail models

| Model | Goodness of fit | Discriminatory value |
|---|---|---|
| Gail | 0.48 (95% CI 0.37–0.64) | 0.735 (95% CI 0.666–0.803) |
| Claus | 0.56 (95% CI 0.43–0.75) | 0.716 (95% CI 0.648–0.784) |
| IBIS | 0.81 (95% CI 0.62–1.08) | 0.762 (95% CI 0.700–0.824) |

Adapted from [51]

overestimate breast cancer risk in women with atypical hyperplasia [101] and premenopausal women with a low BMI [102]. Moreover, two separate studies showed that the IBIS model does not predict *BRCA* mutation status as well as some of the other models [91, 93]. In addition to some of the practical issues with IBIS model mentioned above (e.g., does not include male breast cancer, up to two aunts with ovarian cancer can be included), the IBIS model does not adjust to non-Caucasian women.

## Empiric Model for Cowden Syndrome

### *PTEN* Mutation Risk Calculator

Until recently, the *BRCA1/2* genes were the only hereditary breast cancer genes that had risk models available for risk stratification. In 2011, Tan et al. published the first risk model to assess for Cowden syndrome, one of the conditions collectively referred to as the PTEN hamartoma tumor

the prevalence in the general population. Phenotypic features strongly suggestive of Cowden syndrome (e.g., trichilemmomas and extreme macrocephaly) with the highest relative risks were assigned the highest weight (i.e., 10) whereas features with the lowest relative risks (e.g., fibrocystic breast disease) were assigned the lowest weight (i.e., 1). For features that their group believed to contribute to the potential referral bias, they adjusted the weights down one level (e.g., a diagnosis of thyroid cancer between the ages of 20–29 had a relative risk of ~46–48 and should have been given a weight of 6, but given the potential for referral bias, a weight of 4 was used). An individual's score is generated as the sum of the weights of features from a given individual. The score is then used for the calculation of a point pretest probability of harboring a *PTEN* mutation. Tan et al. recommend *PTEN* genetic testing be pursed when the pretest probability is 3% or greater (an overall score of ≥10); at this cutoff level, 90% of individuals who carry *PTEN* mutations will be identified. The risk calculator can be found online at http://www.lerner.ccf.org/gmi/ccscore.

In addition to the limitation of a potential referral bias, they were unable to validate extreme macrocephaly and gastrointestinal polyp number against the Ohio State cohort; they had to omit extreme macrocephaly completely and they matched polyp presence with multiple polyp status. Further and most importantly, validation of the tool needs to be done on a population-based sampling approach to know that it works in the community setting. Given these limitations, the *PTEN* risk calculator is very helpful in the clinic setting when one is trying to determine when to offer patients genetic for the *PTEN* gene for Cowden syndrome.

## References

1. Saslow D, Boetes C, Burke W, et al. American Cancer Society guidelines for breast screening with MRI as an adjunct to mammography. CA Cancer J Clin. 2007;57:75–89.
2. NCCN Clinical Practice Guidelines in Oncology (NCCN Guidelines™). Breast Cancer Screening and Diagnosis. Version 1.2011. http://www.nccn.org. Accessed 30 Jan 2012.
3. NCCN Clinical Practice Guidelines in Oncology (NCCN Guidelines™). Breast cancer risk reduction. Version 3.2011. http://www.nccn.org. Accessed 30 Jan 2012.
4. U.S. Preventive Services Task Force. Genetic risk assessment and *BRCA* mutation testing for breast and ovarian susceptibility: recommendation statement. Ann Intern Med. 2005;143:355–61.
5. NCCN Clinical Practice Guidelines in Oncology (NCCN Guidelines™). Genetic/familial high-risk assessment: breast and ovarian. Version 1.2011. http://www.nccn.org. Accessed 30 Jan 2012.
6. Antoniou AC, Easton DF. Risk prediction models for familial breast cancer. Future Oncol. 2006;2:257–74.
7. Amir E, Freedman OC, Seruga B, Evans DG. Assessing women at high risk of breast cancer: a review of risk assessment models. J Natl Cancer Inst. 2010;102:680–91.
8. Freedman AN, Seminara D, Gail MH, et al. Cancer risk prediction models: a workshop on development, evaluation and application. J Natl Cancer Inst. 2005;97:715–23.
9. Euhus DM. Understanding mathematical models for breast cancer risk assessment and counseling. Breast J. 2001;7:224–32.
10. CancerGene. http://www8.utsouthwestern.edu/utsw/cda/dept47829/files/65844.html. Accessed 26 Feb 2012.
11. The Breast Cancer Risk Assessment Tool. http://www.cancer.gov/bcrisktool/default.aspx. Accessed 19 Feb 2012.
12. Gail MH, Brinton LA, Byar DP, et al. Projecting individualized probabilities of developing breast cancer for white females who are being examined annually. J Natl Cancer Inst. 1989;81:1879–86.
13. Baker LH. Breast cancer detection demonstration project: five year summary report. CA Cancer J Clin. 1982;32:194–225.
14. Gail MH, Benichou J. Assessing the risk of breast cancer in individuals. In: Devita Jr VT, Hellman S, Rosenberg SA, editors. Cancer prevention. Philadelphia, PA: Lippincott; 1992. p. 1–15.
15. Spiegelman D, Colditz GA, Hunter D, Hertzmark E. Validation of the Gail et al. model for predicting individualized breast cancer risk. J Natl Cancer Inst. 1994;86:600–7.
16. Bondy ML, Lustbader ED, Halabi S, Ross E, Vogel VG. Validation of a breast cancer risk assessment model in women with a positive family history. J Natl Cancer Inst. 1994;86:620–5.
17. Anderson SJ, Ahn S, Duff K. NSABP Breast Cancer Prevention Trial risk assessment program, version 2. NSABP Biostatistical Center Technical Report, 12 Aug 1992.
18. Fisher B, Costantino JP, Wickerham DL, et al. Tamoxifen for the prevention of breast cancer: report of the National Surgical Adjuvant Breast and Bowel Project P-1 study. J Natl Cancer Inst. 1998;90:1371–88.

19. Costantino JP, Gail MH, Pee D, et al. Validation studies of the models projecting the risk of invasive and total breast cancer incidence. J Natl Cancer Inst. 1999;91:1541–8.
20. Rockhill B, Spiegelman D, Byrne C, Hunter DJ, Colditz GA. Validation of the Gail et al. model of breast cancer risk prediction and implications for chemoprevention. J Natl Cancer Inst. 2001;93:358–66.
21. Gail MH, Costantino JP, Pee D, et al. Projecting individualized absolute invasive breast cancer risk in African American women. J Natl Cancer Inst. 2007;99:1782–92.
22. Matsuno RK, Costantino JP, Ziegeler RG, et al. Projecting individualized absolute invasive breast cancer risk in Asian and Pacific Island American women. J Natl Cancer Inst. 2011;103:951–61.
23. Gail MH, Costantino JP, Bryant J, et al. Weighing the risks and benefits of tamoxifen treatment for preventing breast cancer. J Natl Cancer Inst. 1999;91:1829–11846.
24. Gail MH. Discriminatory accuracy from single-nucleotide polymorphisms in models to predict breast cancer risk. J Natl Cancer Inst. 2008;100:1037–41.
25. Gail MH. Value of adding single-nucleotide polymorphism genotypes to a breast cancer risk model. J Natl Cancer Inst. 2009;101:959–63.
26. Mealiffe ME, Stokowski RP, Rhees BK, Prentice RL, Pettinger M, Hinds DA. Assessment of clinical validity of a breast cancer risk model combining genetics and clinical information. J Natl Cancer Inst. 2010;102:1618–27.
27. Couch FJ, DeShano ML, Blackwood MA, et al. *BRCA1* mutations in women attending clinics that evaluate the risk of breast cancer. N Engl J Med. 1997;336:1409–15.
28. Lindor NM, Lindor RA, Apicella C, et al. Predicting *BRCA1* and *BRCA2* gene mutation carriers: comparison of LAMBDA, BRCAPRO, Myriad II and modified Couch models. Fam Cancer. 2007;6:473–82.
29. Parmigiani G, Chen S, Iversen ES, et al. Validity of models predicting *BRCA1* and *BRCA2* mutations. Ann Intern Med. 2007;147:441–50.
30. Lindor NM, Johnson KJ, Harvey H, et al. Predicting *BRCA1* and *BRCA2* gene mutation carriers: comparison of PENN II model to previous study. Fam Cancer. 2010;9:495–502.
31. Werness BA, Ramus SJ, Whittemore AS, et al. Histopathology of familial ovarian tumors in women from families with and without germline *BRCA1* mutations. Hum Pathol. 2000;31:1420–4.
32. Pal T, Permuth-Wey J, Betts JA, et al. *BRCA1* and *BRCA2* mutations account for a large proportion of ovarian carcinoma cases. Cancer. 2005;104:2807–16.
33. Shattuck-Eidens D, Oliphant A, McClure M, et al. *BRCA1* sequence analysis in women at high risk for susceptibility mutations: risk factor analysis and implications for genetic testing. JAMA. 1997;278(15):1242–50.
34. Frank TS, Manley SA, Olopade OI, et al. Sequence analysis of *BRCA1* and *BRCA2*: Correlation of mutations with family history and ovarian cancer risk. J Clin Oncol. 1998;16(7):2417–25.
35. Frank TS, Deffenbaugh AM, Reid JE, et al. Clinical characteristics of individuals with germline mutations in *BRCA1* and *BRCA2*: analysis of 10,000 individuals. J Clin Oncol. 2002;20:1480–90.
36. James PA, Doherty R, Harris M, et al. Optimal selection of individuals for *BRCA* mutation testing: a comparison of available methods. J Clin Oncol. 2006;24:707–15.
37. Barcenas CH, Monawar Hosain GM, Arun B, et al. Assessing *BRCA* carrier probabilities in extended families. J Clin Oncol. 2006;24:354–60.
38. Hartge P, Struewing JP, Wacholder S, Brody LC, Tucker MA. The prevalence of common *BRCA1* and *BRCA2* mutations among Ashkenazi Jews. Am J Hum Genet. 1999;64(4):963–70.
39. Hopper JL, Jenkins MA. Modeling the probability that Ashkenazi Jewish women carry a founder mutation in *BRCA1* or *BRCA2*. Am J Hum Genet. 1999;65:1771–5.
40. Wacholder S, Hartge P. Response to letters from Hopper and Jenkins and Foulkes et al. Am J Hum Genet. 1999;65:1775.
41. Foulkes WD, Brunet JS, Warner E, et al. The importance of family history of breast cancer in predicting the presence of a *BRCA* mutation. Am J Hum Genet. 1999;65:1776–8.
42. Struewing JP, Hartge P, Wacholder S, et al. The risk of cancer associated with specific mutations of *BRCA1* and *BRCA2* among Ashkenazi Jews. N Eng J Med. 1997;336:141–1408.
43. Apicella C, Andrews L, Hodgson SV, et al. Log odds of carrying an ancestral mutation in *BRCA1* and *BRCA2* for a defined personal and family history in an Ashkenazi Jewish woman (LAMBDA). Breast Cancer Res. 2003;5(6):R206–16.
44. Nelson HD, Huffman LH, Fu R, Harris EL. U.S. Preventive Services Task Force. Genetic risk assessment and *BRCA* mutation testing for breast and ovarian susceptibility: systematic evidence review for the U.S. Preventive Services Task Force. Ann Intern Med. 2005;143:362–79.
45. Hodgson SV, Heap E, Cameron J, et al. Risk factors for detecting germline *BRCA1* and *BRCA2* founder mutations in Ashkenazi Jewish women with breast or ovarian cancer. J Med Genet. 1999;36:369–73.
46. Apicella C, Dowty JG, Dite GS, et al. Validation study of the LAMBDA model for predicting the *BRCA1* or *BRCA2* mutation carrier status of North American Ashkenazi Jewish women. Clin Genet. 2007;72:87–97.
47. Claus EB, Risch N, Thompson WD. Autosomal dominant inheritance of early-onset breast cancer: implications for risk prediction. Cancer. 1994;73:643–51.
48. Claus EB, Risch N, Thompson WD. Genetic analysis of breast cancer in the cancer and steroid hormone study. Am J Hum Genet. 1991;48:232–42.

49. McGuigan KA, Ganz PA, Breant C. Agreement between breast cancer risk estimation methods. J Natl Cancer Inst. 1996;88:1315–7.
50. McTiernan A, Kuniyuki A, Yasui Y, et al. Comparisons of two breast cancer risk estimates in women with a family history of breast cancer. Cancer Epidemiol Biomarkers Prev. 2001;10:333–8.
51. Amir E, Evans DG, Shenton A, et al. Evaluation of breast cancer risk assessment packages in the family history evaluation and screening programme. J Med Genet. 2003;40:807–14.
52. Bellcross C. Approaches to applying breast cancer risk prediction models in clinical practice. Commun Oncol. 2009;6:373–9.
53. Claus EB, Schildkraut J, Iversen Jr ES, Berry D, Parmigiani G. Effect of *BRCA1* and *BRCA2* on the association between breast cancer risk and family history. J Natl Cancer Inst. 1998;90:1824–9.
54. Claus EB, Risch N, Thompson WD. The calculation of breast cancer risk for women with a first degree family history of ovarian cancer. Breast Cancer Res Treat. 1993;28:115–20.
55. van Asperen CJ, Jonker MA, Jacobi CE, et al. Risk estimation for healthy women from breast cancer families: new insights and new strategies. Cancer Epidemiol Biomarkers Prev. 2004;13:87–93.
56. Jonker MA, Jacobi CE, Hoogendoorn WE, Nagelkerke NJD, de Bock GH, van Houwelingen JC. Modeling familial clustered breast cancer using published data. Cancer Epidemiol Biomarkers Prev. 2003;12:1479–85.
57. Murphy EA, Mutalik GS. The application of Bayesian Methods in genetic counseling. Hum Hered. 1969;19:126–51.
58. Berry DA, Parmigiani G, Sanchez J, Schildkraut J, Winer E. Probability of carrying a mutation of breast-ovarian cancer gene *BRCA1* based on family history. J Natl Cancer Inst. 1997;89:227–38.
59. Parmigiani G, Berry DA, Aguilar O. Determining carrier probabilities for breast cancer-susceptibility genes *BRCA1* and *BRCA2*. Am J Hum Genet. 1998;62:145–58.
60. Chen S, Wang W, Broman KW, Katki HA, Parmigiani G. BayesMendel: an R environment for Mendelian risk prediction. Stat Appl Genet Mol Biol. 2004;3(1):Article 21.
61. BayesMendel Lab. http://www.astor.som.jhmi.edu/BayesMendel/. Accessed 12 Feb 2012.
62. Burstein HJ, Polyak K, Wong JS, Lester SC, Kaelin CM. Ductal carcinoma in situ of the breast. N Engl J Med. 2004;350:1430–41.
63. Easton DF, Ford D, Bishop DT. Breast Cancer Linkage Consortium. Breast and ovarian cancer incidence in *BRCA1*-mutation carriers. Am J Hum Genet. 1995;56:265–71.
64. Easton DF, Steele L, Fields P, et al. Cancer risks in two large families linked to *BRCA2* on chromosome 13q12-13. Am J Hum Genet. 1997;61:120–8.
65. Struewing JP, Hartge P, Wacholder S, et al. The risk of cancer associated with specific mutations of *BRCA1* and *BRCA2* among Ashkenazi Jews. N Engl J Med. 1997;336:1401–8.
66. Ford D, Easton DF, Stratton M, et al. Genetic heterogeneity and penetrance analysis of the *BRCA1* and *BRCA2* genes in breast cancer families. The Breast Cancer Linkage Consortium. Am J Hum Genet. 1998;62:676–89.
67. Chen S, Iversen ES, Friebel T, et al. Characterization of *BRCA1* and *BRCA2* mutations in a large United States sample. J Clin Oncol. 2006;24:863–71.
68. Chen S, Parmigiani G. Meta-analysis of *BRCA1* and *BRCA2* penetrance. J Clin Oncol. 2007;25: 1329–33.
69. Katki HA. Incorporating medical interventions into carrier probability estimation for genetic counseling. BMC Med Genet. 2007;8:13–23.
70. Domchek SM, Friebel TM, Singer CF, Evans DG, Lynch HT, Isaacs C. Association of risk-reducing surgery in *BRCA1* or *BRCA2* mutation carriers with cancer risk and mortality. JAMA. 2010;304:967–75.
71. Tai YC, Chen S, Parmigiani G, Klein AP. Incorporating tumor immunohistochemical markers in *BRCA1* and *BRCA2* carrier prediction. Breast Cancer Res. 2008;10:401–2.
72. Biswas S, Tankhiwale N, Blackford A, et al. Assessing the added value of breast tumor markers in genetic risk prediction model BRCAPRO. Breast Cancer Res Treat. Published online 24 Jan 2012. doi: 10.1007/s10549-012-1958-z
73. Bellcross CA, Lemke AA, Pape LS, Tess AL, Meisner LT. Evaluation of a breast/ovarian cancer genetics referral screening tool in a mammography population. Genet Med. 2009;11:783–9.
74. Marroni F, Aretini P, D'Andrea E, et al. Evaluation of widely used models for predicting *BRCA1* and *BRCA2* mutations. J Med Genet. 2004;41:278–85.
75. Ready KJ, Vogel KJ, Atchley DP, et al. Accuracy of the BRCAPRO model among women with bilateral breast cancer. Cancer. 2009;115:725–30.
76. Zanna I, Rizzolo P, Sera F, et al. The BRCAPRO 5.0 model is a useful tool in genetic counseling and clinical management of male breast cancer cases. Eur J Hum Genet. 2010;18:856–8.
77. Nanda R, Schumm LP, Cummings S, et al. Genetic testing in an ethnically diverse cohort of high risk women: a comparative analysis of *BRCA1* and *BRCA2* mutations in American families of European and African ancestry. JAMA. 2005;294:1925–33.
78. Vogel KJ, Atchley DP, Erlichman J, et al. *BRCA1* and *BRCA2* genetic testing in Hispanic patients: mutation prevalence and evaluation of the BRCAPRO risk assessment model. J Clin Oncol. 2007;25:4635–41.
79. Kurian AW, Gong GD, Chun NM, et al. Performance of *BRCA1/2* mutation prediction models in Asian Americans. J Clin Oncol. 2008;26:4752–8.
80. Chen S, Blackford AL, Parmigiani G. Tailoring BRCAPRO to Asian-Americans. J Clin Oncol. 2009;27:642–3.
81. Huo D, Senie RT, Daly M, et al. Prediction of *BRCA* mutations using the BRCAPRO model in clinic-

based African American, Hispanic and other minority families in the United States. J Clin Oncol. 2009;27:1184–90.

82. Kurian AW, Gong GD, John EM, et al. Performance of prediction models for *BRCA* mutation carriage in three racial/ethnic groups: findings from the Northern California breast cancer family registry. Cancer Epidemiol Biomarkers Prev. 2009;18:1084–91.
83. Antoniou AC, Pharoah PDP, McMullan G, Day NE, Ponder BAJ, Easton D. Evidence for further breast cancer susceptibility genes in addition to *BRCA1* and *BRCA2* in a population-based study. Genet Epidemiol. 2001;21:1–18.
84. Antoniou AC, Pharoah PDP, McMullan G, et al. A comprehensive model for familial breast cancer incorporating *BRCA1*, *BRCA2*, and other genes. Br J Cancer. 2002;86:76–83.
85. Antoniou AC, Pharoah PDP, Smith P, Easton DF. The BOADICEA model of genetic susceptibility to breast and ovarian cancer. Br J Cancer. 2004;91:1580–90.
86. Antoniou AC, Cunningham AP, Peto J, et al. The BOADICEA model of genetic susceptibility to breast and ovarian cancers: update and extensions. Br J Cancer. 2008;98:1457–66.
87. Antoniou AC, Pharoah PDP, Narod S, et al. Average risks of breast and ovarian cancer associated with *BRCA1* and *BRCA2* mutations detected in case series unselected for family history: a combined analysis of 22 studies. Am J Hum Genet. 2003;72:1117–30.
88. Mavaddat N, Rebbeck TR, Lakhani SR, Easton DF, Antoniou A. Incorporating tumour pathology information in breast cancer risk prediction algorithms. Breast Cancer Res. 2010;12:R28.
89. The BOADICEA model. www.srl.cam.au.uk/genepi/boadicea/boadicea_home.html. Accessed 21 Feb 2012.
90. Roudgardi H, Miedzybrodzka ZH, Haites NE. Probability estimation models for prediction of *BRCA1* and *BRCA2* mutation carriers: COS compared favourably with other models. Fam Cancer. 2008;7:199–212.
91. Panchal SM, Ennis M, Ganon S, Bordeleai LJ. Selecting a *BRCA* risk assessment model for use in a familial cancer clinic. BMC Med Genet. 2008;9:116–24.
92. Antoniou AC, Durocher F, Smith P, Simard J. INHERIT BRCAs program members, Easton DF. *BRCA1* and *BRCA2* mutation predictions using the BOADICEA and BRCAPRO models and penetrance estimation in high-risk French-Canadian families. Breast Cancer Res. 2006;8:R3.
93. Antoniou AC, Hardy R, Walker L, et al. Predicting the likelihood of carry a *BRCA1* or *BRCA2* mutation: validation of BOADICEA, BRCAPRO, IBIS, Myriad and the Manchester scoring system using data from UK genetics clinics. J Med Genet. 2008;45:425–31.
94. Collaborative Group in Hormonal Factors in Breast Cancer. Familial breast cancer: collaborative reanalysis of individuals date from 52 epidemiological studies including 58,209 women with breast cancer and 101,986 women without disease. Lancet. 2001; 358:1389–99.
95. Jacobi CE, de Bock GH, Siegerink B, van Asperen CJ. Differences and similarities in breast cancer risk assessment models in clinical practice: which model to choose? Breast Cancer Res Treat. 2009;115:381–90.
96. Tyrer J, Duffy SW, Cuzick J. A breast cancer prediction model incorporating familial and personal risk factors. Stat Med. 2004;23:1111–30.
97. Anderson H, Bladström A, Olsson H, Möller TR. Familial breast and ovarian cancer: a Swedish population-based register study. Am J Epidemiol. 2000; 152(12):1154–63.
98. Page DL, Dupont WD. Anatomic indicators (histologic and cytologic) of increased breast cancer risk. Breast Cancer Res Treat. 1993;28(2):157–66.
99. de Bock GH, Jacobi CE, Jonker MA, Nagelkerke NJD, van Houwelingen JC. Letter to the editor—a breast cancer risk prediction tool. Stat Med. 2005; 24:1610–2.
100. Ready K, Litton JK, Arun BK. Clinical application of breast cancer risk models. Future Oncol. 2010; 6(3):355.
101. Boughey JC, Hartmann LC, Anderson SS, et al. Evaluation of the Tyrer-Cuzick (International Breast Cancer Intervention Study) model for breast cancer risk prediction in women with atypical hyperplasia. J Clin Oncol. 2010;28:3591–6.
102. van den Brandt PA, Spiegelman D, Yuan SS, et al. Pooled analysis of prospective cohort studies on height, weight and breast cancer risk. Am J Epidemiol. 2000;152:514–27.
103. Hobert JA, Eng C. PTEN hamartoma tumor syndrome: an overview. Genet Med. 2009;11:687–94.
104. Tan MH, Mester J, Peterson C, et al. A clinical scoring system for selection of patients for PTEN mutation testing is proposed on the basis of a prospective study of 3042 probands. Am J Hum Genet. 2011; 88:42–56.
105. Pilarski R, Eng C. Will the real Cowden syndrome please stand up (again)? Expanding mutations and clinical spectra of the PTEN hamartoma tumor syndrome. J Med Genet. 2004;41:323–6.
106. Nelen MR, Padberg GW, Peeters EA, et al. Localization of the gene for Cowden disease to chromosome 10q22-23. Nat Genet. 1996;13:114–6.
107. Eng C. Will the real Cowden syndrome please stand up: revised diagnostic criteria. J Med Genet. 2000; 37:828–30.
108. PTEN Hamartoma Tumor Syndrome on Genereviews.org. http://www.ncbi.nlm.nih.gov/books/NBK1488/. Accessed 29 Feb 2012.

# 2 Genetic and Genomic Factors in Breast Cancer

Lee P. Shulman

## Introduction

Breast cancer is the result of a complex interaction of genetic, genomic, and environmental factors that result in the initiation and progression of malignancy. While certain germline (germinal) inherited genes have been identified that, when altered or mutated, predispose that individual to develop breast cancer and other associated malignancies such as ovarian epithelial cancer (OEC), the majority of breast cancer cases, even those occurring in women with multiple affected family members, are not associated with mutations of genes currently linked to cancer predisposition syndromes. Of interest is that women who develop breast cancer and have identified germinal gene mutations generally do not have a vastly different disease course or prognosis than those who develop sporadic breast cancer and have no detectable gene mutations. However, specific alterations of the somatic genome (i.e., the genome of the actual tumor tissue as opposed to the germinal genome found in all the nucleated cells of an individual) have been identified that better predict prognosis and the relative success or failure of specific therapeutic interventions.

Risk assessment for breast cancer in unaffected women continues to rely on a careful and detailed assessment of personal and family histories within a risk assessment algorithm with the offering of genetic testing to women (and some men) who are found to have an increased likelihood of being a carrier of a deleterious mutation in a cancer susceptibility gene. Accordingly, genetics and genomics have become a central aspect of clinical breast cancer, from risk assessment to prognosis and management. In this chapter, our current understanding of genetic and genomic factors in the assessment of breast cancer risk and prognosis will be presented, recognizing the central role of genetic counseling in cancer risk assessment and the expanding capabilities of genetic and genomic analyses to better delineate risk for developing breast cancer, assess prognosis in affected individuals, and identify more effective preventative and therapeutic interventions.

Some of the material presented in this work is adapted from: Shulman LP. Hereditary breast and ovarian cancer (HBOC). Clinical features and counseling for *BRCA1 and 2*, Lynch syndrome, Cowden syndrome, and Li-Fraumeni syndrome. Obstet Gynecol Clin North Am. 2010;37:109–33.

L.P. Shulman, M.D. (✉)
Division of Clinical Genetics, Feinberg School of Medicine of Northwestern University, Chicago, IL, USA

Northwestern Ovarian Cancer Early Detection and Prevention Program, Feinberg School of Medicine of Northwestern University, Chicago, IL, USA

Cancer Genetics Program, Robert S. Lurie Comprehensive Cancer Center, Feinberg School of Medicine of Northwestern University, Chicago, IL, USA

Department of Obstetrics and Gynecology, Prentice Women's Hospital, Northwestern Memorial Hospital, 250 E. Superior Street, Suite 05-2174, Chicago, IL 60611, USA
e-mail: lps5@cornell.edu

N.M. Hansen (ed.), *Management of the Patient at High Risk for Breast Cancer*,
DOI 10.1007/978-1-4614-5891-3_2, © Springer Science+Business Media New York 2013

## Heritable Breast Cancer

The increased risk for developing cancer in women with mutations in cancer susceptibility genes invariably begins with the inheritance of a germline mutation from either parent. While gynecologic malignancies can only occur in females and the vast majority of breast cancers occur in women, genes that predispose to the development of gynecologic malignancies are mostly autosomal in nature and thus readily inheritable from either parent. This concept is critical when obtaining family history information as both parents can transmit gene mutations; accordingly, obtaining careful and detailed family histories of an individual's maternal and paternal families is vital to estimating accurate risk for cancer development in an individual.

By definition, a germline mutation is present at conception; every cell of the individual will have the gene mutation, a fact that is likely associated with the involvement of multiple organs in many cancer susceptibility syndromes. However, the inheritance of a mutated cancer susceptibility allele is only the *first* step in promoting the development of a malignancy and does not guarantee that an individual will go on to develop a particular malignancy. The development of a heritable cancer, as well as most other cancers, is postulated to be dependent on the occurrence of a second genomic alteration [1]. That an individual has inherited the first "step" serves to explain why such individuals have a considerably higher risk for developing cancer than the general population, as well as why cancer predisposition syndromes are characterized by cancer development at an earlier age and a higher rate of bilaterality than what is observed in the general population.

However, cancer is ultimately a disease of somatic cells; if two (or more) independent events are needed for the cells to become malignant, then inheriting the first step, as opposed to waiting for it to occur through some random events causing a somatic alteration, will surely increase the likelihood of it occurring compared to those individuals who do not inherit such mutations. The second (and any subsequent) step is invariably somatic in nature, also explaining why not everyone who inherits a susceptibility gene develops the malignancy. Molecular studies of cancers in individuals with malignancies arising from hereditary cancer syndromes frequently show a loss of heterozygosity at the genomic position of the tumor suppressor gene in tumor tissue. This loss of heterozygosity is the "second step" in the development of cancer in individuals who have inherited mutated cancer susceptibility genes. Sections describing germinal and somatic mutations that either predispose to or characterize breast cancer will be found later in this chapter; they represent the more current molecular definitions of the first and second "steps" described by Knudson in the early 1970s [2].

There are numerous mechanisms that likely lead to this loss of heterozygosity and the inactivation of the tumor suppressing gene. While such cellular and nuclear events are common and are mostly random processes by which genes and chromosomes are altered, deleted, replaced, or rearranged and not typically associated with organic pathology, such changes in the presence of an inherited mutation in a tumor suppressor gene can lead to the alteration or inactivation of tumor-suppressing gene function and predispose that organ to undergo malignant transformation. This process is known as monoallelic inheritance of a gene mutation with subsequent inactivation of the wild-type allele and loss of heterozygosity. However, it is now recognized that some individuals can inherit mutations in both alleles (either homozygous or compound heterozygous), an uncommon occurrence known as inherited biallelic mutations, which tend to present with a different clinical phenotype, including childhood cancers, to that usually observed with monoallelic (dominant) inheritance of mutations [3].

It is interesting to note that while most hereditary cancer syndromes, including hereditary breast and ovarian cancer syndrome, are mostly transmitted in and present as a classic autosomal dominant inherited condition, the requirement of a second step that inactivates both alleles (biallelic inactivation) makes the *cellular* mechanism necessary for the promotion of carcino-

**Table 2.1** Cancer predisposition genes associated with breast cancer

| Gene (chromosome) | Penetrance | Clinical features |
|---|---|---|
| *BRCA1* (17q21) | High | Breast and epithelial ovarian cancers |
| *BRCA2* (13q12-13) | High | Breast and epithelial ovarian cancers |
| *PTEN* (10q23.3) | High | Cowden syndrome |
| *TP53* (17q13.1) | High | Li-Fraumeni syndrome |
| *RAD51C* (17q23) | High (?) | Breast and epithelial ovarian cancers; Fanconi anemia (subtype-O; biallelic mutation) |
| *CDH1* (16q22.1) | Moderate | Gastric cancer and lobular breast cancer |
| *ATM* (11q22.3) | Moderate | Ataxia-teleangectasia (biallelic mutation) |
| *CHEK2* (22q12.1) | Low | Some association with Li-Fraumeni syndrome |
| *BRIP1* (17q22) | Low | Fanconi anemia (biallelic mutation) |
| *PALB2* (16q12) | Low | Fanconi anemia (biallelic mutation) |
| *KRAS*-variant (12p12.1) | Unknown | Breast cancer, epithelial ovarian, lung cancer, head and neck cancers, GI cancer |

genesis to be recessive in nature. However, the different phenotypes associated with biallelic inheritance compared to monoallelic inheritance bespeak a difference in the molecular biology of these two disease inheritance patterns, and may eventually provide valuable insight into the molecular mechanisms of cancer development.

Nonetheless, most breast cancers, even those associated with considerable family histories, are not associated with germline mutations of known cancer predisposition genes. Accordingly, an alternative mechanism is likely to be responsible for the development of the considerably more cases of cancer than those currently associated with germline mutations of cancer predisposition genes. Fasching et al. proposed that cancer susceptibility may be influenced by relatively common low penetrant genetic polymorphisms, similar to those associated with common adult diseases such as diabetes [4]. It is clear that while the delineation of deleterious mutations in cancer susceptibility genes was a great leap forward in the molecular and clinical delineation of cancer development, we require further investigations into the molecular processes and clinical characteristics of cancer in order to develop more effective screening and diagnostic algorithms and therapeutic interventions that are applicable to more malignancies and considerably more people than are currently impacted by the identification of individuals at high risk for the development of heritable malignancies.

## Molecular Biology of Cancer Predisposition Genes

While most breast malignancies are not associated with an identified germinal mutation, a review of the literature confirms the identification and confirmation of five uncommon but highly penetrant genes (*BRCA1*, *BRCA2*, *PTEN*, *TP53*, *CDH1*) and four rare but moderately penetrant genes (*CHEK2*, ataxia teleangectasia mutated [*ATM*], *BRIP1*, *PALB2*), along with an expanding list of low penetrant genes and putative genes that contribute to the risk of developing breast cancer (Table 2.1). Most of the low penetrant genes have been discovered in genome-wide association studies (GWAS), which are extensive studies of DNA obtained from a large cohort of individuals with a particular condition or disease in search for common genes or genomic sequences that may be associated with development of the disease in question or its prognosis [5]. GWAS studies are becoming an increasingly important tool in identifying cancer- and disease-predisposing germinal genes; however, such studies account for the identification of genes and genomic sequences that account for less than 1/3 of inherited cases of breast cancer [6]. Such studies have also been applied to the detection of somatic gene mutations and genomic sequences in cancer tissue that are associated with disease prognosis and the development of more effective therapeutic interventions.

## Highly Penetrant Susceptibility Cancer Genes

As with other cancer susceptibility genes, those that predispose women and men to develop breast cancer are also likely to increase the risk for developing other cancers in affected individuals. Which organs other than the breast that may be at risk for undergoing malignant transformation resulting from a mutation in a cancer predisposition gene depends on a wide variety of molecular and environmental factors including the specific function(s) of the gene products (RNA, proteins), individual lifestyle issues (e.g., obesity, smoking), and the specific molecular pathway(s) by which the gene mutation increases the likelihood of breast cancer, among other epigenetic and acquired factors. The following genes presented here represent those that convey the highest risk for developing breast cancer as a result of inheriting a deleterious mutation in the specific gene. Inheritance of the gene mutations that result in cancer predisposition syndromes occurs in an autosomal dominant fashion.

## Mechanism of Breast Cancer Susceptibility: Fanconi Anemia (FA) and BRCA Pathway (FA-BRCA)

Mutations of *BRCA1* and *BRCA2* make up the majority of currently detectable germinal mutations associated with a predisposition to breast cancer, with the general mechanism by which this increased risk for breast and ovarian cancer is conferred is believed to be a disruption in the repair of double-stranded DNA resulting from endogenous or exogenous factors. It may be surprising that many of the genes associated with a predisposition to hereditary breast cancer are associated with Fanconi anemia (FA), a rare (approximately 1/350,000 live births), autosomal recessive condition characterized by congenital abnormalities (e.g., short stature, hyperpigmented skin), bone marrow failure, and a predisposition to leukemia (AML) along with solid tumors including vulvar, esophageal, and head and neck malignancies [7, 8].

Fifteen genes currently comprise the FA family of genes with biallelic mutation of these genes resulting in the FA phenotype, as would be expected in any autosomal recessive Mendelian disorder. Not surprisingly, monoallelic mutation of some of these 15 genes results in a different phenotype, one that is characterized by a predisposition to breast cancer and, in some cases, other malignancies such as OEC [9]. In addition to the association of these 15 genes with FA, they also play important roles in the repair of DNA interstrand crosslinks (ICLs) and have come to be characterized as the FA-BRCA pathway. Indeed, it is this repair function that links these genes to an increased risk of breast and other cancers. Adverse affects on DNA repair and homologous recombination, a process which maintains genomic integrity by repairing endogenous and exogenous DNA double strand breaks, are the mechanisms by which *BRCA1*/*BRCA2* mutations, as well as mutations of other cancer predisposition genes such as *ATM*, *BRIP1*, and *PALB2* (all of which are either directly or indirectly associated with the FA-BRCA pathway), are believed to increase the risk for breast and other malignancies [10].

The FA-BRCA pathway provides a strong pathophysiological basis for the delineation of molecular mechanisms associated with the development of breast cancer and associated malignancies. While not all genes in the FA-BRCA pathway are associated with an increased risk for hereditary breast cancer, the study of the FA-BRCA pathway provides important information concerning potential mechanisms of tumorigenesis. Mutations of the genes associated with the multistep mismatch repair (MMR) pathway are associated with Lynch syndrome, a cancer predisposition syndrome not typically associated with a considerable increased risk for breast cancer. However, Williams et al. showed that FANCD2, one of the 15 FA genes, interacts with two of the MMR proteins (MSH2 and MLH1) [8]. With an earlier demonstration of the interaction of *BRIP1* (*FANCJ*) with the MMR complex MutLα, these findings suggest an important role for MMR proteins in the activation of the FA-BRCA pathway and the repair of ICLs, all of which are integral to the process that prevents or predisposes an individual to hereditary breast cancer. With regard to somatic changes associated with the FA-BRCA pathway, a study by Rudland et al. found that the absence of the FA protein FANCD2 was strongly associated with malignant breast cancer specimens, with negative staining being strongly correlated with the presence of metastatic-inducing proteins such as S100A4, S100P, osteopontin, and AGR2 [11]. Such information will be critical for the development of novel and effective therapies that will utilize molecular and protein information from FA-BRCA pathway for the development of effective screening algorithms and therapeutic interventions.

## *BRCA1/BRCA2*

*BRCA1* and *BRCA2* are two separate and distinct tumor suppressor genes that account for approximately 5% of all breast cancer cases [12] and 85% of all cases of hereditary breast and OEC [13], although these two genes account for a smaller percentage of isolated familial breast cancer cases in the absence of EOC [14]. In addition to breast and OECs, individuals with mutations in *BRCA1/2* also demonstrate an increased risk for other cancers including pancreas, stomach, prostate, and colon [15].

*BRCA1* is located on chromosome 17q21, contains 22 coding exons, and spans 80 kb DNA while *BRCA2* is located on chromosome 13q12-13, contains 26 coding exons, and spans 70 kb DNA [16]. These disparate genes are part of the DNA breakage repair pathway and function as tumor-suppressor genes, with mutations resulting in a highly penetrant susceptibility to the development of breast cancer and EOC. Both genes are involved in DNA repair by activating the repair of double strand breaks and initiating homologous recombination [12]. *BRCA1* is a gatekeeper of genomic integrity with multiple roles including homologous repair, checkpoint control, spindle regulation, and transcriptional regulation [17]. *BRCA2* appears to have a more singular role in the DNA repair process through its strict interaction with RAD51 filament formation, which likely serves as a regulatory step in recombination repair [12].

Mutations of *BRCA1* and *BRCA2* associated with the development of breast and associated malignancies are found throughout the coding regions and at splice sites, with most of these mutations being small insertions or deletions that lead to frameshift mutations, nonsense mutations, or splice site alterations. All of these genetic alterations invariably lead to premature protein termination and altered or absent proteins that result in reduced or absent DNA repair and the elimination of suppression of the development of malignancies in breast and ovarian epithelial tissues. In addition to these mutations and some missense mutations, large deletions and rearrangements not detectable by standard PCR have been identified and are now part of the molecular testing provided to those undergoing genetic testing for BRCA mutations. Palma et al. reported that genomic rearrangements, detected by an analysis separate from conventional gene sequencing and aimed at detecting large gene rearrangements not amenable to detection by conventional analyses (e.g., BART analysis), accounted for 18% of *BRCA1/2* mutations in non-Ashkenazi Jewish probands with no such rearrangements being detected in Ashkenazi Jewish probands [18].

The frequency of *BRCA1* and *BRCA2* mutations in the general population is estimated to be 1/300 to 1/800 [19], though a study by Risch et al. in Canada suggests that these frequencies may be considerably higher at 1/140 to 1/300 [20]. However, some populations and communities have a higher frequency of certain *BRCA1/2* mutations than the general population. In the United States, *BRCA1/2* mutations are found in approximately 1 of every 40 individuals of

Eastern European (Ashkenazi) Jewish ancestry. What also distinguishes this community is that three mutations (185delAG and 5382insC in *BRCA1* and 6174delT in *BRCA2*) account for approximately 98% of all mutations detected [21]. In Iceland, the 999del5 mutation in *BRCA2* accounts for approximately 7% of all cases of epithelial ovarian cancer occurring in Icelanders [22]. These mutations are known as "founder mutations," so named because in certain populations begun by a small ancestral group isolated by societal behavior or geography, certain genes in the original "founders" of a community or population can become far more common in succeeding generations than would be expected to occur in the general population because of that geographical or social isolation. The identification of founder mutations allows for more facile screening of individuals of those groups associated with these mutations. As such, evaluating individuals of Eastern European Jewish ancestry at increased risk for a *BRCA1* or *BRCA2* mutation based on family history is now accomplished by first determining the presence of one of these three mutations unless analysis of an affected relative shows that the *BRCA1/2* mutation in the family is not one of these three mutations. Evaluating for these three mutations in high-risk members of the Ashkenazi Jewish community is not only easier than gene sequencing but also less costly. However, even in some clinical scenarios in which a single putative *BRCA1/2* mutation is of interest in the risk assessment process, a "single site" analysis would potentially be augmented with a founder mutation analysis or even full gene sequencing if the family history indicates that another mutation may be present, possibly from the other parental lineage. For individuals from populations associated with founder mutations who are at increased risk for *BRCA1/2* mutations based on family history and found not to have one of the founder mutations, gene sequencing and rearrangement analysis can be offered after a "negative" founder mutation result in order to provide a complete and thorough molecular evaluation [16].

While the clinical aspects of *BRCA1/BRCA2* germinal mutations are well described, there are clinical implications of the somatic changes associated with *BRCA1/BRCA2* breast and ovarian cancers that impact prognosis and the use of certain therapeutic interventions that go beyond the considerable increased risk for developing cancer among those women and men who inherited such mutations. These advancements are associated with use of poly(ADP-ribose) polymerase 1 (PARP1) inhibitors, which provide a new approach to therapies for women and men with *BRCA1/BRCA2*-related cancers by impacting the DNA repair mechanism that is adversely affected in *BRCA1/BRCA2*-related malignancies. A more detailed description will be provided in the section "Somatic Genes."

## Cowden Syndrome

Cowden syndrome, or multiple hamartoma syndrome, is an autosomal dominant condition characterized by the formation of multiple hamartomas in any organ of the body and an increased risk for certain malignancies. Pathognomonic features of Cowden syndrome include facial trichilemmomas, acralkeratoses, and oral papillomatous papules Individuals with Cowden syndrome are at increased risk for developing a variety of benign and malignant conditions, with over 90% of individuals demonstrating mucocutaneous lesions [23]. Germline mutations in PTEN (*P*hosphatase and *TEN*sin homologue deleted on chromosome *TEN*), located at 10q23.3, have been found in 85% of individuals with Cowden syndrome as well as in people with other rare and unrelated conditions such as Bannayan-Riley-Ruvalcaba syndrome and Proteus syndrome. However, these syndromes do share some common phenotypic features that have led to the characterization of these conditions under the common classification of PHTS (PTEN hamartoma tumor syndrome) [24].

In addition to the hamartomas and dermatological conditions, Cowden syndrome is associated with an increased risk of a variety of malignancies. Lifetime risk for nonmedullary thyroid cancer is approximately 10%, with benign thyroid conditions also markedly increased in prevalence among affected individuals. Lhermitte-Duclos disease (dysplastic gangliocytoma of the cerebellum) and renal cell carcinoma have also been reported to be components of Cowden syndrome, although the exact frequency of these two conditions among individuals with Cowden syndrome has yet to be well delineated.

An increased risk of breast cancer has been reported among men with Cowden syndrome, with women with Cowden syndrome having an approximate 75% risk for benign breast disease such as fibromas, fibroadenomas, and fibrocystic changes, as well as an over 50% lifetime risk for breast cancer [25]. In addition, women with Cowden syndrome have a 5–10% lifetime risk of endometrial cancer and an increased risk of developing uterine fibroids [26].

Diagnosis of Cowden syndrome is achieved by demonstrating major and minor criteria as put forth in the International Cowden Syndrome Consortium Operational Criteria for the Diagnosis of Cowden Syndrome [27]. Approximately 80% of individuals who meet the diagnostic criteria are found to have mutations in *PTEN*. Because of the considerable and varied increased risk for cancer development in individuals with Cowden syndrome, surveillance should be undertaken to detect malignancies at an earlier and more treatable stage. Such screening may include a baseline thyroid examination and ultrasound assessment at 18-years-old with an annual thyroid exam thereafter. A family history of renal cancer should prompt an annual urinalysis and urine cytology along with a renal ultrasound. Women with Cowden syndrome should begin annual clinical breast exams at age 18 with semiannual exams beginning at age 25. Mammography should be offered at approximately 25–30 years of age, or 10 years earlier than the youngest affected female in the family. In addition, women with Cowden syndrome should be offered an annual breast MRI upon initiation of annual mammographic exams. Men with Cowden syndrome should have annual clinical breast exams starting at age 25–30, with further evaluation based on the finding of palpable lesions. Annual endometrial biopsies should be performed starting at age 35–40, or 10 years earlier than the youngest affected individual in the family. This can also be augmented by an annual endovaginal ultrasound examination in postmenopausal women [23]. Endometrial cancer is amenable to risk reduction, and conservative approaches to prevention (e.g., copper T 380A, levonorgestrel intrauterine system, oral contraceptives) should be discussed with affected women during their reproductive years. Definitive preventative measures for endometrial cancer, such as hysterectomy, should also be discussed, but should be reserved for women who have completed their childbearing as conservative preventative measures such as combination oral contraceptive and intrauterine contraceptive devices are highly effective in preventing endometrial cancer [28].

## Li-Fraumeni Syndrome

Li-Fraumeni syndrome (LFS) is a rare cancer predisposition syndrome estimated to account for approximately 1% of hereditary breast cancer cases. Mutations in *TP53*, a tumor suppressor gene located on 17p13.1, are the primary cause of LFS, which is transmitted in an autosomal dominant fashion. In addition, families with classic LFS phenotypes have also been found to have mutations in the *CHEK2* gene, found on 22q12.2. Unlike *TP53*, *CHEK2* encodes for a serine/threonine protein kinase that phosphorylates p53, leading to cessation of mitosis and allowing DNA repair; *CHEK2* mutations thus promote the development of malignancy by inhibiting DNA repair, similar to the MMR genes associated with Lynch syndrome.

LFS is characterized by early-onset breast cancer, soft-tissue sarcomas, adrenocortical tumors, brain tumors, and leukemias. In some families with LFS, brain tumors, adrenocortical tumors, and sarcomas may present in childhood. Additional tumors reported in LFS families include ovary, pancreas, lung, stomach, melanoma, and Wilms' tumor [23]. Similar to other cancer susceptibility conditions, LFS appears to increase the risk of early development of cancer, with a 50% risk of cancer by age 40 and a 90% risk of cancer by age 60 [29]. Screening and management of patients at risk for LFS is challenging given the variety of early-onset malignancies associated with this condition. In women, annual clinical breast examinations, including MRI and mammography, should start at age 20, and consideration of oral contraception use is warranted to reduce the risk of ovarian cancer, along with an annual pelvic and abdominal ultrasound examination. However, there are no published guidelines for screening LFS patients; clinicians should strongly consider genetic counseling and testing (*TP53* and *CHEK2*) for individuals and family members with a considerable history of sarcomas and early-onset cancers.

## Hereditary Diffuse Gastric Cancer

Gastric cancer is a common cause of cancer worldwide and estimated to become the tenth leading cause of mortality by the year 2030 [30]. As with breast and ovarian cancers, the vast majority of gastric cancers occur sporadically, with only 1–3% of gastric cancers being associated with an inherited cancer predisposition syndrome. Such cases are referred to as hereditary diffuse gastric cancer (HDGC) [31]; with approximately 1/3 of families fulfilling criteria for HDGC will have a mutation in *CDH1* (E-cadherin; 16q22). Mutations in *CDH1* are highly penetrant, resulting in an 80% lifetime risk for developing gastric cancer, similar to the risk of developing breast cancer in women with *BRCA1/2* mutations [31].

Inheriting a mutation in *CDH1* is also associated with a high risk for developing lobular breast cancer in women, with *CDH1* mutations conveying an approximate lifetime risk of 60%. The *CDH1* locus (16q22) is frequently associated with a loss of heterozygosity in breast cancers and is associated with a poor clinical prognosis. Accordingly, inheriting a mutation in *CDH1* ("first step") would markedly increase the likelihood of breast cancer by increasing the likelihood of a loss of heterozygosity if the "second step" occurs. The molecular mechanism by which this occurs appears to be associated with aberrant promoter hypermethylation, an event observed in cancers and in this clinical situation, associated with a loss of expression and function of E-cadherin, a protein related to tissue integrity [32, 33]. Accordingly, the striking increase in breast cancer risk among women who carry a *CDH1* mutation is associated with a loss of heterozygosity that prevents the normal production of E-cadherin which serves to maintain tissue integrity and suppress the development of breast cancer.

## Other Susceptibility Genes in Breast Cancer

Similar to the aforementioned genes, other genes predispose to the development of breast cancers and other malignancies by similar mechanisms; specifically, an altered gene that essentially reduces or removes the inhibition of abnormal cell growth and development in breast tissue and other organs. What differentiates these genes from the others previously described is that these genes are not as highly penetrant; that is, inheriting the gene by an individual does not increase the likelihood of breast cancer development to the same degree as that associated with more highly penetrant genes. The likely reason for this is that there are other genes or epigenetic factors, thus far unidentified, which are required to initiate the development of breast and extramammary malignancies. The epidemiological impact of mutations in the *CHEK2* gene (see below) may be an example of a gene that when mutated can present with a novel phenotype associated with other cancer predisposing genes (*TP53*). Perhaps the actual mechanism affected by the gene mutation (i.e., *CHEK2* mutations apparently inhibit DNA repair similar to the MMR genes of Lynch syndrome) determines whether the gene mutation has a singular clinical impact, as with *BRCA1/2* mutations, or rather functions more like a modifier gene that exerts a deleterious effect only in the presence of other genetic, genomic, or epigenetic factors.

### *RAD51C*

Germline mutations in genes involved in homologous recombination have been associated with a variety of human genetic disorders and malignancies. Homologous recombination maintains genomic integrity by repairing endogenous and exogenous DNA double strand breaks, failure of which can lead to aberrant genetic rearrangements and a variety of chromosomal structural alterations associated with Mendelian syndromes (e.g., Fanconi anemia, Bloom syndrome) and a predisposition to the development of a number of malignancies [34]. With the recognition that *BRCA1* and *BRCA2* are known to regulate homologous recombination, other genes that adversely affect homologous recombination can be associated with an increased likelihood of genetic disorders and cancer development.

An apparently highly penetrant gene for breast and ovarian cancer, *RAD51C*, has recently been identified and is found on chromosome 17q23. RAD51C is involved in two specific complexes and has multiple functions in DNA damage response and the maintenance of genomic stability [35, 36]. Similar to *PRIB1* and *PALB2*, biallelic mutations of *RAD51C* are associated with Fanconi anemia (subtype-O), whereas monoallelic mutations are associated with a predisposition to hereditary breast cancer. RAD51 function appears to be regulated by both BRCA1 and BRCA2, although BRCA2 has regions that directly interact with RAD51 for the mobilization of RAD51 in response to DNA damage.

Initial studies have demonstrated that *RAD51C* may be mutated in 1.5–4.0% of all families predisposed to breast and ovarian cancer [37]. Despite the initial scientific and clinical support for *RAD51C* as a cancer susceptibility gene, others have not found a high prevalence of *RAD51C* mutations in at-risk breast-ovarian cancer cohorts [38] or may not be as highly penetrant as has been demonstrated in some studies [39]. As the actual frequency of *RAD51C* has not yet been precisely delineated as well as the effect of the various identified germline mutations on the risk of breast and ovarian cancers in women and men carrying such mutations, further studies are needed in order to determine whether *RAD51C* should be included in a universal or targeted genetic screening panel for women with family histories of breast and ovarian cancer. Further studies of the mechanism of *RAD51C* mutations in the initiation and development of breast and ovarian cancers, especially its molecular interaction with *BRCA2*, will help determine the precise role of *RAD51C* in risk and prognosis determination for breast and ovarian cancers in low- and high-risk populations.

## Other Putative and Less Penetrant Cancer Susceptibility Genes

While there are likely highly penetrant genes that are responsible for the development of breast and other malignancies that have not yet been identified as a result of their very low frequency among women and families with breast and ovarian cancer, the presence of mild to moderately penetrant genes is likely responsible for a considerable percentage of breast and other organic malignancies. The following listing of genes is by no means exhaustive, but does represent some of the more commonly evaluated genes associated with cancer predisposition.

### *ATM*

The ataxia teleangectasia mutated gene, or *ATM*, is located on chromosome 11q22.3 and encodes a checkpoint kinase intrinsic to DNA repair. Biallelic mutations of this gene are associated with the autosomal recessive disease known as ataxia-teleangectasia. Heterozygotes that carry a single mutation do not express the phenotype of ataxia-teleangectasia, but do have a 2–5-fold increase in the risk for breast cancer [12].

### *CHEK2*

The checkpoint kinase-2 gene (*CHEK2*) is located on chromosome 22q12.1 and encodes a checkpoint kinase that is a key mediator in DNA damage response. Mutations of *CHEK2* were initially associated with LFS (see above); however, studies found some *CHEK2* germline variants (e.g., 1000delC, 1157T) were not associated with LFS or an LFS-like syndrome but only with an increased risk for breast cancer [40]. *CHEK2* seems to be a low penetrant gene; the 1000delC variant incurs a twofold increase in the risk of breast cancer in women and a tenfold increase in men [12].

## *BRIP1* (BRCA1-Interacting Protein-Terminal Helicase 1)

*BRIP1*, also known as *FANCJ* or *BACH1*, is found on chromosome 17q22 and along with *PALB2* and *RAD51C*, encodes for proteins that participate in the FA pathway and are involved in the maintenance of DNA stability. Biallelic mutations in these genes are associated with FA phenotypes while monoallelic mutations of these genes are associated with a predisposition to hereditary breast cancer [41].

Cantor et al. first detected *BRIP1* mutations in two individuals with early onset breast cancer and family histories of breast cancer [42]. However, the exact mechanism by which *BRIP1* mutations may increase the risk for breast cancer, or whether or not all *BRIP1* mutations predispose to hereditary breast cancer, remains unclear. Seal et al. found that *BRIP1* mutations conferred a twofold increase in the risk for breast cancer among mutation carriers [43].

Indeed, the relationship between specific *BRIP1* and *BRCA1* mutations and their role in the development and progression of breast cancer remains unclear with further delineation of this genetic "relationship" potentially providing important information regarding tumorigenesis in *BRCA1* and *BRIP1* mutation carriers [10]. Until further clinical and molecular studies are undertaken, it is best to describe *BRIP1* as a low to moderately penetrant gene with an as yet undefined impact on the risk for breast cancer.

## *PALB2*

As opposed to BRIP1, the literature concerning *PALB2* provides for a stronger association between mutations in this gene and a predisposition to hereditary breast cancer. In a small study from Australia, Wong et al. found that mutations in *PALB2* were responsible for 2.8% of hereditary breast cancer cases [41], a frequency comparable (1.1%) to that reported by Rahman et al. in a larger UK study in which there were no *PALB2* mutations detected among the 1,084 subjects in the comparator control group [9].

*PALB2*, which is derived from the phrase "partner and localizer of BRCA2," is located on 16p12. Because of its interaction with BRCA2, it is not surprising that biallelic mutations of *PALB2* result in a Fanconi anemia phenotype similar to that found in individuals with biallelic *BRCA2* mutations and different from the phenotype associated with biallelic mutations of the other FA genes. It is also not surprising that *PALB2* mutations are not only associated with an increase in the risk for breast cancer in women but also in men. To this end, Rahman et al. found that mutations in this gene conferred an increased risk of almost exclusively breast cancer and that the magnitude of the increase in women was 2.3-fold with an increased, though not specified, risk of breast cancer in men with *PALB2* mutations [9]. In all, *BRCA1*, *BRCA2*, and *TP53* account for approximately 15–20% of the familial risk for breast cancer; *PALB2* mutations are estimated to add an additional 2–3% to the characterization of familial risk for breast cancer. However, the mechanisms by which *PALB2* and the other FA-BRCA pathway gene mutations predispose women and men to breast cancer are complex and still not well delineated. *PALB2*, along with *BRCA2* and *BRIP1*, are all cancer susceptibility genes that are not part of the FA core complex but are the only FA genes that act downstream of FANCD2, a FA protein associated with an increased risk for sporadic breast cancer [44].

## *KRAS*-Variant

While the aforementioned cancer susceptibility genes increase the risk of malignancy as a result of mutations of tumor suppressor genes, an oncogene may result in increased cancer susceptibility through a completely different pathway.

The *KRAS*-variant is a functional variant in a *let-7* microRNA (miRNA) complementary site in the 3′-untranslated region of the *KRAS* oncogene (rs61764370). miRNA are a class of approximately 22-nucleotide noncoding RNAs that are evolutionarily conserved and function by negatively regulating gene expression by binding to partially complementary sites in the 3′-untranslated regions (3′ UTR) of target mRNAs. miRNAs are aberrantly expressed in virtually all cancers, where they function as a novel class of oncogenes or tumor suppressors [45]. Because miRNAs are global gene regulators, even small aberrations in miRNA levels or their target sites can lead to important cellular changes. In support of this concept, emerging evidence shows that SNPs within miRNAs or miRNA binding sites can be functional and act as powerful biomarkers of cancer risk when one allele alters miRNA function or binding characteristics [46]. The variant is relatively uncommon with a minor allele frequency of about 7% in populations of European descent, is uncommon in Africans, and almost absent in East Asians and Native Americans [46, 47].

Ratner et al. reported the *KRAS*-variant to be associated with 28% of unselected cases of OEC and 61% of cases of HBOC syndrome not characterized by *BRCA1/2* mutations [46]. Another study found a significant increased association of the *KRAS*-variant among women with triple-negative (i.e., estrogen and progesterone receptor negative and HER2 negative) [48]. However, similar to *RAD51C* and other putative cancer predisposition genes, not all studies have found a significant or clinically relevant association of the *KRAS*-variant among women with ovarian cancer or a personal or family history of HBOC syndrome [49]. Nonetheless, a recent study by Cerne et al. may shed light on the novel attributes of the *KRAS*-variant and the risk of breast and ovarian cancer [50]. In this study from Slovenia, the authors found results similar to that of Pharoah et al. [49]; specifically, that among 530 sporadic cases of postmenopausal breast cancer and 165 cases of familial breast cancer cases, including 29 cases characterized by *BRCA1/2* mutations, there was no increased incidence of *KRAS*-variant when compared to 270 matched postmenopausal controls. However, they did find that among postmenopausal women using estrogen-based hormone therapy, the presence of the *KRAS*-variant was associated with HER2-positive tumors and tumors that were more poorly differentiated, both characteristics indicative of a poorer prognosis and suggestive of a potentially novel mechanism that may involve an estrogen pathway or receptor in the development and progress of breast cancer among women with *KRAS*-variant.

## Somatic Genes

Breast cancer is a heterogeneous disease. Initially, prognosis for breast cancer was based on tumor size alone; however, this approach was not accurate given the novel and unique prognostic and therapeutic aspects attributable to breast malignancies regardless of tumor size. Later on, a histological classification system was developed, dividing breast cancer into groups distinguished by the histological appearance of the tumor. While this represented an improvement over the previous classification system, it too failed to provide an accurate assessment of prognosis. The most widely used classification system of breast cancer currently combines histomorphological information (such as histological subtype and grading) as well as TNM staging information [tumor size (T) together with lymph node (N) and distant metastasis occurrence (M)] [51, 52].

The aforementioned genes presented in this chapter characterize germline or heritable mutations that are found in each and every cell of an individual but increase the risk of malignancy in only specific organs. The development of cancer invariably results in a profound alteration of the genetic material in tumor cells when compared to similar cells that have not undergone malignant transformation. While many of these changes within the cancer genome are random and represent the disruptive effect of the malignant transformative process on the nuclear, cellular, and even mitochondrial functions within the cell, studies have shown that there are certain changes within the affected cellular genome, or somatic changes, that occur in a nonrandom manner and may be representative of novel processes that are associated with malignant transformation. In this regard, analysis of the somatic nature of breast cancer tissue has been found to be very useful in providing for a more accurate estimation of prognosis and the development therapeutic interventions that target novel molecular pathways in the cancer tissue and provide for the development of more effective treatment modalities.

A more recent approach to better classify breast cancer subgroups is that of gene expression profiling which seeks to characterize the somatic changes within the tumor tissue. This molecular characterization of breast cancer tissue has become commonplace in cancer centers worldwide. Malignancies are now routinely characterized by the positivity or negativity of the molecular expression of estrogen (ER) and progesterone receptors (PR), as well as for the overexpression of the oncogene HER-2. The implication of the positivity or negativity of any of these three somatic findings is covered in greater detail elsewhere in this book. However, one particular result of these three assays deserves discussion in this chapter: triple negative breast cancer (TNBC). TNBC is defined as the absence of estrogen receptors (ER), progesterone receptors (PR), and the absence of HER-2 overexpression and accounts for approximately 15% of all breast cancer tumors, and occurs at a higher frequency among premenopausal women and women of African descent [53]. TNBC is also associated with obesity and high parity, instead of the low parity more commonly associated with other types of breast cancer [53]. Regardless of the demographic distribution of TNBC cancers, these malignancies are associated with a poorer prognosis than non-TNBC breast cancers, with a higher rate of metastatic spread to brain and lungs and early recurrence, with few effective therapeutic options available in cases of recurrence [17, 52, 54].

Sørlie et al. categorized breast cancers into five gene expression subtypes: Luminal A, Luminal B, HER-2 Enriched, Basal-like, and Normal-like, each of which have been associated with unique clinical characteristics [55]. TNBC tumors have a basal-like morphology, expressing myoepithelial-cell-type cytokeratins CK5, CK14, CK17, frequent mutations in *TP53*, cadherin, and epidermal growth factor receptor similar to that found in basal epithelial layer cells [56]. *BRCA1*-associated tumors are also frequently associated with basal-like morphology and commonly display a TNBC phenotype [54]. Somatic mutations in *BRCA1/2* rarely occur in cases of sporadic breast cancer, but a high incidence (20%) of *BRCA1/2* mutations are found in cases of TNBC. While not all basal-type tumors or *BRCA1*-associated tumors are triple negative malignancies, the molecular mechanisms associated with the development of breast cancer in women with *BRCA1* mutations clearly underlie the somatic changes found in sporadic TNBC cancers [17]. Of further interest is that among those cases of TNBC not associated with *BRCA1* mutations, there appears to be an inhibition of BRCA1 expression through other mechanisms including "gene silencing" in which methylation resulting from carcinogenesis effectively blocks expression of *BRCA*-related proteins and renders the cell to be similar to a *BRCA1/2* mutated cell without any of the germline mutations typically associated with the loss of *BRCA* gene expression [57]. These unique tumor characteristics have been described as "BRCAness" and represent the considerable similarities between *BRCA1*-related cancers and TNBC. However, the similarities described herein do not apply to *BRCA2*-related malignancies, which appear to be a far more heterogenous group of cancers than *BRCA1*-related cancers.

It is the spectrum of molecular and cellular similarities of TNBCs to *BRCA1*-related breast cancers that provides the potential for development of more effective therapeutic interventions for these more aggressive tumors. Inactivating mutations in genes involved in the DNA damage response pathways are associated with increased risk for cancer susceptibility and occur both as germline or somatic mutations with increasing evidence of epigenetic gene silencing as an additional cause of loss of protein function. Loss of function by any mechanism of the aforementioned gene products in a tumor cell precursor clone leads to an accelerated mutation acquisition and underpins the initiation and development of the malignancy [58]. A potentially new strategy that has emerged for treatment of *BRCA1*- and *BRCA2*-related tumors is the use of poly(ADP-ribose) polymerase 1 (PARP1) inhibitors.

The human genome is continuously exposed to exogenous (e.g., exposure to genotoxic compounds) and endogenous (e.g., recombination aberrations) deleterious events that have the potential to destabilize the genome. It is the DNA repair pathways that serve to maintain genome stability and integrity, and as such have been found to be tumor suppressor in nature with mutations in the genes that make up these pathways being associated with cancer predisposition syndromes, as has been previously described with *BRCA1* and *BRCA2*, both of which are involved in DNA double strand break repair. There are currently 16 members of the PARP family of which only PARP1 and PARP2 are involved in DNA repair [59]. PARP is involved in base excision repair, a key pathway in the repair of DNA single strand break. PARP activity in cells is typically low, but is stimulated by DNA strand breaks. PARP1 and PARP2 form homodimers and heterodimers at DNA break sites and serve to recruit other needed proteins for the repair process as well as activating other necessary cellular processes needed for DNA repair. The absence of PARP leads to spontaneous single strand breaks that collapse replication forks into double strand breaks, triggering homologous recombination for repair. However, with the loss of functional BRCA1 or BRCA2, cells will be sensitized to inhibit PARP activity, apparently leading to the persistence of the DNA lesions which are usually repaired by homologous recombination. When both pathways are defective this will result in chromosomal instability, cell cycle arrest, and finally apoptosis. Cell survival assays show that cell lines lacking wildtype BRCA1 or BRCA2 were extremely sensitive to PARP inhibitors compared to heterozygous mutant or the wildtype cells [60]. These results suggest the potential use of PARP inhibitors in the treatment of *BRCA1*- and *BRCA2*-related breast and ovarian cancers with recent and ongoing clinical trials showing promising results and clinical outcomes [61].

Given the similarities of TNBC and *BRCA-1* related cancers, its stands that PARP inhibitors could have a similar beneficial effect on TNBC. Indeed, early studies showed promise with addition of iniparib to a chemotherapeutic regimen provided to women with TNBC. However, a more robust phase 3 trial recently showed no clinical benefit with iniparib in women with TNBC [62]. However, it should be noted that iniparib is different from other PARP inhibitors, so that the findings with iniparib should not necessarily be considered to be representative of all PARP inhibitors.

With our increasing understanding of the complex network that is the DNA damage response, pathways already recognized to be critical to the establishment of the cancer phenotype are thus gaining additional roles as controllers of DNA repair and subjects of clinical study as putative sites for therapeutic agents. The initial success with PARP-1 and PARP-2 in *BRCA1/2*-related cancers has been shown to target tumor deficiencies in DNA repair as well sensitizing to DNA damaging therapeutics such as radiation and chemotherapy. Further identification of relevant somatic changes and the implication of these changes in tumorigenesis will likely be the approach that we use to develop new and more effective diagnostic and therapeutic modalities.

## Cancer Risk Assessment

The past two decades have witnessed the identification of several genes that have been associated with hereditable breast and gynecologic cancers, thereby promoting the development of and need for cancer genetic counseling. Similar to conventional genetic counseling for pediatric and prenatal conditions, cancer genetic counseling is geared to identifying individuals with mutated cancer predisposition genes as well as those family and personal histories that impact the overall risk for development of cancer. However, unlike conventional genetic counseling in which most individuals or fetuses with a particular phenotype are likely to possess a deleterious gene or abnormal chromosome complement, most cases of cancer, even those associated with considerable family histories in individuals of high-risk ethnic and racial groups, are not associated with the inheritance of cancer predisposition genes. Indeed, no more than 10% of most types of cancer are associated with increased heritability [63]. Nonetheless, counseling has become a central part of the risk assessment process, provided not only to identify those individuals with mutations in cancer predisposition genes, but also to provide accurate information and emotional support to those individuals who have not inherited deleterious mutations found in parents or siblings as well as to those individuals who have not inherited specific mutations but still may be at an increased risk for developing cancer.

Cancer risk assessment is a process by which individuals are identified who are at increased risk for a hereditary or familial cancer and are offered a different approach to prevention and screening than that which is offered to individuals in the general population. Such altered interventions for high-risk individuals can range from an earlier initiation of screening, such as the initiation of mammography before the age of 40 in women with a *BRCA1/2* mutation, to the incorporation of screening protocols not offered to non-high risk individuals, such as the use of regular breast MRI examinations in women with *BRCA1/2* mutations. The detection of a deleterious mutation may also prompt a more novel or extreme approach to prevention, such as the consideration of prophylactic mastectomy to reduce the risk for breast cancer in women with *BRCA1/2* mutations. However, not all preventative measures offered to high-risk individuals are necessarily extreme or extirpative in nature; for example, women at increased risk for epithelial ovarian cancer are likely to be encouraged to breastfeed or consider bilateral tubal ligation once childbearing has been completed as a way to reduce the risk for EOC without increasing the risk for breast cancer [14, 64]. What is clear is that the identification of high-risk individuals, whether as a result of inheriting a deleterious mutation or because of an extensive family history of cancer, allows for the offering of risk reducing strategies that have been shown to prolong lives and improve quality-of-life for high-risk individuals [65].

Assessing risk for hereditable cancers involves a variety of tools and tests that a counselor can use depending on the personal and family history of the individual presenting for counseling and risk assessment. Nonetheless, obtaining medical records and pathology reports is critical to provide accurate counseling and risk assessment, as many individuals may not be aware of the actual information concerning their own medical history or that of family members. While genetic testing provides definitive information in individuals with deleterious mutations, most individuals at risk for a heritable cancer will not test positive for a deleterious mutation, which will most likely be the result if an individual is actually not at risk for the malignancy associated with the tested mutation as a result of an inaccurate family history.

Assuming one has provided accurate personal and family histories, counselors can use a variety of approaches to assess risk for developing heritable cancers. Qualitative and quantitative risk assessments are used to determine an individual's risk for possessing a deleterious mutation in a cancer susceptibility gene and for developing cancer. Qualitative risk assessment primarily uses family and personal histories to determine an individual's risk. Such risk analysis also incorporates a variety of other factors including, where applicable and not exclusively, environmental factors including exposure to toxic substances, use of medications, pathology reports, and lifestyle issues (e.g., number of pregnancies, length of time breastfeeding, etc.). An accurate qualitative assessment includes a detailed personal and family history, supported by corroborated details of the individual's personal and family history. Such details will include, but are not limited to, the age of patient and family members, reproductive histories, histories of genetic disorders and major illnesses, causes of death, and lifestyle issues (e.g., obesity, oral contraceptive use) that

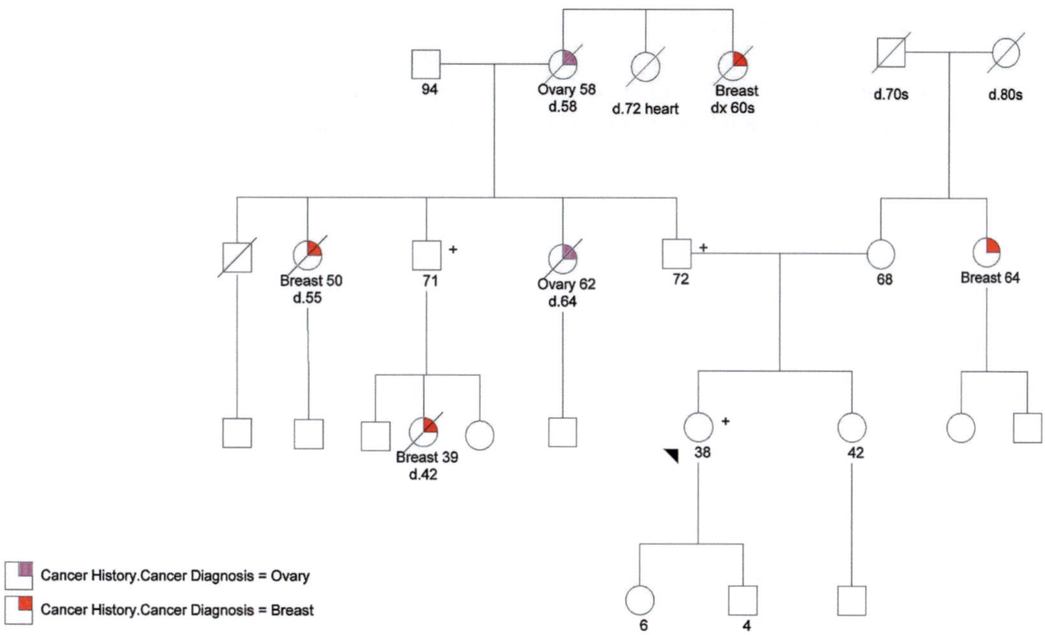


**Fig. 2.1** Pedigree of woman with *BRCA2* mutation (6174delT; *arrowhead*). Transmission is through paternal side of family; paternal uncle was the individual initially tested and was found to carry the deleterious mutation. All individuals in the family with the mutation are denoted with a [+] symbol

could impact morbidity and mortality as well as increasing or decreasing risk for cancer development. In addition, for family members with cancer, further detail is needed including age of diagnosis, staging and grading of tumor, and years of survival. Optimally, this information should be obtained from operative and pathology reports as well as medical records. All of this information can be included into a pedigree (Fig. 2.1) that provides an easy-to-access overview of the proband and his/her family. Such information is critical even in the absence of genetic testing outcomes.

Quantitative risk assessment employs risk assessment models to ascertain an individual's risk for developing cancer or for carrying a deleterious mutation in a cancer susceptibility gene. While risk assessment models are widely used to assess risk for certain cancers such as breast cancer, not all malignancies are amenable to risk assessment by a model [66]. As such, counselors usually use qualitative and quantitative approaches to determine an individual's risk for carrying a deleterious cancer susceptibility gene and provide nondirective counseling concerning the decision to undergo genetic testing or to initiate particular screening, diagnostic, or preventative measures.

Counselors also perform a psychosocial assessment of their patients, as patients frequently face emotional stress and psychological upset based on the findings of the counseling and genetic testing. Counselors should obtain information from patients prior to counseling and risk assessment concerning their expectations for the counseling session, the personal impact of the cancer(s) in question, the economic impact of undergoing counseling and testing and the potential clinical outcomes, their relationship with relatives and the ability to obtain information from those relatives as well as the desire to alter their lifestyle and initiate preventative measures in case an increased risk for cancer is determined. Equally important is the sense of the patient concerning the personal and familial implications of positive or negative genetic testing results. Olaya et al. found that 50% of individuals at increased risk for carrying a *BRCA1/2* mutation chose not to undergo genetic testing, with insurance coverage playing little to no role in the decision to undergo or forego such testing [67]. In this study, the authors sought to develop counseling instruments that would better explain the benefits of testing to unaffected high-risk individuals and to target those with a high school level education as a strategy to improve testing rates. One should consider that those individuals who chose to forego genetic testing in this study did choose to undergo genetic counseling because of an increased risk for developing cancer. This study thus clearly demonstrates that a variety of psychosocial factors play a major role in determining not only decisions to obtain counseling and testing, but also specific choices in this informational process. Accordingly, counselors must be aware of and incorporate these psychosocial issues into their counseling process if they are to provide effective counseling and empower their patients to obtain all the information that they seek and to respect the patient's desire to not obtain certain information.

While testing an individual for an autosomal dominant deleterious mutation that occurs in a parent is a relatively straightforward process, the emotional implications of either a positive or negative results should be addressed prior to testing as the emotional impact of the testing outcomes may not necessarily be easy to predict. A good example of this is found in the movie "In The Family" (J. Rudnick, Producer, Kartemquin Films, 2008), a film that documents the life of a woman who carries a *BRCA1* mutation and details the lives of other individuals at risk for or with heritable breast and ovarian malignancies. In one scene, three daughters are finding out their *BRCA1* mutation status, having decided to get testing because their mother has a deleterious *BRCA1* mutation. Two daughters are found to have inherited the mutation while the other was found to not carry the gene. Surprisingly, it is the unaffected sibling who is most upset at the findings of the genetic testing. Genetic risk assessment and testing may provide qualitative and quantitative analysis to individuals at increased risk for developing cancer; however, the perception of that risk by patients is driven by emotional and psychological factors that are considerably impacted by the individual's experience with cancer. The delineation and acceptance of psychosocial factors such as coping mechanisms, behavior modifications, and emotional reactions to medical and nonmedical events can greatly assist the counselor in providing accurate information that is best used by the patient.

Finally, not everyone who undergoes genetic testing receives a definitive result indicating the presence or absence of a deleterious mutation. Of those undergoing testing for *BRCA1/2* mutations, approximately 5–10% are found to have a variant of uncertain clinical significance (VUS) [68]. VUS are usually missense or potential splice site changes that have not, as yet, been shown to be definitively associated with adverse clinical outcomes. More than 1,500 VUS have been identified and are frequently identified in individuals of minority ethnic population. Most VUS have only been reported in one to two individuals, making further analysis of the clinical impact of VUS challenging [69]. Once a VUS is identified, further analyses such as segregation analysis or study variants in multiple unrelated individuals are applied in an attempt to characterize the VUS as clinically relevant (favor deleterious) or irrelevant (favor polymorphism). However, small sibships and family sizes as well as few individuals with any particular VUS impede the mathematical estimation needed to better characterize the clinical impact of a specific VUS [69].

The finding of a VUS is obviously a difficult clinical outcome that can lead to considerable emotional distress and angst concerning the unknown clinical implication of the genetic test result. In such situations, counselors must use their skills to provide a clear and measured overview of the meaning and implication of the test and provide emotional support for a patient who may be distraught because of the inability to obtain a definitive assessment of her risk for developing cancer [70].

## Conclusions

The recognition of the increasing role of genetics and genomics in the development, assessment, and treatment of cancer requires professionals to be able to integrate current scientific and clinical evidence with an ability to obtain critical information from patients so as to provide the necessary support to facilitate the process by which individuals at high risk are identified and offered appropriate screening, diagnostic, and preventative interventions to reduce the risk of cancer and improve overall clinical outcomes. As we learn more about the molecular mechanisms of cancer initiation, development, and metastasis, the assessment of the tumor genome and exome will not only better characterize the prognostic and therapeutic aspects of each malignancy, but allow for the development of targeted and more effective preventative and therapeutic interventions. Given the heterogeneity of breast cancer, it is unlikely that a single laboratory assay, imaging procedure or historical vignette will provide sufficient information to adequately screen the population. Accordingly, cancer risk assessment will remain our most important tool in assessing the risk of each individual woman to develop breast cancer and thus to determine the best approach to screening for that individual person.

For those found to be at high risk for developing breast cancer, counseling is the process by which high-risk women are provided with the information and emotional support needed to facilitate their decision-making process concerning further testing and preventative interventions. Although technological advances will likely alter the cancer genetic counseling process in the future, for now and the foreseeable future this is how patients will best be served in their search for answers concerning their risks for developing cancer, and in the delineation of improved interventions to prevent and treat breast cancer, a widespread cause of morbidity and mortality among all women regardless of race, ethnicity, or socioeconomic status.

## References


1. Knudson Jr AG. Two genetic hits (more or less) to cancer. Nat Rev Cancer. 2001;1:157–62.
2. Knudson Jr AG. Heredity and human cancer. Am J Pathol. 1974;77:77–84.
3. Rahman N, Scott RH. Cancer genes associated with phenotypes in monoallelic and biallelic mutation carriers: new lessons from old players. Hum Mol Genet. 2007;16(Spec No. 1):R60–6.
4. Fasching PA, Gayther S, Pearce L, et al. Role of genetic polymorphisms and ovarian cancer susceptibility. Mol Oncol. 2009;3:171–81.
5. Zhang B, Beeghly-Fadiel A, Long J, Zheng W. Genetic variants associated with breast cancer risk: comprehensive field synopsis, meta-analysis, and epidemiologic evidence. Lancet Oncol. 2011;12:477–88.
6. Turnbull C, Ahmed S, Morrison J, et al. Genome-wide association study identifies five new breast cancer susceptibility loci. Nat Genet. 2010;42:504–7.
7. Rosenberg PS, Greene MH, Alter BP. Cancer incidence in persons with Fanconi anemia. Blood. 2003; 101:822–6.
8. Williams SA, Wilson JB, Clark AP, et al. Functional and physical interaction between the mismatch repair and FA-BRCA pathways. Hum Mol Genet. 2011;20: 4395–410.
9. Rahman N, Seal S, Thompson D, et al. *PALB2*, which encodes a BRCA2-interacting protein, is a breast cancer susceptibility gene. Nat Genet. 2007;39:165–7. doi:10.1038/ng1959.
10. Cantor SB, Guillemette S. Hereditary breast cancer and the BRCA1-associated FANCJ/BACH1/BRIP1. Future Oncol. 2011;7:253–61. doi:10.2217/fon.10.191.
11. Rudland PS, Platt-Higgins AM, Davies LM, et al. Significance of the Fanconi anemia FANCD2 protein in sporadic and metastatic human breast cancer. Am J Pathol. 2010;176:2935–47.
12. van der Groep P, van der Wall E, van Diest PJ. Pathology of hereditary breast cancer. Cell Oncol. 2011;34:71–88.
13. Lynch HT, Casey MJ, Snyder CL, et al. Hereditary ovarian carcinoma: heterogeneity, molecular genetics, pathology, management. Mol Oncol. 2009;3:97–137.
14. Kjaer SK, Mellemkjaer L, Brinton LA, et al. Tubal sterilization and risk of ovarian, endometrial and cervical cancer. A Danish population-based follow-up study of more than 65,000 sterilized women. Int J Epidemiol. 2004;33:596–602.
15. Friedenson B. BRCA1 and BRCA2 pathways and the risk of cancers other than breast and ovarian. MedGenMed. 2005;7:60.
16. Shulman LP. Hereditary breast and ovarian cancer (HBOC). Clinical features and counseling for *BRCA1 and 2*, Lynch syndrome, Cowden syndrome, and Li-Fraumeni syndrome. Obstet Gynecol Clin North Am. 2010;37:109–33.

17. Shuen AY, Foulkes WD. Inherited mutations in breast cancer genes-risk and response. J Mammary Gland Biol Neoplasia. 2011;16:3–15.
18. Palma MD, Domchek SM, Stopfer J, et al. The relative contribution of point mutations and genomic rearrangements in BRCA1 and BRCA2 in high-risk breast cancer families. Cancer Res. 2008;68:7006–14.
19. Whittemore AS, Gong G, Imyre J. Prevalence and contribution of BRCA1 mutations in breast cancer and ovarian cancer: results from 3 US population-based case-control studies of ovarian cancer. Am J Hum Genet. 1997;60:496–504.
20. Risch HA, McLaughlin JR, Cole DEC, et al. Population BRCA1 and BRCA2 mutation frequencies and cancer penetrances: a Kin-Cohort Study in Ontario, Canada. J Natl Cancer Inst. 2006;98:1694–706.
21. Metcalfe KA, Poll A, Royer R, et al. Screening for founder mutations in BRCA1 and BRCA2 in unselected Jewish women. J Clin Oncol. 2010;28:387–91.
22. Mikaelsdottir EK, Valgeirsdottir S, Eyfjord JE, et al. The Icelandic founder mutation BRCA2 999del5: analysis of expression. Breast Cancer Res. 2004;6:284–90.
23. Allain DC. Genetic counseling and testing for common hereditary breast cancer syndromes. J Mol Diagn. 2008;10:383–95.
24. Orloff MS, Eng C. Genetic and phenotypic heterogeneity in the PTEN hamartomas tumour syndrome. Oncogene. 2008;27:5387–97.
25. Tan MH, Mester JL, Ngeow J, et al. Lifetime cancer risks in individuals with germline PTEN mutations. Clin Cancer Res. 2012;18:400–7.
26. Blumenthal GM, Dennis PA. PTEN hamartoma tumor syndromes. Eur J Hum Genet. 2008;16:1289–300.
27. Eng C. Will the real Cowden syndrome please stand up: revised diagnostic criteria. J Med Genet. 2000; 37:828–30.
28. Shulman LP. Advances in female hormonal contraception: current alternatives to oral regimens. Treat Endocrinol. 2003;2:247–56.
29. Lustbader ED, Williams WR, Bondy ML, et al. Segregation analysis of cancer in families of childhood soft-tissue-sarcoma patients. Am J Hum Genet. 1992;51:344–56.
30. Mathers CD, Loncar D. Projections of global mortality and burden of disease from 2002 to 2030. PLoS Med. 2006;3:e442.
31. Fitzgerald RC, Hardwick R, Huntsman D, et al. Hereditary diffuse gastric cancer: updated consensus guidelines for clinical management and directions for future research. J Med Genet. 2011;47:436–44.
32. Caldeira JR, Prando EC, Quevedo FC, et al. CDH1 promoter hypermethylation and E-cadherin protein expression in infiltrating breast cancer. BMC Cancer. 2006;6:48.
33. Sproul D, Nestor C, Culley J. Transcriptionally repressed genes become aberrantly methylated and distinguish tumors of different lineages in breast cancer. Proc Natl Acad Sci USA. 2011;108:4364–9.
34. Somyajit K, Subramanya S, Hagaraju G. *RAD51C*: a novel cancer susceptibility gene is linked to Fanconi anemia and breast cancer. Carcinogenesis. 2010;31: 2031–8.
35. Smeenk G, de Groot AJ, Romeijn RJ, et al. Rad51C is essential for embryonic development and haploinsufficiency causes increased DNA damage sensitivity and genomic instability. Mutat Res. 2010;689:50–8.
36. Clague J, Wilhoite G, Adamson A, et al. *RAD51C* germline mutations in breast and ovarian cancer cases from high-risk families. PLoS One. 2011;6(9):e25632. doi:10.1371/journal.pone.0025632.
37. Meindl A, Hellebrand H, Wick C, et al. Germline mutations in breast and ovarian cancer pedigrees establish RAD51C as a human cancer susceptibility gene. Nat Genet. 2010;42:410–4.
38. De Leeneer K, Van Bockstal M, De Brouwer S, et al. Evaluation of *RAD51C* as cancer susceptibility gene in a large breast-ovarian cancer patient population referred for genetic testing. Breast Cancer Res Treat. 2012;133(1):393–8.
39. Johnson J, Healey S, Khanna KK, et al. Mutation analysis of RAD51L1 (RAD51B/REC2) in multiple-case, non-BRCA1/2 breast cancer families. Breast Cancer Res Treat. 2011;129:255–63.
40. Vahteristo P, Bartkova J, Eerola H, et al. A *CHEK2* genetic variant contributing to a substantial fraction of familial breast cancer. Am J Hum Genet. 2002;71:432–8.
41. Wong MW, Nordfors C, Mossman D, et al. BRIP1, PALB2, and RAD51C mutation analysis reveals their relative importance as genetic susceptibility factors for breast cancer. Breast Cancer Res Treat. 2011;127:853–9.
42. Cantor SB, Bell DW, Ganesan S, et al. BACH1, a novel helicase-like protein, interacts directly with BRCA1 and contributes to its DNA repair function. Cell. 2001;105(1):149–60.
43. Seal S, Thompson D, Renwick A, et al. Truncating mutations in the Fanconi anemia J gene BRIP1 are low-penetrance breast cancer susceptibility alleles. Nat Genet. 2006;38:1239–41.
44. Barroso E, Pita G, Arias JI, et al. The Fanconi anemia family of genes and its correlation with breast cancer susceptibility and breast cancer features. Breast Cancer Res Treat. 2009;118:655–60.
45. Esquela-Kerscher A, Slack FJ. Oncomirs: microRNAs with a role in cancer. Nat Rev Cancer. 2006;6:259–69.
46. Ratner E, Lu L, Boeke M, et al. A *KRAS*-variant in ovarian cancer acts as a genetic marker of cancer risk. Cancer Res. 2010;70:6509–15.
47. Chin L, Ratner E, Leng S, et al. A SNP in a let-7 microRNA complementary site in the KRAS 3′UTR increases non-small cell cancer risk. Cancer Res. 2008;68:8535–40.
48. Paranjape T, Heneghan H, Lindner R, et al. A 3′-untranslated region *KRAS* variant and triple-negative breast cancer: a case-control and genetic analysis. Lancet Oncol. 2011;12:377–86.
49. Pharoah PDP, Palmieri RT, Ramus SJ, et al. The role of KRAS rs61764370 in invasive epithelial ovarian cancer: implications for clinical testing. Clin Cancer Res. 2011;17:3742–50.

50. Cerne JZ, Stegel V, Gersak K, Novakovic S. KRAS rs61764370 is associated with HER2-overexpressed and poorly-differentiated breast cancer in hormone replacement therapy users: a case control study. BMC Cancer. 2012;12:105.
51. Greene FL, Sobin LH. The staging of cancer: a retrospective and prospective appraisal. CA Cancer J Clin. 2008;58:180–90.
52. De Ruijter TC, Veeck J, de Hoon JPJ, et al. Characteristics of triple-negative breast cancer. J Cancer Res Clin Oncol. 2011;137:183–92.
53. Peddi PF, Ellis MJ, Ma C. Molecular basis of triple negative breast cancer and implications for therapy. Int J Breast Cancer. 2012, Article ID 217185, 7 pages. doi:10.1155/2012/217185.
54. Foulkes WD, Smith IE, Reis-Filho JS. Triple negative breast cancer. N Engl J Med. 2010;363:1938–48.
55. Sørlie T, Perou CM, Tibshirani R, et al. Gene expression patterns of breast carcinomas distinguish tumor subclasses with clinical implications. Proc Natl Acad Sci U S A. 2001;98:10869–74.
56. Nielson TO, Hsu FD, Jensen K, et al. Immunohistochemical and clinical characterization of the basal-like subtype of invasive breast carcinoma. Clin Cancer Res. 2004;10:5367–74.
57. Galizia E, Giorgetti G, Piccinini G, et al. BRCA1 expression in triple negative sporadic breast cancers. Anal Quant Cytol Histol. 2010;32:24–9.
58. Glendenning J, Tutt A. PARP inhibitors—current status and the walk towards early breast cancer. Breast. 2011;20 Suppl 3:S12–9.
59. Schreiber V, Dantzer F, Ame JC, De Murcia G. Poly(ADP-ribose): novel functions for an old molecule. Nat Rev Mol Cell Biol. 2006;7:517–28.
60. Farmer H, McCabe N, Lord J, et al. Targeting the DNA repair defect in BRCA mutant cells as a therapeutic strategy. Nature. 2005;434:917–21.
61. Plummer R. Poly(ADP-ribose) polymerase inhibitor: a new direction for *BRCA* and triple negative breast cancer? Breast Cancer Res. 2011;13:218–24.
62. Javie M, Curtin MJ. The potential for poly(ADP-ribose) polymerase inhibitors in cancer therapy. Ther Adv Med Oncol. 2011;3:257–67.
63. Kinsler KW, Vogelstein B. Lessons from hereditary colorectal cancer. Cell. 1996;87:159–70.
64. Jordan SK, Siskind V, Green C, et al. Breastfeeding and risk of epithelial ovarian cancer. Cancer Causes Control. 2010;21:109–16.
65. Kurian AW, Sigal BM, Plevritis SK. Survival analysis of cancer risk reduction strategies for BRCA1/2 mutation carriers. J Clin Oncol. 2010;28:222–31.
66. Prucka SK, McIlvried DE, Korf BR. Cancer risk assessment and the genetic counseling process: using hereditary breast and ovarian cancer as an example. Med Princ Pract. 2008;17:173–89.
67. Olaya W, Esquivel P, Wong JH, et al. Disparities in BRCA testing: when insurance coverage is not a barrier. Am J Surg. 2009;198:562–5.
68. Murray ML, Cerrato F, Bennett RL, Jarvik GP. Follow-up of carriers of BRCA1 and BRCA2 variants of unknown significance: variant reclassification and surgical decisions. Genet Med. 2011;13:998–1005.
69. Miller-Samuel S, MacDonald DJ, Weitzel JN, et al. Variants of uncertain significance in breast cancer-related genes: real-world implications for a clinical conundrum. Part one: clinical genetics recommendations. Semin Oncol. 2011;38:469–80.
70. Petrucelli N, Lazebnik N, Huelsman KM, Lazebnik RS. Clinical interpretation and recommendations for patients with a variant of uncertain significance in BRCA1 or BRCA2: a survey of genetic counseling practice. Genet Test. 2002;6:107–13.

# 3 BRCA Mutation

Ashley N. Hardy, Elizabeth Tarasewicz,
and Jacqueline S. Jeruss

## Introduction: What Are BRCA Mutations?

Breast cancer is the most common malignancy affecting women in the United States and the second leading cause of cancer-related deaths. According to the National Cancer Institute, approximately 200,000 women are diagnosed with breast cancer each year in the United States and 40,000 die of the disease [1]. Although the vast majority of breast cancers are diagnosed in women without known risk factors, 5–10% of newly diagnosed cases can be traced to hereditary gene mutations that significantly increase the likelihood of developing breast and other malignancies [2].

Approximately 80% of these hereditary breast cancers are the result of germline mutations in the Breast Cancer Susceptibility Genes, BRCA1 and BRCA2, which are inherited in an autosomal dominant fashion. BRCA1, which is located on chromosome 17q12-21, and BRCA2, located on chromosome 13q12-13, are tumor suppressor genes that are essential for DNA repair, transcriptional regulation, and cell cycle control [3]. As a result, mutation of these genes (the majority being frameshift or nonsense mutations resulting from small insertions or deletions) [4] leads to an elevated lifetime risk of developing breast cancer as well as other malignancies.

BRCA1 is activated and phosphorylated by CHK2 and ataxia telangiectasia mutated (ATM) kinase in response to DNA damage. BRCA1 then binds Rad51, a protein required for homologous recombination of double-strand breaks [5], which allows it to cooperate with BRCA2 to facilitate DNA repair. BRCA1 also exerts its effects on DNA repair through its interaction with various other proteins, which bind specifically to its BRCT (BRCA1 C-termini) domain to promote activation of critical $G_2$/M phase cell cycle checkpoints. If mutations occur within this domain, BRCA1 is unable to bind to its partners, allowing damaged DNA to escape repair [3] (Fig. 3.1). In terms of transcriptional regulation and cell cycle control, upon phosphorylation by ATM [6], the normal BRCA1 protein can regulate the expression of the GADD45 and p21 genes, ultimately inducing cell cycle arrest in response to DNA damage caused by ionizing radiation [7, 8]. Note that p53, another well-known tumor suppressor gene, has been demonstrated to exert the same effects with BRCA1 acting as a co-activator, helping to explain why mutations of the BRCA1 gene can inhibit p53 transcription [9, 10] (Fig. 3.2).

It is estimated that, in the general population, mutations of the BRCA1 and BRCA2 genes occur in 1 in every 300–500 people [11]. However, in certain populations the frequency of these mutations is higher, notably in those individuals

A.N. Hardy, M.D. (✉) • E. Tarasewicz, B.S.
• J.S. Jeruss, M.D., Ph.D.
Department of Surgery, Northwestern Memorial Hospital, Chicago, IL 60611, USA
e-mail: ashley.nicole.hardy@gmail.com; etarasewicz@u.northwestern.edu; jjeruss@nmh.org

N.M. Hansen (ed.), *Management of the Patient at High Risk for Breast Cancer*,
DOI 10.1007/978-1-4614-5891-3_3, © Springer Science+Business Media New York 2013

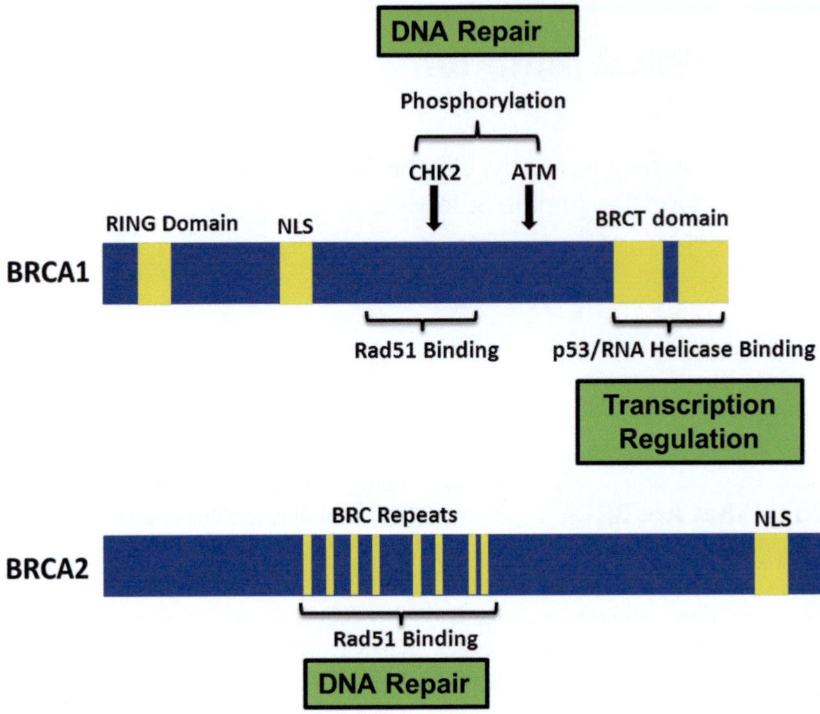


**Fig. 3.1** Characteristics of the BRCA1 and BRCA2 proteins. BRCA1: Features of the BRCA1 protein include the N-terminal RING domain, nuclear localization signals (NLS), and the two C-terminal BRCT domains (*yellow*). Sites of phosphorylation by CHK2 and ATM are indicated (*black arrows*) along with the site of Rad51 binding (*bracket*). BRCA2: Rad51 binds to six of the eight BRC repeats present in the BRCA2 protein (*bracket*). (Adapted from Venkitaraman (2001) with the permission of Elsevier Science Ltd)

of Ashkenazi Jewish descent, in which the incidence of BRCA mutations is 1 in 40 [12]. Three mutations (185delAG and 5382insC in BRCA1 and 6174delT in BRCA2) account for over 90% of the BRCA mutations found in the Ashkenazi Jewish population [13]. Additional founder mutations have been traced to other groups, most commonly of Icelandic, Polish, French Canadian, and Italian origin [14].

## Clinical Implications of BRCA Mutations

Women with BRCA1 or BRCA2 mutations have a substantially increased risk of developing breast cancer compared to non-BRCA mutation carriers, with a 76–84% chance of developing breast cancer by age 70 (compared with a 13% likelihood for noncarriers) [15, 16]. In addition, carriers of either mutation are more likely to be diagnosed at an earlier age, tend to present with tumors of higher histologic grade, and are more likely to develop cancer in the contralateral breast compared to sporadic controls [17]. Despite these similarities, there are a number of differences that exist between the two genes that are important to consider (Table 3.1).

Specifically, BRCA1 breast tumors tend to be of a higher grade as a result of higher mitotic rates and nuclear polymorphisms and display elevated levels of cyclin E expression [18, 19]. This is in contrast to BRCA2-related tumors, which are more likely to overexpress cyclin D1 and in which the higher grade observed in these tumors is the result of decreased tubule formation [18, 20].

Differences between BRCA1 and BRCA2 also exist with respect to hormone receptor status. The majority of BRCA1 breast tumors have a triple-negative phenotype as they lack expression

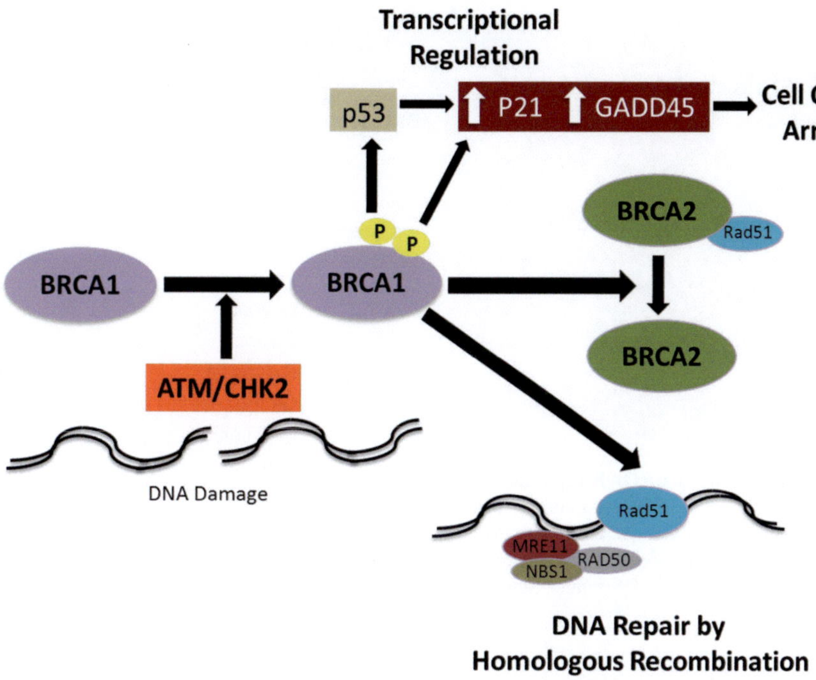


**Fig. 3.2** The role of BRCA proteins in DNA repair, transcriptional regulation, and cell cycle control. Upon exposure to a DNA damaging agent, ATM or CHK2 phosphorylates BRCA, upregulating the expression of proteins that mediate cell cycle arrest (p21, GADD45) directly, or through transcription of p53. Phosphorylated BRCA1 also promotes DNA repair in cooperation with BRCA2 and Rad51. (Adapted from Venkitaraman (2001) with the permission of Elsevier Science Ltd)

**Table 3.1** Comparison of the BRCA genes and associated breast cancer characteristics

| Characteristics | BRCA1 | BRCA2 |
|---|---|---|
| Inheritance pattern | Autosomal dominant | Autosomal dominant |
| Chromosomal locale | 17q12-21 | 13q12-13 |
| Cellular functions | DNA repair | DNA repair |
| | Transcriptional regulation | Transcriptional regulation |
| | Cell cycle control | Cell cycle control |
| Breast cancer risks | 45% of Hereditary breast cancer | 35% of Hereditary breast cancer |
| | 71% Risk by age 70 (95% CI 53–82%) | 84% Risk by age 70 (95% CI 43–95%) |
| Breast cancer characteristics | Early age of onset | Early age of onset |
| | High grade | High grade |
| | High mitotic rate | Decreased tubule formation |
| | Nuclear polymorphisms | |
| | Increased incidence of ER/PR negativity | Increased incidence of ER/PR positivity |
| | HER2/neu negative | HER2/neu negative |
| | Cyclin E overexpression | Cyclin D1 overexpression |
| | Increased risk of bilateral cancer | Increased risk of bilateral cancer |
| Other (non-breast) associated cancer risks | Ovarian cancer (26–36% by age 70) | Ovarian cancer (10–27% by age 70) |
| | Cervical, uterine, pancreatic, colorectal | Gastric, pancreatic, gallbladder, bile duct, skin (melanoma, basal cell) |
| | Males: prostate | Males: breast, prostate |

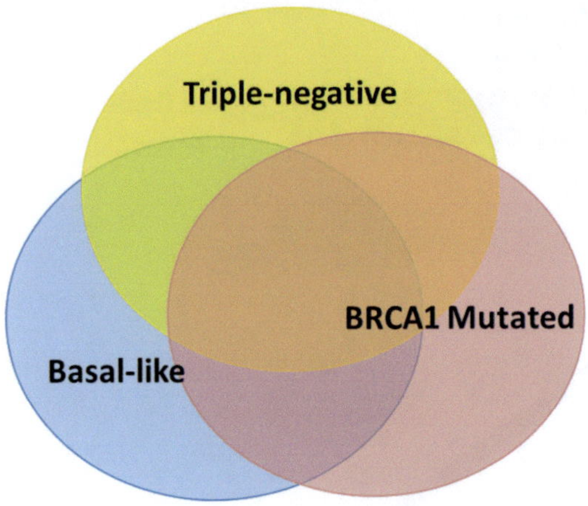


**Fig. 3.3** Relationship between BRCA1, triple-negative, and basal-like breast cancers. BRCA1-mutated breast cancer often phenotypically overlaps with both triple-negative and basal-like breast cancers. (Adapted from Pal et al. (2011) with the permission of Springer Science + Business Media)

of the estrogen (ER) and progesterone receptors (PR) and are HER2/neu negative. Additionally the majority of BRCA1 tumors have morphologic features similar to those described in basal-like cancers as they have been shown to express the markers CK5/6 and EGFR [21, 22] (Fig. 3.3). In comparison, BRCA2 tumors exhibit ER positivity in 60–90% of cases and PR positivity in 40–80%, similar to the expression patterns found in sporadic controls [23, 24]. Altogether, the differences that exist between the two mutations may affect treatment strategies and may account for the differences in survival times, which are shorter for patients with BRCA1 mutations [25].

The mutations also confer an increased chance of developing other cancers, most frequently ovarian cancer, with a lifetime risk ranging from 26–36% and 10–27% for BRCA1 and BRCA2 carriers, respectively [26]. BRCA1 mutations are also associated with cervical, uterine, pancreatic, and colon cancer while BRCA2 mutations are affiliated with cancers of the stomach, pancreas, gallbladder, bile duct, and skin (melanoma and basal cell carcinoma) [27, 28]. Men carrying BRCA1 mutations are at elevated risk for testicular and early-onset (prior to age 55) prostate cancer while those with BRCA2 mutations are at risk for developing male breast cancer [29] (Table 3.2).

**Table 3.2** Relative risks of cancers (non-breast) associated with BRCA mutations [28, 67, 68]

| | Associated cancers | Relative risk |
|---|---|---|
| BRCA1 | Ovarian | 13 |
| | Cervical | 3.7 |
| | Uterine | 2.7 |
| | Pancreatic | 2.3 |
| | Colorectal | 1.5 |
| | Prostate | 1.8 |
| BRCA2 | Ovarian | 21 |
| | Gastric | 2.6 |
| | Pancreatic | 3.5 |
| | Gallbladder and bile duct | 5.0 |
| | Melanoma | 2.6 |
| | Male breast | 1.7 |
| | Prostate | 4.7 |

Given the clinical implications of being a BRCA carrier, genetic testing to assess for the presence of these mutations has been implemented into clinical practice in much of the developed world [30].

## Screening Guidelines for BRCA Mutations

Although not standardized, according to the US Preventive Services Task Force, the following high-risk patient scenarios should prompt a recommendation for BRCA mutation testing [31]:

- ≥ 2 First-degree relatives diagnosed with breast cancer, with at least one diagnosis made at age 50 or younger
- ≥ 3 First- or second-degree relatives diagnosed with breast cancer at any age
- First-degree relatives with bilateral breast cancer
- First- or second-degree relative diagnosed with both breast and ovarian cancer at any age
- Several first- and second-degree relatives diagnosed with breast and ovarian cancer
- ≥ 2 First- or second-degree relatives with an ovarian cancer diagnosis at any age
- Male relative with breast cancer
- Women of Ashkenazi Jewish descent with a first-degree relative diagnosed with breast or ovarian cancer or with ≥ second-degree relatives (maternal or paternal) with a breast or ovarian cancer diagnosis

**Table 3.3** Breast and ovarian cancer surveillance strategies for BRCA mutation carriers based on National Cancer Comprehensive Network (NCCN) guidelines

| | Screening modality | Recommended frequency |
|---|---|---|
| Breast cancer | Self breast exam (SBE) | Monthly starting at age 18 |
| | Clinical breast exam (CBE) | Every 6 months starting at age 25 or 5–10 years prior to the earliest breast cancer diagnosis |
| | Mammography | Annually beginning at age 25–30 or 5–10 years prior to the earliest breast cancer diagnosis |
| | Magnetic resonance imaging (MRI) | Annually beginning at age 25–30 or 5–10 years prior to the earliest breast cancer diagnosis |
| Ovarian cancer | Transvaginal ultrasonography | Every 6–12 months beginning at age 25–35 or 5–10 years prior to earliest ovarian cancer diagnosis |
| | Serum CA-125 measurements | Every 6–12 months beginning at age 25–35 or 5–10 years prior to earliest ovarian cancer diagnosis |

## Surveillance Options for BRCA Mutation Carriers

For individuals found to be carriers of BRCA1 or BRCA2 mutations, attempts should be made to ensure that if cancer develops, it is detected early, or ideally, prevented from developing at all (Table 3.3). Surveillance strategies for BRCA patients include the performance of monthly self-breast exams (SBE), clinical breast exams (CBE) every 6 months, imaging of the breast with yearly mammograms and magnetic resonance imaging (MRI) starting between 25 and 30 years of age or before the earliest diagnosis of breast cancer was made in the affected family [32]. Although SBE and CBE may add little to cancer detection rates in BRCA carriers, they are recommended as they allow patients to gain a greater sense of familiarity with their breast tissue, and in the case of CBE, provides patients with the opportunity to connect to their health care provider [33].

In a prospective study comparing the various breast cancer surveillance modalities for BRCA mutation carriers, MRI had a sensitivity of 77% for detecting breast cancers compared to the 36–33% sensitivity achieved by mammography and ultrasound, respectively. The sensitivity approached 95% when the modalities were combined [34]. Despite the expense and the potential for false positive findings, MRI has been proven to be cost-effective for BRCA mutation carriers as demonstrated in a study by Plevritus et al. This study estimated that combined annual screening with MRI and mammography would provide an additional 2 life years for women with BRCA1 mutations and 18 months for those with BRCA2 mutations [35].

Although transvaginal ultrasound and serum CA 125 level testing have limited sensitivity and specificity for the detection of early stage ovarian cancer, because of the significant risk, the American College of Obstetricians and Gynecologists (ACOG) recommends that BRCA carriers undergo annual or semiannual screening with these tests beginning at 25–35 years of age or 5–10 years prior to the earliest familial ovarian cancer diagnosis [36].

## Prevention Strategies for BRCA Mutation Carriers

Several strategies exist to reduce cancer risk in patients with BRCA mutations, ranging from prophylactic surgery, chemoprevention, and lifestyle modifications (Table 3.4). One of the largest multicenter prospective studies, the Prevention and Observation of Surgical End Points (PROSE), determined that prophylactic bilateral mastectomy conferred a 90% risk reduction in BRCA1 and BRCA2 mutation carriers after a mean follow-up of 6.4 years [37].

In recent years, nipple-sparing mastectomy (NSM) has evolved as an option for women undergoing mastectomy given the excellent cosmetic results and psychological benefit achieved, especially for young cancer patients [38]. Despite these benefits, concern exists regarding the oncologic

**Table 3.4** Risk-reducing strategies for BRCA mutation patients and other factors that may impact a patient's likelihood of developing hereditary breast or ovarian cancer

| | Strategy | Influence on risk |
|---|---|---|
| Prophylactic surgery | Prophylactic bilateral mastectomy (PBM) | 90% Risk reduction |
| | Prophylactic bilateral | 53% Risk reduction in breast cancer |
| | Salpingo-oophorectomy (PBSO) | 96% Risk reduction in ovarian cancer |
| Chemoprevention | Selective estrogen receptor modulators (SERMs) | 50–58% Risk reduction |
| | Oral contraceptives (OCPs) | 70% Risk reduction in ovarian cancer<br>Potential increased breast cancer risk |
| Other factors | Hormone replacement Therapy (HRT) | No influence with short-term use |
| | Breast feeding | 40% Risk reduction after 1 year for BRCA1 |
| | High parity | Reduced risk for BRCA1<br>Potential increased risk for BRCA2 |

safety of this operation, notably for BRCA mutation carriers and others with elevated cancer risk, given the possibility of nipple involvement by the tumor [39]. To date, there appears to be a low probability of nipple involvement by premalignant lesions (i.e., atypical hyperplasia and carcinoma in situ) or invasive carcinoma in the nipple areola complex (NAC) of BRCA carriers as demonstrated by a study examining the presence of such lesions in women with BRCA mutations that underwent prophylactic mastectomy over a time course of 22 years [40]. Further research needs to be done in this area given the fact that more women are choosing to pursue NSM. Currently, intraoperative retroareolar frozen sections are obtained to assess for the presence of cancer involving the NAC prior to proceeding with nipple-sparing surgery.

Bilateral prophylactic salpingo-oophorectomy (PBSO) has been associated with a reduction in the risk for both ovarian and breast cancer for BRCA mutation carriers. This was also demonstrated by the PROSE study, which reported a 96% reduction in ovarian cancer risk and a 53% reduction in breast cancer risk among BRCA carriers undergoing PBSO compared to matched controls [41]. Studies have shown that this risk reduction was greatest if performed by age 40 or upon the cessation of childbearing [42]. In addition to providing a reduction in the incidence of breast and ovarian cancer, a prospective multicenter cohort found a reduction in all-cause mortality (hazard ratio, HR = 0.40, 9%% CI, 0.26–0.61) that was both ovarian (HR = 0.44, 95% CI, 0.26–0.76) and breast cancer-specific (HR = 0.21, 95% CI, 0.06–0.80) in BRCA patients [43].

Nonsurgical prevention strategies for BRCA-positive patients include chemoprevention, lifestyle modifications, and close surveillance. The incomplete penetrance of mutations of the BRCA1 and BRCA2 genes supports the idea that various hormonal and reproductive factors can influence the risk of cancer development within this patient population.

Several studies have investigated the impact of chemoprevention with tamoxifen on the development of breast cancer in BRCA mutation carriers. Tamoxifen, a selective estrogen receptor modulator (SERM), is routinely used in the treatment of estrogen receptor-positive breast cancers.

In the National Surgical Adjuvant Breast and Bowel Project (NSABP)-P1 trial, a subgroup analysis concluded that although tamoxifen was able to reduce the incidence of breast cancer for women with a BRCA2 mutation, women with a BRCA1 mutation were not conferred the same benefit. This appeared to correlate with the observation that the majority of BRCA1 tumors are ER-negative while BRCA2 tumors are predominately ER-positive [23, 24], yet the study's small sample size (8 women with BRCA1 and 11 with BRCA2 mutations) prevents any definitive conclusion for this analysis [44]. Conversely, in a case–control study examining 285 BRCA1/2 mutation carriers with bilateral breast cancer and 751 mutation carriers with unilateral cancer, the use of tamoxifen conferred a reduction in the risk for the development of contralateral cancer for both BRCA1 and BRCA2 mutation carriers by 50 and 58%, respectively. Thus, these findings suggest that risk reduction with tamoxifen therapy may be independent of hormone receptor status for BRCA patients [45].

Although the protective effect of oral contraceptives in BRCA1/2 mutation carriers for the prevention of ovarian cancer has been established, with a risk reduction of 34% for new oral contraceptive users and a 70% risk reduction for those with 6 or more years of use [46], the impact of oral contraceptives on the risk of breast cancer in this patient population is controversial. In one case–control study of 1,311 pairs of BRCA mutation carriers, those with a history of oral contraceptive use was associated with an increased risk of breast cancer among those with BRCA1 mutations (OR = 1.20; 95% CI = 1.02–1.40). An increased risk, however, was not observed among those with BRCA2 mutations (OR = 0.94; 95% CI = 0.72–1.24) [47]. Despite these findings, other population-based studies have failed to demonstrate an association between oral contraceptive use and the development of breast cancer in BRCA mutation patients [48, 49].

Investigations have also been conducted to determine the effect that hormone replacement therapy (HRT) might have on subsequent breast cancer risk in BRCA mutation carriers, particularly for those who use short-term HRT to combat menopausal symptoms (vaginal dryness, hot flashes, decreased libido, fatigue, memory and cognitive changes) after undergoing PBSO. In a multicenter prospective cohort study of BRCA1/BRCA2 mutation carriers that underwent PBSO with or without HRT, short-term HRT did not counteract the risk reduction associated with PBSO [50].

Breastfeeding is thought to be protective against the development of breast cancer as a result of favorable alteration of the hormonal milieu [51], delay in the reestablishment of ovulatory cycles [52], and induction of extended terminal differentiation [53]. A case–control study examining the impact of breastfeeding showed that BRCA1 mutation carriers who breastfed for more than 1 year had a 40% cancer risk reduction compared to those patients that breastfed for a shorter duration or chose not to breastfeed at all. Note that similar results were not observed for BRCA2 carriers, which may be explained by the smaller study sample size of those along with the different biology associated with BRCA2 mutation carriers [54].

Parity has been evaluated as a potential modifier of breast cancer risk in BRCA mutation carriers in several studies with largely mixed results. Although pregnancy appears to provide protection against the development of breast cancer before age 35 for the general population, there are concerns that the opposite may be true for those harboring a BRCA mutation, who are more likely to develop cancers prior to age 40. These concerns were initially supported by the findings from Jernstrom et al., who observed that the risk of breast cancer increased with each additional pregnancy in BRCA mutation carriers prior to age 40, particularly for those with BRCA2 mutations [55]. However, in subsequent studies by Cullinane et al. and McLaughlin et al., parity was associated with a reduced risk of developing breast cancer among BRCA1 mutation carriers (OR = 0.67; 95% CI = 0.46–0.96; $p = 0.03$), but an increased risk for BRCA2 patients (OR = 2.74; 95% CI = 1.18–6.41; $p = 0.02$) [56], and appeared to increase by 17% with each additional birth [57].

## Breast Cancer Treatment Strategies for BRCA Mutation Carriers

While many aspects of breast cancer treatment for BRCA patients are similar to those of non-mutation carriers, the underlying biology of these tumors and the additional risks they confer affect their management (Fig. 3.4). Because of the increased risk of recurrence and of developing cancer in the contralateral breast, many BRCA mutation carriers may choose to undergo bilateral mastectomy as part of their initial therapy. In fact, there is an estimated 20–42% 10-year risk of developing contralateral breast cancer in women with BRCA-positive tumors compared to a 5–6% risk observed in sporadic controls [58]. Prophylactic mastectomy of the

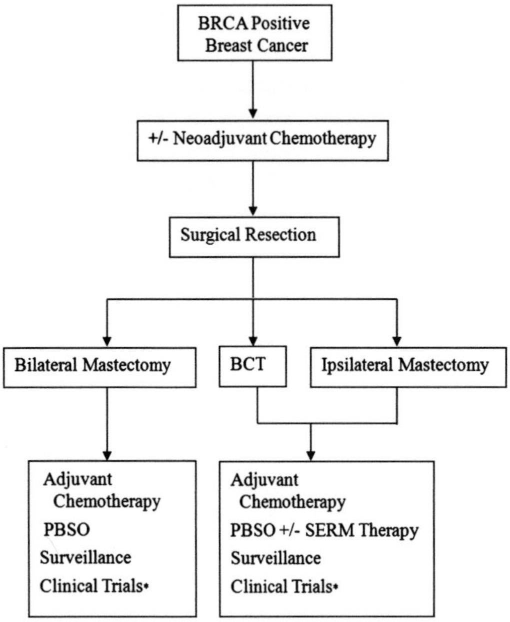


**Fig. 3.4** Treatment algorithm for BRCA mutation carriers diagnosed with unilateral breast cancer. *BCT* breast conservation surgery; *PBSO* prophylactic bilateral salpingo-ophorectomy; *SERM* selective estrogen receptor modulator. *Asterisk* patients may benefit from enrollment in clinical trials using PARP and Cdk inhibitors

unaffected, contralateral breast may decrease the risk of developing subsequent cancer in that breast by 90% although it has not been shown to improve survival when used as monotherapy [59].

For those BRCA patients who instead choose to pursue breast conservation therapy (BCT or lumpectomy combined with radiation therapy), there should be recognition that as with sporadic controls, there is a higher risk of ipsilateral tumor recurrence compared with those that undergo mastectomy. However, focusing on BCT alone, several studies have demonstrated that the risk of recurrence was similar between BRCA mutation carriers and sporadic controls. Note that this is particularly the case when BCT is followed by either PBSO or tamoxifen therapy as observed in a study by Pierce et al., which showed that the rates of ipsilateral recurrence were twice as high in those of BRCA patients who did not undergo PBSO. Furthermore, there was a 31% rate of recurrence in those BRCA mutation carriers who did not take tamoxifen following BCT compared to no recurrences amongst those that had taken the medication over a 15-year period [60]. Thus, these findings suggest that for those BRCA patients choosing to undergo BCT, strong consideration should be placed on following this with PBSO and/or tamoxifen therapy given the impact on reduced breast cancer recurrence. Finally, as previously mentioned, PBSO is associated with an approximate 96% risk reduction in ovarian cancer development in BRCA mutation carriers [41].

As BRCA-positive tumors tend to be of higher grade, hormone receptor negative (notably BRCA1 tumors), and at an advanced stage at the time of diagnosis [17], the majority of patients with these tumors are candidates for chemotherapy. Recent studies have suggested that specific chemotherapeutic agents, notably platinum-based agents, may have greater efficacy in patients with BRCA-mutated tumors based on their mechanism of action. Although not routinely used in the treatment of breast cancer in general, defects in DNA repair render BRCA-positive tumors more sensitive to the DNA damaging effects of cisplatin and other agents in this class [61]. In fact, in a mouse model of BRCA1 breast cancer, 100% of those mice treated with high doses of cisplatin exhibited a complete pathologic response whereas those treated with doxorubicin were refractory [62].

Studies have also suggested that BRCA-mutated tumors may be resistant to the effects of paclitaxel, another chemotherapeutic agent widely used in the treatment of breast cancer, by impairing the mitotic spindle assembly checkpoint and overriding the mitotic arrest normally induced by the paclitaxel and other taxanes [63].

In addition to the more conventional therapies, new classes of medications, including the poly (ADP-ribose) polymerase (PARP) inhibitors and cyclin-dependent kinase (Cdk) inhibitors, have shown promise for the treatment of BRCA1 and BRCA2-positive breast cancers in the preclinical setting. These tumors are susceptible to PARP inhibitors as DNA damage exerted by PARP inhibition is unable to be repaired by BRCA-mediated homologous recombination [64]. Utilizing such therapies may obviate the need for such highly toxic doses of chemotherapy in the treatment of patients with BRCA-positive tumors [65].

Thus far, a phase 1 study utilizing single-agent olaparib, an oral PARP inhibitor, demonstrated a favorable therapeutic index and clinical response in 64% of BRCA mutation carriers. In contrast, patients with sporadic cancers failed to show any response [66].

Recently, a study by Johnson et al. evaluated the combined effect of PARP and Cdk inhibition, given the fact that Cdk1 is necessary for BRCA-mediated homologous recombination. As a result, by inhibiting the activity of Cdk1, BRCA-positive tumors appeared to be more sensitive to the effects of PARP inhibition both *in vitro* and *in vivo* [65].

## Summary

In summary, BRCA1 and BRCA2 genes are classified as tumor suppressors given their roles in DNA repair, transcriptional regulation, and cell cycle control [3]. Mutations in these genes therefore increase the susceptibility for cancer development, namely of the breast and ovaries, accounting for 5–10% and 10–15% of all newly diagnosed breast and ovarian cancers, respectively [2]. BRCA-mutated breast cancers are typically diagnosed at an earlier age, can be bilateral, and of higher histologic grade [17]. Given the clinical implications of being a BRCA carrier, patients with high-risk personal and family history characteristics should undergo testing to assess for the presence of these mutations. Risk-reducing strategies for BRCA mutation carriers range from prophylactic mastectomy and oophorectomy, to chemoprevention with SERMs and lifestyle modifications. Cancer treatment options for these patients are similar to sporadic controls although their underlying biology may make the use of platinum-based chemotherapy more efficacious [61, 62]. Finally, although PARP and Cdk inhibitors have shown promise in phase 1 clinical trials for the treatment of BRCA-mutated tumors [66], there remains a need for more targeted therapies to treat these extremely complex, highly penetrant breast cancers.

## References

1. Jemal A, Siegel R, Xu J, Ward E. Cancer statistics, 2010. CA Cancer J Clin. 2010;60(5):277–300.
2. Campeau PM, Foulkes WD, Tischkowitz MD. Hereditary breast cancer: new genetic developments, new therapeutic avenues. Hum Genet. 2008;124(1):31–42.
3. Venkitaraman AR. Chromosome stability, DNA recombination and the BRCA2 tumour suppressor. Curr Opin Cell Biol. 2001;13(3):338–43.
4. Kais Z, Chiba N, Ishioka C, Parvin JD. Functional differences among BRCA1 missense mutations in the control of centrosome duplication. Oncogene. 2012;31(6):799–804.
5. Shinohara A, Ogawa H, Ogawa T. Rad51 protein involved in repair and recombination in S. cerevisiae is a RecA-like protein. Cell. 1992;69(3):457–70.
6. Xu B, Kim S, Kastan MB. Involvement of Brca1 in S-phase and G(2)-phase checkpoints after ionizing irradiation. Mol Cell Biol. 2001;21(10):3445–50.
7. MacLachlan TK, Somasundaram K, Sgagias M, et al. BRCA1 effects on the cell cycle and the DNA damage response are linked to altered gene expression. J Biol Chem. 2000;275(4):2777–85.
8. Somasundaram K, Zhang H, Zeng YX, et al. Arrest of the cell cycle by the tumour-suppressor BRCA1 requires the CDK-inhibitor p21WAF1/CiP1. Nature. 1997;389(6647):187–90.
9. Zhang H, Somasundaram K, Peng Y, et al. BRCA1 physically associates with p53 and stimulates its transcriptional activity. Oncogene. 1998;16(13):1713–21.
10. Zheng L, Li S, Boyer TG, Lee WH. Lessons learned from BRCA1 and BRCA2. Oncogene. 2000;19(53):6159–75.
11. Roukos DH, Briasoulis E. Individualized preventive and therapeutic management of hereditary breast ovarian cancer syndrome. Nat Clin Pract Oncol. 2007;4(10):578–90.
12. Tonin P, Weber B, Offit K, et al. Frequency of recurrent BRCA1 and BRCA2 mutations in Ashkenazi Jewish breast cancer families. Nat Med. 1996;2(11):1179–83.
13. Phelan CM, Kwan E, Jack E, et al. A low frequency of non-founder BRCA1 mutations in Ashkenazi Jewish breast-ovarian cancer families. Hum Mutat. 2002;20(5):352–7.
14. Ferla R, Calo V, Cascio S, et al. Founder mutations in BRCA1 and BRCA2 genes. Ann Oncol. 2007;18 Suppl 6:vi93–8.
15. Easton DF, Ford D, Bishop DT. Breast and ovarian cancer incidence in BRCA1-mutation carriers. Breast Cancer Linkage Consortium. Am J Hum Genet. 1995;56(1):265–71.
16. Ford D, Easton DF, Peto J. Estimates of the gene frequency of BRCA1 and its contribution to breast and ovarian cancer incidence. Am J Hum Genet. 1995;57(6):1457–62.

17. Metcalfe K, Lynch HT, Ghadirian P, et al. Contralateral breast cancer in BRCA1 and BRCA2 mutation carriers. J Clin Oncol. 2004;22(12):2328–35.
18. Hedenfalk I, Duggan D, Chen Y, et al. Gene-expression profiles in hereditary breast cancer. N Engl J Med. 2001;344(8):539–48.
19. Chappuis PO, Donato E, Goffin JR, et al. Cyclin E expression in breast cancer: predicting germline BRCA1 mutations, prognosis and response to treatment. Ann Oncol. 2005;16(5):735–42.
20. Lakhani SR, Jacquemier J, Sloane JP, et al. Multifactorial analysis of differences between sporadic breast cancers and cancers involving BRCA1 and BRCA2 mutations. J Natl Cancer Inst. 1998;90(15):1138–45.
21. Tischkowitz MD, Foulkes WD. The basal phenotype of BRCA1-related breast cancer: past, present and future. Cell Cycle. 2006;5(9):963–7.
22. Pal SK, Mortimer J. Triple-negative breast cancer: novel therapies and new directions. Maturitas. 2009;63(4):269–74.
23. Lakhani SR, Van De Vijver MJ, Jacquemier J, et al. The pathology of familial breast cancer: predictive value of immunohistochemical markers estrogen receptor, progesterone receptor, HER-2, and p53 in patients with mutations in BRCA1 and BRCA2. J Clin Oncol. 2002;20(9):2310–8.
24. Eerola H, Heikkila P, Tamminen A, Aittomaki K, Blomqvist C, Nevanlinna H. Histopathological features of breast tumours in BRCA1, BRCA2 and mutation-negative breast cancer families. Breast Cancer Res. 2005;7(1):R93–100.
25. Lee EH, Park SK, Park B, et al. Effect of BRCA1/2 mutation on short-term and long-term breast cancer survival: a systematic review and meta-analysis. Breast Cancer Res Treat. 2010;122(1):11–25.
26. Rebbeck TR, Kauff ND, Domchek SM. Meta-analysis of risk reduction estimates associated with risk-reducing salpingo-oophorectomy in BRCA1 or BRCA2 mutation carriers. J Natl Cancer Inst. 2009;101(2):80–7.
27. Thompson D, Easton DF. Cancer incidence in BRCA1 mutation carriers. J Natl Cancer Inst. 2002;94(18):1358–65.
28. The Breast Cancer Linkage Consortium. Cancer risks in BRCA2 mutation carriers. J Natl Cancer Inst. 1999;91(15):1310–6.
29. Liede A, Karlan BY, Narod SA. Cancer risks for male carriers of germline mutations in BRCA1 or BRCA2: a review of the literature. J Clin Oncol. 2004;22(4):735–42.
30. Narod SA, Foulkes WD. BRCA1 and BRCA2: 1994 and beyond. Nat Rev Cancer. 2004;4(9):665–76.
31. Nelson HD, Huffman LH, Fu R, Harris EL. Genetic risk assessment and BRCA mutation testing for breast and ovarian cancer susceptibility: systematic evidence review for the U.S. Preventive Services Task Force. Ann Intern Med. 2005;143(5):362–79.
32. Daly MB, Axilbund JE, Buys S, et al. Genetic/familial high-risk assessment: breast and ovarian. J Natl Compr Canc Netw. 2010;8(5):562–94.
33. Spiegel TN, Hill KA, Warner E. The attitudes of women with BRCA1 and BRCA2 mutations toward clinical breast examinations and breast self-examinations. J Womens Health (Larchmt). 2009;18(7):1019–24.
34. Warner E, Plewes DB, Hill KA, et al. Surveillance of BRCA1 and BRCA2 mutation carriers with magnetic resonance imaging, ultrasound, mammography, and clinical breast examination. JAMA. 2004;292(11):1317–25.
35. Plevritis SK, Kurian AW, Sigal BM, et al. Cost-effectiveness of screening BRCA1/2 mutation carriers with breast magnetic resonance imaging. JAMA. 2006;295(20):2374–84.
36. American College of Obstetricians and Gynecologists; ACOG Committee on Practice Bulletins—Gynecology; ACOG Committee on Genetics; Society of Gynecologic Oncologists. ACOG practice bulletin no. 103: hereditary breast and ovarian cancer syndrome. Obstet Gynecol. 2009;113(4):957–66.
37. Rebbeck TR, Friebel T, Lynch HT, et al. Bilateral prophylactic mastectomy reduces breast cancer risk in BRCA1 and BRCA2 mutation carriers: the PROSE Study Group. J Clin Oncol. 2004;22(6):1055–62.
38. Didier F, Radice D, Gandini S, et al. Does nipple preservation in mastectomy improve satisfaction with cosmetic results, psychological adjustment, body image and sexuality? Breast Cancer Res Treat. 2009;118(3):623–33.
39. Vlajcic Z, Zic R, Stanec S, Lambasa S, Petrovecki M, Stanec Z. Nipple-areola complex preservation: predictive factors of neoplastic nipple-areola complex invasion. Ann Plast Surg. 2005;55(3):240–4.
40. Reynolds C, Davidson JA, Lindor NM, et al. Prophylactic and therapeutic mastectomy in BRCA mutation carriers: can the nipple be preserved? Ann Surg Oncol. 2011;18(11):3102–9.
41. Rebbeck TR, Lynch HT, Neuhausen SL, et al. Prophylactic oophorectomy in carriers of BRCA1 or BRCA2 mutations. N Engl J Med. 2002;346(21):1616–22.
42. Eisen A, Lubinski J, Klijn J, et al. Breast cancer risk following bilateral oophorectomy in BRCA1 and BRCA2 mutation carriers: an international case–control study. J Clin Oncol. 2005;23(30):7491–6.
43. Domchek SM, Friebel TM, Singer CF, et al. Association of risk-reducing surgery in BRCA1 or BRCA2 mutation carriers with cancer risk and mortality. JAMA. 2010;304(9):967–75.
44. King MC, Wieand S, Hale K, et al. Tamoxifen and breast cancer incidence among women with inherited mutations in BRCA1 and BRCA2: National Surgical Adjuvant Breast and Bowel Project (NSABP-P1) Breast Cancer Prevention Trial. JAMA. 2001;286(18):2251–6.
45. Gronwald J, Tung N, Foulkes WD, et al. Tamoxifen and contralateral breast cancer in BRCA1 and BRCA2 carriers: an update. Int J Cancer. 2006;118(9):2281–4.
46. Narod SA, Risch H, Moslehi R, et al. Oral contraceptives and the risk of hereditary ovarian cancer. Hereditary Ovarian Cancer Clinical Study Group. N Engl J Med. 1998;339(7):424–8.

47. Vessey M, Painter R. Oral contraceptive use and cancer. Findings in a large cohort study, 1968–2004. Br J Cancer. 2006;95(3):385–9.
48. Lee E, Ma H, McKean-Cowdin R, et al. Effect of reproductive factors and oral contraceptives on breast cancer risk in BRCA1/2 mutation carriers and noncarriers: results from a population-based study. Cancer Epidemiol Biomarkers Prev. 2008;17(11):3170–8.
49. Milne RL, Knight JA, John EM, et al. Oral contraceptive use and risk of early-onset breast cancer in carriers and noncarriers of BRCA1 and BRCA2 mutations. Cancer Epidemiol Biomarkers Prev. 2005;14(2):350–6.
50. Rebbeck TR, Friebel T, Wagner T, et al. Effect of short-term hormone replacement therapy on breast cancer risk reduction after bilateral prophylactic oophorectomy in BRCA1 and BRCA2 mutation carriers: the PROSE Study Group. J Clin Oncol. 2005;23(31):7804–10.
51. Petrakis NL, Wrensch MR, Ernster VL, et al. Influence of pregnancy and lactation on serum and breast fluid estrogen levels: implications for breast cancer risk. Int J Cancer. 1987;40(5):587–91.
52. Henderson BE, Pike MC, Casagrande JT. Breast cancer and the oestrogen window hypothesis. Lancet. 1981;2(8242):363–4.
53. Russo J, Tay LK, Russo IH. Differentiation of the mammary gland and susceptibility to carcinogenesis. Breast Cancer Res Treat. 1982;2(1):5–73.
54. Jernstrom H, Lubinski J, Lynch HT, et al. Breast-feeding and the risk of breast cancer in BRCA1 and BRCA2 mutation carriers. J Natl Cancer Inst. 2004;96(14):1094–8.
55. Jernstrom H, Lerman C, Ghadirian P, et al. Pregnancy and risk of early breast cancer in carriers of BRCA1 and BRCA2. Lancet. 1999;354(9193):1846–50.
56. McLaughlin JR, Risch HA, Lubinski J, et al. Reproductive risk factors for ovarian cancer in carriers of BRCA1 or BRCA2 mutations: a case–control study. Lancet Oncol. 2007;8(1):26–34.
57. Cullinane CA, Lubinski J, Neuhausen SL, et al. Effect of pregnancy as a risk factor for breast cancer in BRCA1/BRCA2 mutation carriers. Int J Cancer. 2005;117(6):988–91.
58. Bordeleau L, Panchal S, Goodwin P. Prognosis of BRCA-associated breast cancer: a summary of evidence. Breast Cancer Res Treat. 2010;119(1):13–24.
59. van Sprundel TC, Schmidt MK, Rookus MA, et al. Risk reduction of contralateral breast cancer and survival after contralateral prophylactic mastectomy in BRCA1 or BRCA2 mutation carriers. Br J Cancer. 2005;93(3):287–92.
60. Pierce LJ, Levin AM, Rebbeck TR, et al. Ten-year multi-institutional results of breast-conserving surgery and radiotherapy in BRCA1/2-associated stage I/II breast cancer. J Clin Oncol. 2006;24(16):2437–43.
61. Tassone P, Tagliaferri P, Perricelli A, et al. BRCA1 expression modulates chemosensitivity of BRCA1-defective HCC1937 human breast cancer cells. Br J Cancer. 2003;88(8):1285–91.
62. Shafee N, Smith CR, Wei S, et al. Cancer stem cells contribute to cisplatin resistance in Brca1/p53-mediated mouse mammary tumors. Cancer Res. 2008;68(9):3243–50.
63. Chabalier C, Lamare C, Racca C, Privat M, Valette A, Larminat F. BRCA1 downregulation leads to premature inactivation of spindle checkpoint and confers paclitaxel resistance. Cell Cycle. 2006;5(9):1001–7.
64. McCabe N, Turner NC, Lord CJ, et al. Deficiency in the repair of DNA damage by homologous recombination and sensitivity to poly(ADP-ribose) polymerase inhibition. Cancer Res. 2006;66(16):8109–15.
65. Johnson N, Li YC, Walton ZE, et al. Compromised CDK1 activity sensitizes BRCA-proficient cancers to PARP inhibition. Nat Med. 2011;17(7):875–82.
66. Fong PC, Boss DS, Yap TA, et al. Inhibition of poly(ADP-ribose) polymerase in tumors from BRCA mutation carriers. N Engl J Med. 2009;361(2):123–34.
67. Risch HA, McLaughlin JR, Cole DE, et al. Population BRCA1 and BRCA2 mutation frequencies and cancer penetrances: a kin-cohort study in Ontario, Canada. J Natl Cancer Inst. 2006;98(23):1694–706.
68. Niell BL, Rennert G, Bonner JD, Almog R, Tomsho LP, Gruber SB. BRCA1 and BRCA2 founder mutations and the risk of colorectal cancer. J Natl Cancer Inst. 2004;96(1):15–21.

# High Risk Breast Lesions and Pathologic Evaluation

4

Thomas J. Lawton

## Lobular Neoplasia

Foote and Stewart were the first to use the term lobular carcinoma in situ (LCIS) in 1941 describing a proliferation of cells within breast lobules that were cytologically similar to invasive lobular carcinoma [1]. Later, other authors deemed lesions with similar cells but with less involvement of a lobule as atypical lobular hyperplasia (ALH) [2]. Since the cells of ALH and LCIS are identical (Fig. 4.1) and it appeared it was just the extent of involvement of a lobule by lobular neoplastic cells, the term lobular neoplasia (LN) was coined in 1978 by Haagensen to encompass atypical lobular hyperplasia (ALH) and lobular carcinoma in situ (LCIS) [3].

Histologically, LN (which includes ALH and LCIS) in the classic form is composed of discohesive, small, relatively uniform cells with round to oval nuclei with scanty cytoplasm. The cells generally lack nucleoli and there are rare mitotic figures. These were originally described as Type A cells. Type B cells (often found in the same terminal ductal lobular unit (TDLU) as Type A cells) were described as larger than Type A cells, they had less uniformity, more cytoplasm, and often prominent nucleoli. There are also varying morphologies of the cells of LN including apocrine differentiation and signet ring (when the cells have intracytoplasmic vacuoles containing mucin).

The cells of LN often extend up from the lobular unit into the terminal ducts in what is termed "pagetoid" extension. This can often make it difficult to distinguish LN from solid low grade ductal carcinoma in situ (DCIS) which may have extended down into the lobules (so-called cancerization of lobules). The characteristic growth pattern along terminal ducts by LN cells which "undermine the overlying epithelium" as well as the discohesive nature of the constituent cells can aid in this differential. In difficult cases, an e-cadherin immunohistochemical stain can be useful as it is nearly always absent in cases of LN [4, 5].

Since LCIS and ALH are composed of similar cells the diagnostic distinction between them is based on the extent of involvement of breast lobules. Pathologists use different criteria to distinguish these two entities but the most commonly used criteria are of that by Page et al. [6]. For a diagnosis of LCIS, the involved lobules should have lobular neoplastic cells that fill and distend at least 50% of the acinar units. The criteria for "distention" were subsequently described as eight or more lobular neoplastic cells spanning an acinar unit [2]. If fewer than 50% of the acinar units in a lobule are "filled and distended," then a diagnosis of ALH is made (Fig. 4.2). While the term lobular neoplasia (LN) is often used to encompass both of these entities, based on these histologic criteria and follow-up epidemiologic studies routinely

T.J. Lawton, M.D. (✉)
Pacific Breast Pathology Medical Corporation,
101 Calypso Shores, Novato, CA 94949, USA
e-mail: thomaslawton@mac.com

N.M. Hansen (ed.), *Management of the Patient at High Risk for Breast Cancer*,
DOI 10.1007/978-1-4614-5891-3_4, © Springer Science+Business Media New York 2013

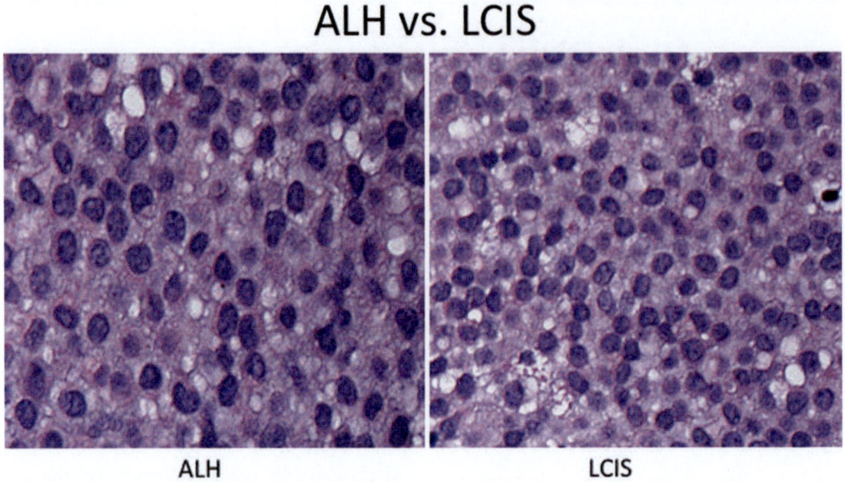


**Fig. 4.1** The cells of atypical lobular hyperplasia (ALH) and lobular carcinoma in situ (LCIS) are identical. They are discohesive, have small, round to oval nuclei, and generally lack nucleoli

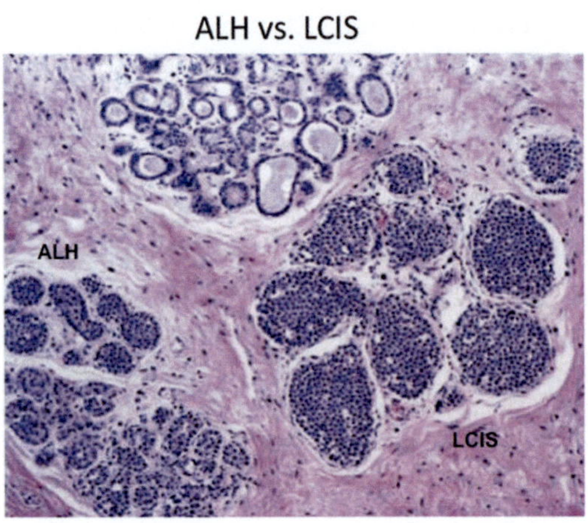


**Fig. 4.2** ALH and LCIS in the same biopsy. This image shows the distinction between the two entities. For a diagnosis of LCIS, at least 50% of the acinar units in a lobule should be "filled and distended" with lobular neoplastic cells

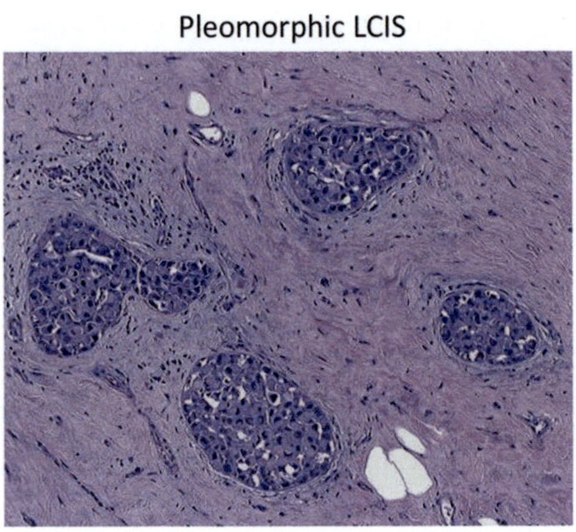


**Fig. 4.3** In pleomorphic lobular carcinoma in situ (pLCIS), the lobular neoplastic cells are still discohesive but there is greater nuclear pleomorphism than in classic LCIS

showing a lower rate in the incidence of the subsequent development of invasive carcinoma for ALH vs. LCIS, pathologists generally recommend maintaining the two entities as separate [2, 6–8].

In the past decade or so, some variants of LCIS have been described including lesions with central necrosis and others with high grade cytology called pleomorphic LCIS (pLCIS) [4, 5, 9–11]. In pLCIS the cells have a similar growth pattern and remain discohesive as in classic LCIS, but they have far more nuclear pleomorphism than the monomorphic cytology seen in classic LCIS (Fig. 4.3). Often, pLCIS and classic LCIS occur in the same biopsy (Fig. 4.4).

It can often be difficult to distinguish pLCIS from high grade DCIS. Several features can be helpful as the cells of pLCIS will remain discohesive unlike those of high grade DCIS. As in classic LN, pathologists can use immunohistochemistry in difficult cases to distinguish pLCIS from high

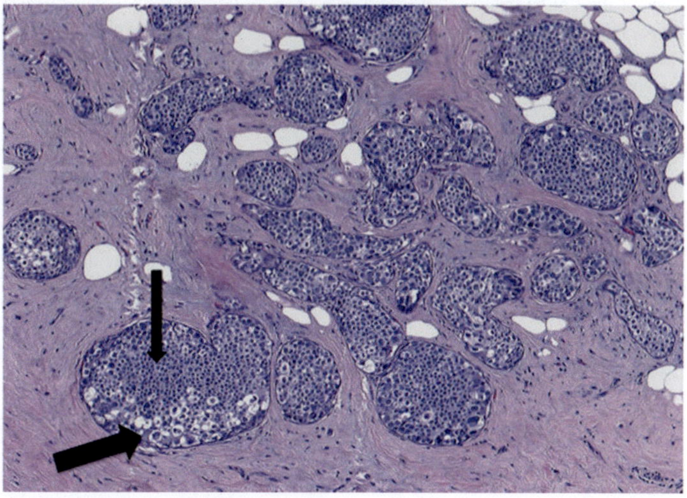


**Fig. 4.4** This image shows both classic LCIS and pLCIS in the same ducts and lobules involving an area of adenosis. The *thicker arrow* shows the pLCIS while the *thinner arrow* shows classic LCIS

grade DCIS, as DCIS and normal ducts will maintain e-cadherin membrane expression whereas LN generally will not.

## Columnar Cell Lesions

Columnar cell lesions have been termed variably over the years in the pathology literature including terms such as columnar cell change (CCC), columnar cell hyperplasia (CCH), columnar metaplasia, expanded lobular units with columnar alteration, blunt duct adenosis, atypical lobules type A of minimal severity, hypersecretory hyperplasia, and most recently, columnar alteration with prominent apical snouts and secretions (CAPSS). There are basically three groups of columnar cell lesions: CCC, CCH, and flat epithelial atypia (FEA) [12, 13].

CCC is on the low end of the spectrum of columnar cell lesions. The histology is characterized by variably dilated acinar units in a lobule lined by one to two layers of columnar epithelial cells with uniform, oval to elongated nuclei. In CCC, the cells are oriented in the usual perpendicular fashion to the basement membrane. As in all columnar cell lesions, there are frequently luminal secretions and central calcifications.

CCH has a similar histology to CCC but unlike in CCC where there are only one to two epithelial cells lining the space, there is hyperplasia of the same type of cells which often stratify in CCH.

On the upper end of the spectrum is FEA. The term flat epithelial atypia (FEA) was adopted by the World Health Organization Working Group on the Pathology and Genetics of Tumors of the Breast in 2003 [14]. The typical histology of FEA shows cystically dilated lobular units that are lined by one to a few layers of monomorphic, but enlarged, round to oval epithelial cells with low-grade cytologic atypia which lose their typical perpendicular orientation to the basement membrane (Figs. 4.5 and 4.6). This cytologic atypia and loss of orientation to the basement membrane separate FEA from CCC and CCH. The cells in FEA often have apical "snouts" and as in CCC and CCH frequently there are luminal secretions and central calcifications. In FEA, although the epithelial cells are atypical, there are no architectural changes as seen in atypical ductal hyperplasia (ADH) or low grade DCIS such as micropapillary or cribriform growth patterns. Any of these architectural patterns would exclude a diagnosis of FEA [15].

## Atypical Ductal Hyperplasia

ADH was originally coined to describe an intraductal proliferation that has "some but not all" of the features of low grade DCIS [6]. Practically

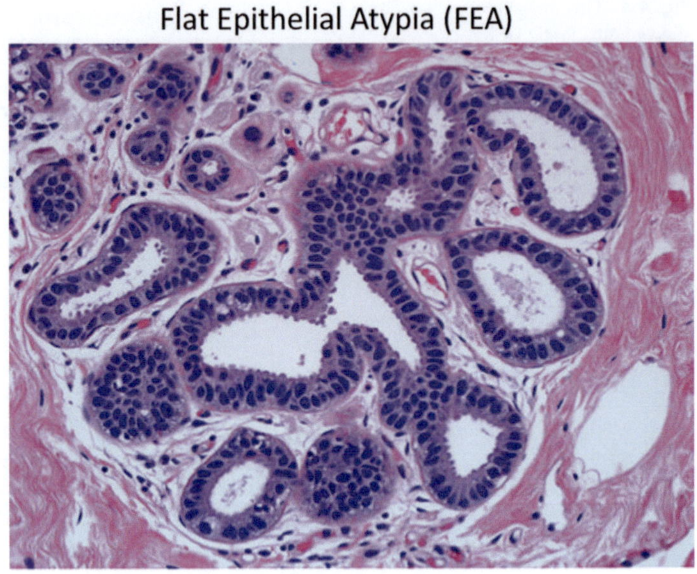


**Fig. 4.5** A medium power view of flat epithelial atypia (FEA). The acini in the involved lobules are distended and the ductal cells have enlarged nuclei with prominent nucleoli not oriented perpendicular to the basement membrane

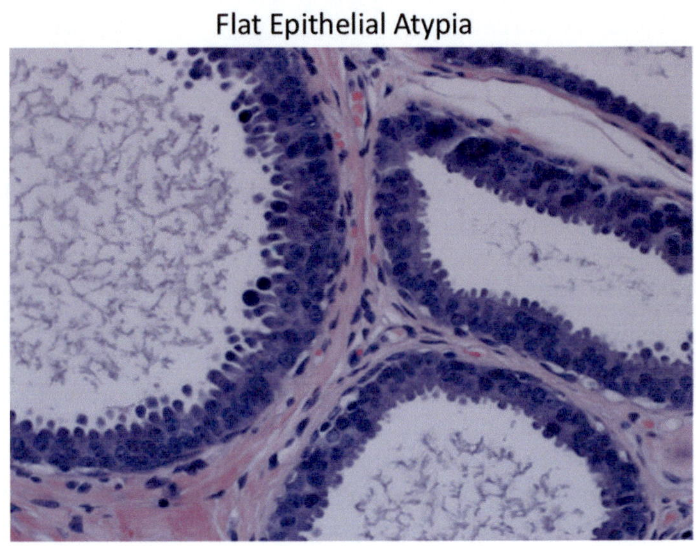


**Fig. 4.6** Higher power view of FEA showing the enlarged cells with prominent nucleoli not oriented perpendicular to the basement membrane. This image also shows the prominent "snouts" and intraluminal secretions often seen in this entity

speaking, this diagnosis is reserved for cases in which the architecture is that of low grade DCIS but the population involved is not monomorphic or the cells are monomorphic but the architecture is not that of low grade DCIS (Fig. 4.7) [16].

In making a diagnosis of ADH, some authors in the literature have suggested using a more quantitative approach. In one of the original papers on the diagnosis of ADH the authors suggested that if fewer than two duct spaces were involved completely by a process that appeared like low grade DCIS then a diagnosis of ADH was made (Fig. 4.8) [17, 18]. Others have suggested a size limit such that if a focus of what appears to be low grade DCIS is seen, if that focus measures less than 0.2 cm then a diagnosis of ADH is made [19]. However, these suggested criteria are based on arbitrary cut-off points.

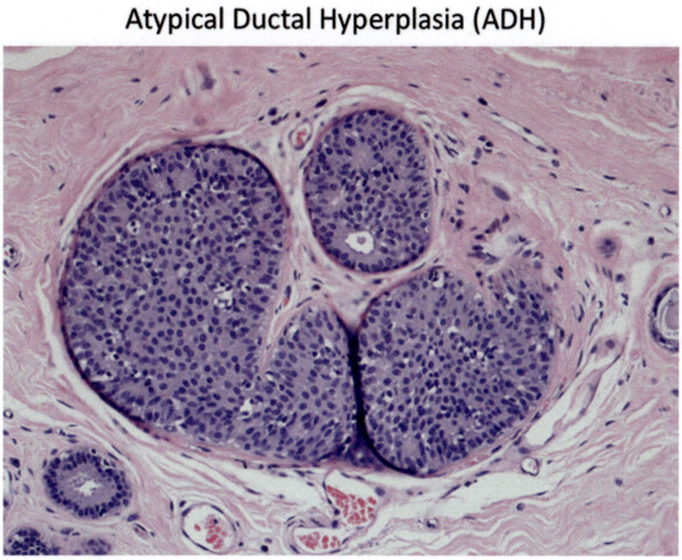


**Fig. 4.7** Atypical ductal hyperplasia (ADH). Several ducts with a relatively monomorphous population of ductal cells with a focal rigid secondary lumen. However, there is an admixed population of myoepithelial cells and many of the cells "overlap" and thus this focus does not fulfill criteria for low grade ductal carcinoma in situ (DCIS)

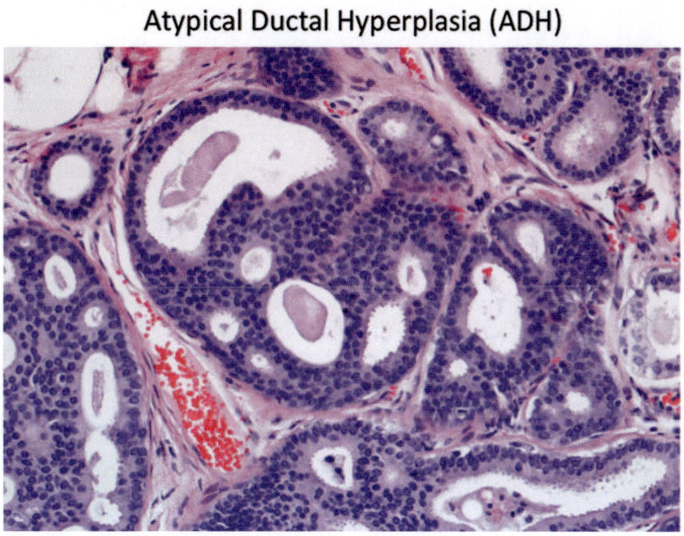


**Fig. 4.8** ADH. There is partial involvement of a duct with a uniform population of cells forming a rigid cribriform architecture. However, a second population of columnar cells lines the remainder of the duct, and therefore this focus does not fulfill criteria for low grade DCIS

Thus the distinction between a high risk lesion such as ADH from DCIS can be very subjective. There are studies in the literature showing how pathologists disagree on the diagnosis of ADH vs. low grade DCIS and even from usual type ductal hyperplasia (UDH) [20]. Since the implications for the relative risk to the patient for the possibility of developing a subsequent carcinoma, criteria need to be better defined between the entities of UDH, ADH, and low grade DCIS.

## Papillary Lesions

Papillomas are benign intraductal proliferations composed of fibrovascular cores lined by a myoepithelial layer over which lies an epithelial layer (Figs. 4.9 and 4.10). Central papillomas (usually subareolar) tend to be solitary but multiple papillomas tend to occur more peripherally in the breast.

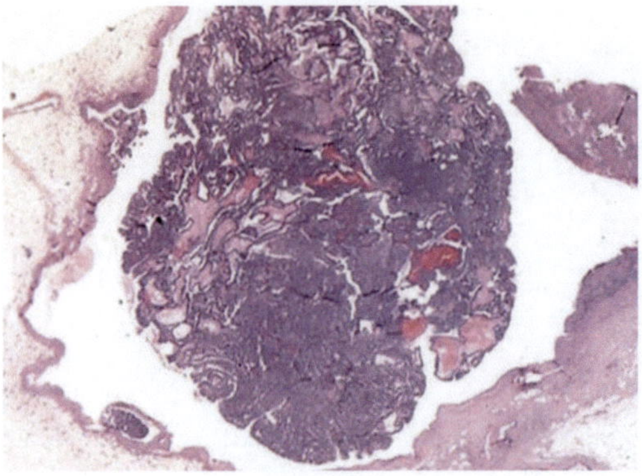


**Fig. 4.9** Solitary intraductal papilloma. An intraductal proliferation of ductal epithelium growing on fibrovascular stalks lined by myoepithelial cells

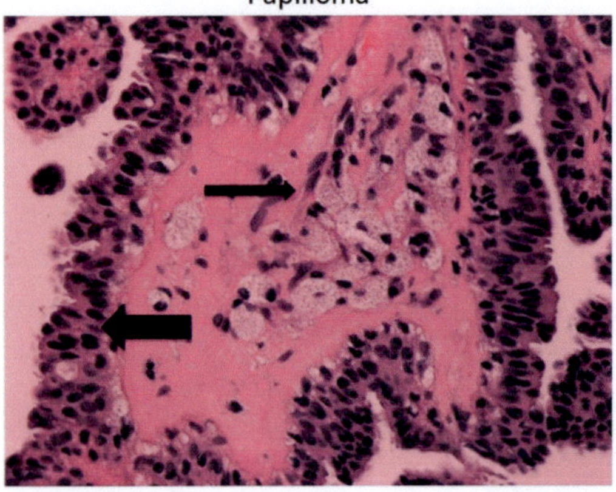


**Fig. 4.10** High power view of an intraductal papilloma. The *thick arrow* shows the ductal epithelium and the *thin arrow* shows the fibrovascular stalks which frequently contain foam cells

The epithelium in an intraductal papilloma often forms just a single layer overlying the myoepithelial layer and fibrovascular core; however, all types of epithelial proliferations that occur in the breast can involve papillomas: usual type hyperplasia (UDH), atypical hyperplasia (ADH and ALH), and carcinoma in situ (DCIS and LCIS). Distinguishing between ADH and DCIS within a papilloma is controversial based on the literature. Some authors believe in size criteria suggesting that if a population of what appears histologically to be low grade DCIS in a papilloma measures less than 3 mm it should be

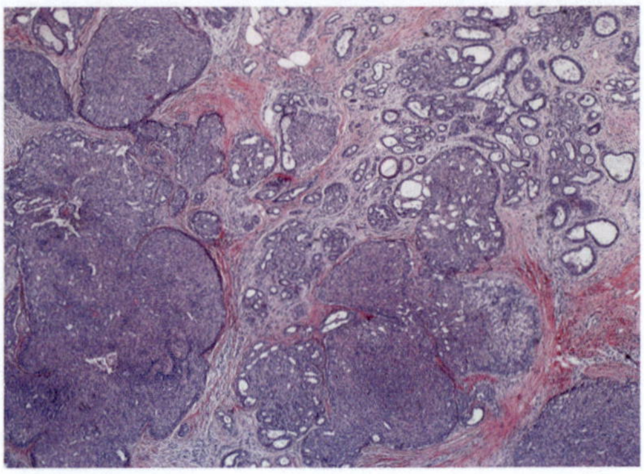


**Fig. 4.11** Multiple papillomas. Unlike a solitary intraductal papilloma, this image shows numerous ducts involved by an intraductal epithelial proliferation with fine fibrovascular stalks

diagnosed as ADH. Others feel that if a similar population occupies less than 30% of the papilloma it should be diagnosed as ADH. Finally, others believe any size focus of what appears to be low grade DCIS within a papilloma should be called DCIS [21, 22].

Finally, there is some data suggesting that solitary intraductal papillomas pose an increased risk to the patient for the development of a subsequent carcinoma, albeit slim; however, data suggests when multiple papillomas are present it appears that risk is increased (Fig. 4.11) [23, 24].

## Radial Scar/Complex Sclerosing Lesion

Radial scar and complex sclerosing lesion are terms used to describe a stellate characteristic pathologic lesion that at low power has a central fibroelastotic stromal area surrounded by irregular ducts and lobules that radiate from this central stromal area (Fig. 4.12). By convention, radial scar refers to a lesion measuring 1 cm or less and complex sclerosing lesion refers to lesions with the same histology but which measure greater than 1 cm [25].

Often, in the central stromal area, there are entrapped benign ducts which can mimic a tubular carcinoma. Benign ducts will maintain their myoepithelial cell layer whereas tubular carcinomas

Radial Scar

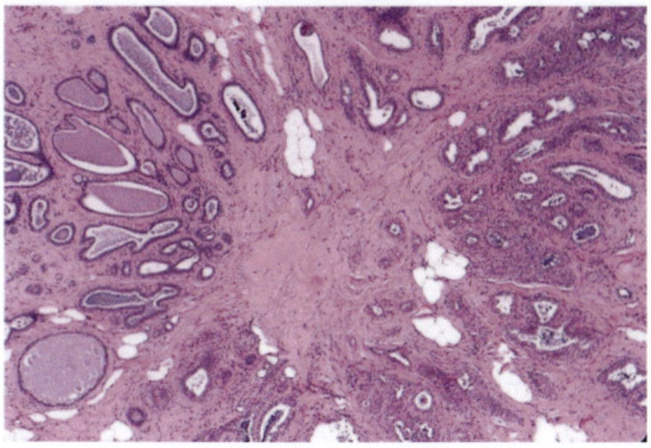

**Fig. 4.12** Radial scar. This image shows a lesion with a central fibroelastotic stromal area (scar) with ducts and lobules radiating from the central stromal area

will not so this is usually not a problem on routine H & E. However, if it is an issue, routine immunohistochemistry for myoepithelial markers (e.g., SMHC, p63, or calponin) can aid in the differential diagnosis.

The ducts and lobules surrounding the central fibroelastotic stromal area can be involved by any type of usual epithelial proliferation seen in the breast including UDH, atypical hyperplasia (ADH and ALH), and in situ carcinoma (DCIS and LCIS).

## References


1. Foote FW, Stewart FW. Lobular carcinoma in situ: a rare form of mammary cancer. Am J Pathol. 1941;17(4):491–496.3.
2. Simpson PT, et al. The diagnosis and management of pre-invasive breast disease: pathology of atypical lobular hyperplasia and lobular carcinoma in situ. Breast Cancer Res. 2003;5(5):258–62.
3. Haagensen CD, et al. Lobular neoplasia (so-called lobular carcinoma in situ) of the breast. Cancer. 1978;42(2):737–69.
4. Jacobs TW, et al. Carcinomas in situ of the breast with indeterminate features: role of E-cadherin staining in categorization. Am J Surg Pathol. 2001;25(2):229–36.
5. Maluf HM, Swanson PE, Koerner FC. Solid low-grade in situ carcinoma of the breast: role of associated lesions and E-cadherin in differential diagnosis. Am J Surg Pathol. 2001;25(2):237–44.
6. Page DL, et al. Atypical hyperplastic lesions of the female breast. A long-term follow-up study. Cancer. 1985;55(11):2698–708.
7. Wheeler JE, et al. Lobular carcinoma in situ of the breast. Long-term followup. Cancer. 1974;34(3):554–63.
8. Rosen PP, et al. Lobular carcinoma in situ of the breast. Detailed analysis of 99 patients with average follow-up of 24 years. Am J Surg Pathol. 1978;2(3):225–51.
9. Georgian-Smith D, Lawton TJ. Calcifications of lobular carcinoma in situ of the breast: radiologic-pathologic correlation. AJR Am J Roentgenol. 2001;176(5):1255–9.
10. Sneige N, et al. Clinical, histopathologic, and biologic features of pleomorphic lobular (ductal-lobular) carcinoma in situ of the breast: a report of 24 cases. Mod Pathol. 2002;15(10):1044–50.
11. Fadare O, et al. Lobular intraepithelial neoplasia [lobular carcinoma in situ] with comedo-type necrosis: a clinicopathologic study of 18 cases. Am J Surg Pathol. 2006;30(11):1445–53.
12. Schnitt SJ, Vincent-Salomon A. Columnar cell lesions of the breast. Adv Anat Pathol. 2003;10(3):113–24.
13. Moinfar F. Flat ductal intraepithelial neoplasia of the breast: a review of diagnostic criteria, differential diagnoses, molecular-genetic findings, and clinical relevance—it is time to appreciate the Azzopardi concept! Arch Pathol Lab Med. 2009;133(6):879–92.
14. Tavassoli FA, et al. Intraductal proliferative lesions. In: Tavassoli FA, Devilee P, editors. World Health Organization Classification of Tumor of the Breast and Female Genital Organs. Lyon: IARC; 2003. p. 63–75.
15. Lerwill MF. Flat epithelial atypia of the breast. Arch Pathol Lab Med. 2008;132(4):615–21.
16. Pinder SE, Ellis IO. The diagnosis and management of pre-invasive breast disease: ductal carcinoma in situ (DCIS) and atypical ductal hyperplasia (ADH)—current definitions and classification. Breast Cancer Res. 2003;5(5):254–7.
17. Page DL, Rogers LW. Combined histologic and cytologic criteria for the diagnosis of mammary atypical ductal hyperplasia. Hum Pathol. 1992;23(10):1095–7.
18. Simpson JF. Update on atypical epithelial hyperplasia and ductal carcinoma in situ. Pathology. 2009;41(1):36–9.
19. Tavassoli FA. Intraductal hyperplasias, ordinary and atypical. In: Tavassoli FA, editor. Pathology of the breast. Norwalk: Appleton & Lange; 1992. p. 155–91.
20. Rosai J. Borderline epithelial lesions of the breast. Am J Surg Pathol. 1991;15(3):209–21.
21. Page DL, et al. Subsequent breast carcinoma risk after biopsy with atypia in a breast papilloma. Cancer. 1996;78(2):258–66.
22. Collins LC, Schnitt SJ. Papillary lesions of the breast: selected diagnostic and management issues. Histopathology. 2008;52(1):20–9.
23. Harjit K, et al. Multiple papillomas of the breast: is current management adequate? Breast. 2006;15(6):777–81.
24. Lewis JT, et al. An analysis of breast cancer risk in women with single, multiple, and atypical papilloma. Am J Surg Pathol. 2006;30(6):665–72.
25. Page D, Anderson T. Radial scars and complex sclerosing lesions. In: Anderson T, editor. Diagnostic histopathology of the breast. Edinburgh: Churchill Livingston; 1987. p. 89–103.

# Management of High-Risk Lesions

# 5

Christine M. Gresik and Seema A. Khan

## Introduction

Although all women are at risk of breast cancer, a particularly high risk is associated with the presence of specific changes in the breast. These include epithelial atypia documented on breast biopsy [1, 2], and extremely dense breast tissue on mammography [3]. Today, these conditions are mainly discovered on imaging and documented with image-guided core needle biopsy. Knowledge of the appropriate management of women with high-risk breast lesions is essential to guide decisions regarding the need for surgical excision, intense surveillance, and preventive interventions, either medical or surgical. This chapter summarizes the risk of malignancy associated with specific high risk lesions as well as the appropriate surveillance and management of such lesions.

Epidemiologic studies over the last 25 years have provided information that allows the classification of benign breast lesions into three broad categories based on the associated breast cancer risk: nonproliferative change, proliferation without atypia, and atypical proliferation. The diagnostic frequency of these categories has changed over the last two decades, as the method of discovery has shifted from physical examination to ever more sensitive imaging techniques. Whereas the large cohort studies that have examined the risk of breast cancer associated with benign lesions have shown that atypical proliferations comprise about 3–4% of all benign biopsies [2, 4, 5], these included surgical biopsies in the pre-core biopsy era. Series of core needle biopsies suggest a higher frequency of atypical lesions, ranging from 5 [6, 7] to 14% [7, 8]. The number of atypical lesions diagnosed on core needle biopsy is therefore increasing, emphasizing the need for rational strategies of clinical management. The reported frequency of the main categories of benign breast lesions that confer increased risk of breast cancer in recent series is shown in Fig. 5.1. In this chapter, we will consider management strategies in three distinct areas: need for surgical excision; optimal surveillance; and preventive interventions.

C.M. Gresik, M.D. (✉)
Lynn Sage Comprehensive Breast Center, Feinberg School of Medicine of Northwestern University, 250 East Superior Street, Prentice 4-420, Chicago, IL 60611, USA
e-mail: cgresik@nmh.org

S.A. Khan, M.D.
Robert H. Lurie Comprehensive Cancer Center, Feinberg School of Medicine of Northwestern University, 303 East Superior Street, Lurie 4-111, Chicago, IL 60611, USA
e-mail: skhan@nmh.org

## Decision for Surgical Excision

The rationale for surgical excision following core biopsy diagnosis of a high-risk lesion is driven by the potential for underdiagnosis, related to the possibility of an adjacent coexisting carcinoma.

N.M. Hansen (ed.), *Management of the Patient at High Risk for Breast Cancer*, DOI 10.1007/978-1-4614-5891-3_5, © Springer Science+Business Media New York 2013

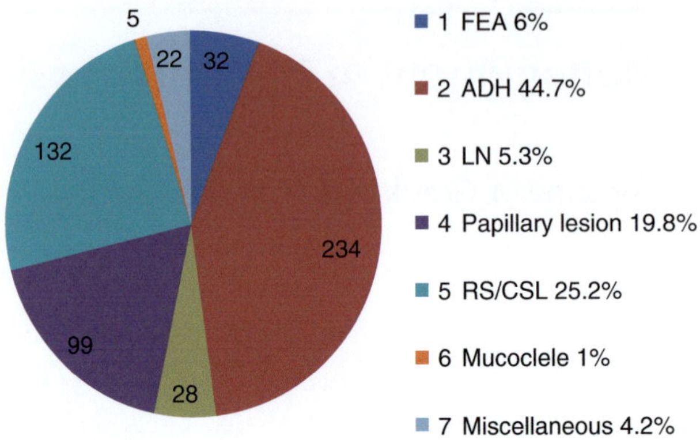


**Fig. 5.1** Frequency of high-risk lesion in 2.6 million screened women—*FEA* flat epithelial atypia, *ADH* atypical ductal hyperplesia (this includes atypical papilloma and ADH mixed with other lesions), *LN* lobular neoplasia (atypical lobular hyperplasia and lobular carcinoma in situ); papillary lesion (without atypia); mucocele-like lesions (Adapted from El-Sayed et al. Histopathology. 2008 53:650–57)

**Table 5.1** Upgrade rates of borderline lesions in a large series of core needle biopsies

| Lesion | *N* | % Excised | N upgraded | PPV % excision | PPV % excision + F/U |
|---|---|---|---|---|---|
| ADH | 141 | 55.3 | 63 | 44.7 | 40.6 |
| LN | 23 | 39.1 | 14 | 60.9 | 58.3 |
| Papillary lesion | 44 | 74.3 | 10 | 22.7 | 15.9 |
| Radial scar | 41 | 83.3 | 7 | 16.7 | 12.3 |
| Phyllodes tumor | 24 | 87.5 | 3 | 12.5 | 12.5 |
| NOS | 5 | 80 | 1 | 20 | 20.3 |
| All | 279 | 64.9 | 98 | 35.1 | 29.9 |

*ADH* atypical duct hyperplasia; *LIN* lobular neoplasia; *NOS* not otherwise specified; *PPV* positive predictive value; F/U follow-up minimum 6 months for masses and 12 months for calcifications (Adapted with permission, Houssami et al. Br J Cancer. 2007;96:1253–1257)

Thus the goal of surgical excision is to rule out the existence of overt malignancy in adjacent tissue and not necessarily to completely excise the entire focus of atypia, although this is often accomplished unless the radiological abnormality is large. Once coexistent malignancy has been excluded, the patient can then be counseled regarding future surveillance, life-style modification, and possible risk-reducing strategies such as chemoprevention.

Lesions for which surgical excision has been recommended are shown in Table 5.1, along with the rates of upgraded diagnosis described in various clinical series. There is a continuum in the risk of diagnostic upgrade for these lesions, ranging from close to 0 to 30% or more. They fall into roughly three groups, with radial scar and papilloma falling at the lower end, and atypical duct hyperplasia (ADH) at the high end. The position of lobular lesions varies according to whether or not they are separated into atypical lobular hyperplasia (ALH) and lobular carcinoma in situ (LCIS), or clumped together into lobular neoplasia (LN). The rationale for

**Table 5.2** Risk estimates of breast cancer based on class of benign breast lesion

| Author followed by ref. no | Relative risk for class of lesion (95% CI) | | | | | | |
|---|---|---|---|---|---|---|---|
| | NP | PDWA | AH/ADH | LN | Biopsy years | Number of women | Number of cases |
| Tamimi 2010 | 1.00 | 1.3 (0.9–1.8) | 3.5 (2.3–5.3) | NA | Pre-1995 | 2,005 | 365 |
| Kabat 2010 | 1.00 | 1.4 (1.1–1.9) | 2.7 (0.5–15.6) | 8.1 (0.9–71) | 1946–1994 | 1,239 | 665 |
| Hartmann 2005 | 1.3 (1.2–1.4) | 1.9 (1.7–2.1) | 4.2 (3.3–5.4) | NA | 1967–1991 | 1,907 | 707 |
| London 1997 | 1.00 | 1.7 (1.2–2.6) | 2.4 (1.3–4.5) | 5.3 (2.7–10.4) | Pre-1988 | 331 | 46 |
| McDivitt 1992 | 1.5 (1.3–1.9) | 1.8 (1.3–2.) | 2.6 (1.6–4.1) | NA | Pre-1990 | 694 | 433 |
| Carter 1988 | 1.5 | 1.9 | 3.0 | NA | Pre-1986 | 16,692 | 485 |
| Dupont 1985 | 1.5 (1.2–1.8) | 1.9 (1.2–2.9) | 5.3 (3.1–8.8) | NA | 1959–1968 | <5,234 | 134 |

*NP* non-proliferative, *PDWA* proliferation without atypia, *AH* atypical hyperplasia (when lobular lesions are not analyzed separately from ductal), *ADH* atypical ductal hyperplasia, *LN* atypical lobular lesions

considering the two together is based on the fact that the distinction between them is quantitative, not qualitative, and therefore a reliable distinction cannot be made based on core needle biopsy material. The upgrade rate for all lesion types also varies with the size of the imaging abnormality (larger lesions are more likely to be underdiagnosed) [9], and the size of the sampling needle (14 gauge cores are associated with higher rates of underdiagnosis) [10]. Although the upgrade rates in Table 5.2 appear higher than in smaller series dedicated to the analysis of specific types of borderline lesions [11, 12], the data are strengthened by the size of the series, and the fact that the entire range of atypical lesions is included, allowing one to get a sense of the relative potential for upgrading when these diagnoses are made on CNB. Additionally, the authors have included women who did not undergo excision, a source of bias in series that include only surgical cases.

Despite multiple attempts to identify features of CNB-diagnosed atypical lesions that would allow the selection of patients who do not require surgical excision, there are no validated criteria that define lesions with a low-enough risk of upgrade that excision can be reliably avoided. However, several studies have identified older age and volume of atypia (i.e., number of atypical foci) as being associated with higher risk of upgrade, in addition to the size of the radiological lesion. In general, older studies using 14 gauge core needles reported rates of upgrade of up to 50% [13–15]. More recent series of vacuum-assisted biopsy have suggested that complete excision of calcifications with vacuum-assisted CNB may allow management with observation alone [16], but this cannot be considered as a validated approach at the moment.

Overall, a consensus governs the need for surgical excision of ductal proliferations with atypia (ADH, papilloma, radial scar, columnar sclerosing lesion) with only a minority of patients with small lesions and complete CNB ablation being *tentatively* eligible for observation without excision. However, there remains ambiguity in the literature regarding the need for excision of lobular lesions, radial scar, and papilloma, particularly if the lesion is small, and has been ablated by CNB, with no residual radiological findings [17–19]. The quality and expertise of local radiology and pathology consultants should clearly guide individual practitioners in their recommendations to patients who may be eligible for observation alone.

## Risk of Future Breast Cancer

Several large cohort studies have defined the risk of breast cancer among women with a history of benign breast biopsy. The risk estimates associated with the three broad categories of lesions are shown in Table 5.3. The findings are fairly consistent in that nonproliferative BBD confers a relative risk of about 1.5 (or 1.0 if it is used as the reference category); proliferation without atypia carries a RR of about 2.0, and atypical hyperplasia is associated with a three- to fivefold increased risk of developing breast cancer. When authors have separated out ADH from lobular lesions, lobular neoplasia appears to carry a higher relative risk than ductal lesions, but this finding cannot be considered to be firm at the moment, given the small numbers in these studies [5, 20]. It is nevertheless a potentially important distinction, since lobular lesions are being detected with greater frequency given the increasing use of MRI, and the greater sensitivity of digital mammography, where they are now being seen as areas of abnormal enhancement and as microcalcifications, in contrast to the classical view that lobular neoplasia tends to be a purely incidental finding.

An emerging model of breast cancer evolution suggests that atypical epithelial proliferation is a risk marker for low-grade malignancy of both ductal and lobular types [21, 22]. This idea has been articulated based on studies of clonality of atypical epithelial lesions and related cancers, and on histological associations between these lesions. This concept is also supported by follow-up data on women with a history of benign breast biopsies, which suggest that subsequent cancers are largely estrogen receptor positive cancer.

**Table 5.3** American Cancer Society recommendations for breast MRI screening as an adjunct to mammography

| |
|---|
| Recommend annual MRI screening (based on evidence*) |
| *BRCA* mutation |
| First-degree relative of *BRCA* carrier, but untested |
| Lifetime risk ~20–25% or greater, as defined by BRCAPRO or other models that are largely dependent on family history |
| Recommend annual MRI screening (based on expert consensus opinion†) |
| Radiation to chest between age 10 and 30 years |
| Li–Fraumeni syndrome and first-degree relatives |
| Cowden and Bannayan–Riley–Ruvalcaba syndromes and first-degree relatives |
| Insufficient evidence to recommend for or against MRI screening‡ |
| Lifetime risk 15–20%, as defined by BRCAPRO or other models that are largely dependent on family history |
| Lobular carcinoma in situ (LCIS) or atypical lobular hyperplasia (ALH) |
| Atypical ductal hyperplasia (ADH) |
| Heterogeneously or extremely dense breast on mammography |
| Women with a personal history of breast cancer, including ductal carcinoma in situ (DCIS) |
| Recommend against MRI screening (based on expert consensus opinion) |
| Women at <15% lifetime risk |

*-1st set of recommendations based on peer reviewed published data
†-2nd set of recommendations based on consensus opinion
‡-3rd set–insufficient evidence to recommend or not recommend MRI

## Specific High-Risk Lesions

### Radial Scar

A radial scar is generally classified as a proliferative lesion, although it can be associated with foci of ADH. It is most commonly identified as an architectural distortion on mammography, with radiating spicules and central lucency which makes it difficult to distinguish from invasive carcinoma based on imaging alone. Excision is recommended unless the lesion is small and ablated by core biopsy; if atypia is present, excision should always be performed. The future risk associated with radial scar without atypia generally reflects that of PDWA [23, 24], although at least one study shows no significant impact of radial scar on breast cancer risk in the absence of atypia [25].

### Papillary Lesions

Papillomas consist of hyperplasic duct epithelium supported by a fibrovascular core of tissue which become friable, producing spontaneous bloody nipple discharge which prompts their clinical presentation [26]. When papillomas are focused peripherally near the terminal duct-lobular unit, they can often be multiple and are referred to as papillomatosis, and are more likely to present as radiological abnormalities. When associated with nipple discharge, ductography can be used to identify a filling defect in the system. Alternatively, ductoscopy may be used to identify the precise location of the lesion and resection will both confirm the diagnosis and alleviate the symptom. Asymptomatic, radiologically detected papillary lesions are associated with DCIS at rates ranging from 10 to 20% [27, 28]. When atypia is present however, the upgrade rate approximates that of ADH [27, 29]. For this reason, it is generally recommended that all papillary lesions identified via core biopsy should be surgically excised to rule out concomitant malignancy; although the need for excision of all papillomata diagnosed on NCB has been questioned recently [19], criteria for safe observation remain to be defined.

Central, solitary papilloma carries a modest increase in breast cancer risk, similar to that of proliferative disease; peripheral, particularly multiple papillomata are associated with an increased risk of subsequent breast cancer which directly correlates with the volume of atypia [30]. If no atypia is identified on final excisional pathology, no further immediate treatment is warranted. However, the finding of associated atypia should prompt the discussion of chemoprevention as a risk-reducing strategy and guide the need for future surveillance.

## Flat Epithelial Atypia

The optimal clinical management of this lesion, which was previously labeled "clinging" DCIS, remains unclear due to the variations in terminology used to describe these lesions and secondary to the limited number of cases that have been studied in a systematic fashion [31]. Flat epithelial atypias (FEA) are often seen in association with DCIS and with some types of invasive breast carcinoma, particularly tubular carcinoma [32, 33]. Upgrade rates for pure FEA in small series are either similar to ADH [33], or lower [34, 35]. In one recent series, none of 33 patients with a diagnosis of pure FEA on core biopsy were upgraded, compared to 3/10 cases when both FEA and ADH were present. This led the authors to conclude that when pure FEA is related to a small radiologic target, surgical excision is not necessary [34]. However, FEA is often admixed with ADH [36], in which case the behavior is similar to ADH. Breast cancer risk following a diagnosis of FEA is also somewhat uncertain again related to small numbers, but appears to be increased [37].

Thus it is likely that FEA represents an indolent, nonobligate precursor to low-grade ductal carcinoma [21]; studies with extended follow-up suggest an increased risk of subsequent cancer are needed to confirm the long-term risk in this group. Until these studies are completed, the standard management of a diagnosis of FEA on core biopsy is surgical excision. When FEA is found to be the dominant lesion in the excisional biopsy or is found to be present at the surgical margin, re-excision is not considered necessary since there is no evidence of a direct progression to carcinoma. Because of its intimate relationship with ADH in many patients, recommendation for chemoprophylaxis and optimal surveillance follows the same lines as ADH, until better data become available.

## Atypical Ductal Hyperplasia

ADH has been extensively studied with regard to the progression to malignancy and therefore its management is somewhat less controversial than that of other high-risk lesions. Surgical excision is universally recommended, since the upgrade rate is reliably 20% or higher [7]. With the widespread use of large-core needle biopsy however, there is emerging data that small lesions (under 6 mm) and less than three foci of ADH may identify a group of women who can be safely observed [38, 39]. However, as with other work in this field, these suggestions are based on retrospective analyses and need to be confirmed before they can be implemented in practice.

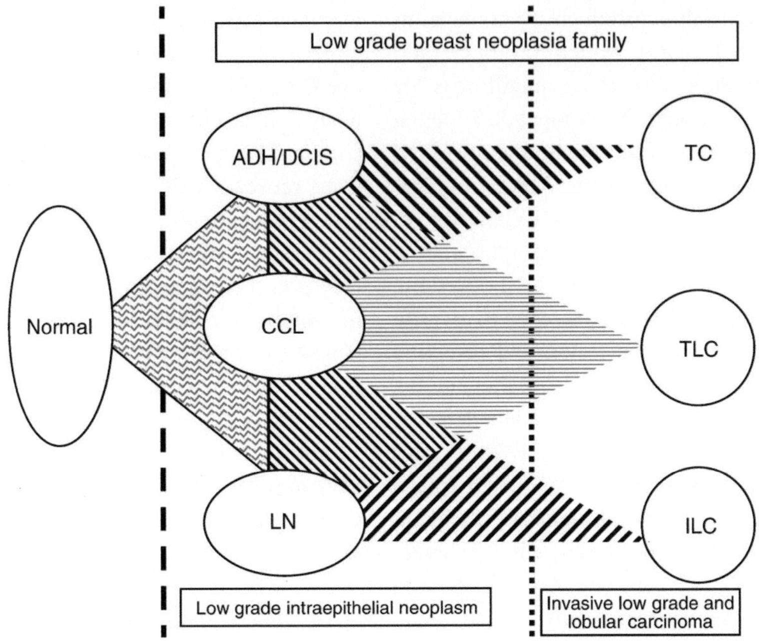


**Fig. 5.2** A schematic diagram to illustrate the evolutionary pathways of low-grade breast in situ and invasive neoplasia. *TC* tubular carcinoma, *TLC* tubulo-lobular carcinoma, *ILC* invasive lobular carcinoma (Reproduced with permission, Ian O Ellis. Mod Pathol. 2010;23)

The relative risk of subsequent cancer in women with ADH is increased from three- to fivefold, as shown in Table 5.3 [2, 5, 40]. The seminal study regarding the risk of subsequent malignancy associated with ADH was published from Vanderbilt University by Dupont and Page [4] who identified 377 atypical hyperplasias (3.6% of 10,542 biopsies); these consisted of ADH in 2.6% and ALH in 1.6% of women. With a mean follow-up of 17 years (range 1.4–24.3 years), 18/150 women with ADH subsequently developed invasive cancer. The relative risk of developing future breast cancer was 4.4-fold the general population, with an absolute risk of 10%. About half of these cancers occurred in the ipsilateral breast and the majority (14/18) developed within 10 years of the atypical biopsy. This theme of approximately fourfold increased risk and equal laterality of subsequent cancer is observed again in the more recent cohort study from the Mayo clinic [2], see Fig. 5.2. However, the waning of risk after 10 years has not been duplicated, and it is likely that risk remains elevated for decades.

The Vanderbilt data showed an interaction of atypical histology and the presence of a family history of breast cancer in a first degree relative, increasing the relative risk to ninefold the general population, and the absolute risk to 20% at 15 years [41]. However the findings from the subsequent, similarly sized cohort assembled at the Mayo Clinic did not show any interaction with family history [2]. Regardless of other features of the risk profile, women with a benign breast biopsy showing atypical hyperplasia should have their risk assessed using a statistical model. Most will meet criteria for counseling regarding risk-reducing medication, and a substantial proportion are willing to accept this (see discussion below of chemoprevention).

## Lobular Neoplasia

The collective term "lobular neoplasia" is commonly used to describe both ALH and LCIS, since the distinction between the two descriptors is quantitative rather than qualitative, with the main criterion being the fraction of the TDLU involved [42, 43]. In ALH, 50% of the lobules are filled with lobular neoplastic cells, while the entire lobule is filled with neoplastic cells in LCIS. Although LCIS appears to carry a higher risk for breast cancer than ALH in cohorts where surgical biopsy material is available [40, 44], their distinction in core biopsy material is less reliable in CNB samples, lending credence to the notion that lobular neoplasia is a more functional label [45]. Notably, the frequency of LCIS is rising, particularly among postmenopausal women [46]; although the reasons for this have not been defined, increased sensitivity of imaging techniques is almost certainly partially responsible.

For lobular neoplasia, as for other high-risk lesions, the first decision facing the clinician and patient is whether or not excision is required; the literature remains mixed in this regard. Even recent, large series show wide variation in the yield of malignant diagnoses upon surgical excision following CNB. These range from under 5% (3/68) for pure LN with concordant imaging [47] to 19% for ALH and 33% for LCIS in a series of 789 LN lesions [48]. Strikingly, series that start with a large denominator population of many thousands of women and drill down to the fraction with lobular neoplasia on CNB show the highest upgrade rates [7, 49, 50]. For example, Brem et al. started with a population of 32,420 core needle biopsies and found lobular neoplasia in 278 (0.9%), of which 164 (59%) continued to surgical excision, with pathological confirmation of cancer in 38 (23%) [50]. The upgrade rate was similar for lesions diagnosed as LCIS (25%, 17 of 67 lesions) vs. ALH (22%, 21 of 97 lesions). Upgrades were significantly more frequent when the lesion prompting CNB was a mass rather than microcalcifications, use of a core biopsy device rather than a vacuum device ($p<0.01$), and obtaining fewer specimens ($p<0.0001$). Thus although small, single institution series may show a low conversion rates for CNB-diagnosed lobular neoplasia, larger series drawn from a well-defined denominator population show consistently higher rates of upgrading. The key for safe observation appears to be (1) incidental finding of LN, (2) no residual radiographic lesion (3) absence of associated ADH or pleomorphic LCIS, and (4) meticulous attention to radiology–pathology correlation with a high level of expertise available in these two areas. If these conditions are met, close clinical follow-up can be considered, although the bulk of the evidence supports excisional biopsy.

With regard to breast cancer risk, ALH continues to be regarded somewhat separately from LCIS since the large cohorts have utilized older surgical biopsy data. The relative risk of breast cancer for patients with a diagnosis of ALH is similar to that of ADH in the Vanderbilt and Mayo cohorts, since these lesions were considered as one category [2, 4], with an approximate fourfold increase in risk. Subsequent, smaller studies that have separated LN from ADH show higher RR for LN, in the range of five- to eightfold [5, 20]. In an analysis of the Nurses' Health Study, stratification by menopausal status was possible, and it appears that ALH in premenopausal women has a significantly stronger association with breast cancer risk (OR=9.6; 95% CI, 3.3–27.8) than in postmenopausal women (OR=3.7; 95% CI, 1.3–10.2)[20].

The laterality of subsequent breast cancer in patients with ALH has been examined by Page et al. [51]. The overall relative risk of developing cancer was 3.1 (95% CI, 2.3–4.3, $P<0.0001$). Of the 252 women reviewed, 68% of 50 subsequent invasive cancers developed in the ipsilateral breast and 24% in the contralateral breast. An additional two women had subsequent bilateral cancer.

The breast cancer risk of LCIS is generally considered to be higher than that of ALH [44]; annual risk of breast cancer is often quoted as ~1% per year, although recent data from Memorial Sloan Kettering Cancer Center suggests a higher annual risk, in the region of 2–3% [52]. Subsequent invasive cancers have either ductal or lobular histology. The laterality distribution is similar to ALH, and like ALH, LCIS is considered to be an indicator of risk rather than a direct precursor to invasive disease [53], although that premise is questioned in the case of lesions with pleomorphic features, as discussed below.

Pleomorphic LCIS (PLCIS) is a recently described entity, characterized by discohesive,

central necrosis and calcifications, both of which are rarely seen with LCIS [54, 55]. The cellular features may make it difficult to distinguish from DCIS, but the hallmark of e-cadherin negativity is easily established with immunohistochemistry [55]. The upgrade rate for pleomorphic LCIS is higher than for the classic variety, and excision is recommended for conclusive diagnosis [17]. The treatment for PLCIS is similar to that of DCIS in the fact that complete excision with tumor-free margins is generally agreed-upon, but no consensus exists regarding the most appropriate treatment as long-term outcomes for this condition are not available. Likewise, the role of radiation therapy following lumpectomy for PLCIS is unclear due to lack of knowledge of the long-term behavior of PLCIS.

## High-Risk Lesions in BRCA Mutation Carriers

Studies comparing the prevalence of histopathologic lesions in prophylactic mastectomy (PM) specimens from women with *BRCA* mutations and in mastectomy specimens obtained at autopsy from an age- and race-matched comparison group without a known cancer predisposition suggest that high-risk lesions also precede cancer development in this population [56]. Kauff et al. compared the prevalence of benign, premalignant, and cancerous lesions from 24 cases and 48 comparison subjects. The results demonstrated an odds ratio of 12.7 (95% confidence interval, 3.1–52.4; $P<0.001$) for the detection of any high-risk lesion (DCIS, LCIS, ADH, or ALH) in specimens from the BRCA mutation group. This finding suggests that hereditary breast carcinoma does have a preinvasive phase that may be detectable with aggressive surveillance and that like sporadic breast carcinoma, *BRCA*-associated breast carcinoma arises from a stepwise, morphologically recognizable progression through atypical hyperplasia to carcinoma in situ and finally invasion. Notably, atypical lesions are as (or more) frequent in PM specimens of women with an autosomal dominant familial breast cancer pattern, but no BRCA mutation [57]. Since there is no information about the time-course of progression from high-risk lesion to cancer, it is not clear how useful information about the presence of high-risk lesions in mutation carriers would be for planning the timing of interventions such as risk-reducing mastectomy. This particular high-risk group clearly merits aggressive screening regardless of whether high-risk lesions are present or not.

## Surveillance

There is no consensus regarding intense surveillance of women at high risk of breast cancer because of biopsy-diagnosis of high-risk epithelial lesions. According to the American Cancer Society guidelines, there is insufficient data to recommend MRI surveillance for women with atypical hyperplasia or LCIS, a lifetime breast cancer probability of 15–20% (estimated using a model that relies largely on family history), or for women with extremely dense breasts [58]. Since these guidelines were published, several single-institution series of MRI surveillance in patients with LCIS have been published, showing an incremental detection of malignancy over that detected on mammography alone. In one such study of 670 MRI exams in 220 women, 14 cancers were found on MRI alone; six were DCIS, three were invasive malignancies that were ablated by the biopsy procedure (no residual cancer at surgery), and the remainder were invasive cancers, ranging in size from 5 mm to 1.3 cm [59]. Given the emerging concepts of high-risk lesions being indicators of low-grade, well-differentiated malignancy, there is a real concern that the cancers being detected at the cost of considerable expense (financial and emotional) may eventually be classified as "idle" cancers, with little if any impact on survival. An earlier study from the same institution which included 252 women with LCIS and 126 women with atypical hyperplasia showed that MRI screening generated more biopsies for a large proportion of patients, and facilitated detection of cancer in only a small highly selected group of patients with LCIS [60]. At the moment, the available evidence does not support the use of MRI surveillance for women with high-risk breast lesions, unless they meet the criterion of >20% lifetime risk estimated by a model that relies mainly on family history. The mainstay of screening following a diagnosis of a high-risk lesion remains annual mammography, although digital mammography appears to have advantages in young women and those with dense breasts [61].

## Prevention

Medical prevention is addressed in full in Chap. 8, but it is worth noting here that women with atypical hyperplasia and LCIS appeared to derive a particularly large benefit from tamoxifen therapy in the P-1 trial of the National Surgical Adjuvant Breast and Bowel Project (NSABP). A total of 6% of the total participants had LCIS and the trial demonstrated a risk reduction of 66% (RR 0.44, 95% CI 0.16–1.06) for this group. For women with atypical hyperplasia, the risk reduction was even greater, with an RR of 0.14 (95% CI 0.03–0.47) [62]. These estimates are not statistically significant because of the small number of breast cancer events in this subset of patients, but the direction is consistent between the two groups, and if pooled, would likely be statistically significant. Other tamoxifen trials did not address this specific issue.

The P-2 trial of the NSABP (Study of Tamoxifen and Raloxifene or STAR) succeeded the P-1 [63]. Eligibility criteria were generally similar to the P-1 trial, but entry was restricted to postmenopausal women because of the lack of safety data for raloxifene in premenopausal women. Of the 19,767 participants, almost 3,000 had a history of LCIS or atypical hyperplasia. The 8-year results of this trial show a slight disadvantage for raloxifene compared to tamoxifen, which was nonsignificant for women with a history of LCIS (RR 1.13, 95% CI 0.76–1.69), but was significant for those with a history of atypical hyperplasia (RR 1.48, 95% CI 1.06–2.09). Thus tamoxifen provides a larger benefit for women with high-risk lesions than for the larger population of high-risk women, and among hysterectomized postmenopausal women, may be superior to raloxifene.

More recently Goss et al. examined the use of the aromatase inhibitor exemestane for the primary prevention of breast cancer in high-risk women [64]. Of the 4,560 participants, 8% were known to have a history of LCIS, ADH, or ALH at entry. The risk reduction for the entire study population was seen as an RR of 0.35 (95% CI 0.18–0.70), whereas for women with prior high-risk lesions it was 0.36 (95% CI 0.11–1.12). Thus there does not appear to be a specifically better benefit for women with high-risk lesions, at least in this early report of this study, with a total of 43 breast cancer events so far.

Another aspect of the implementation of medical prevention strategies for breast cancer is the fact that women who have had a recent abnormal mammogram, followed by a breast biopsy with atypical findings, are more receptive to counseling regarding the use of drugs like tamoxifen [65]. It is therefore worthwhile to provide women with high-risk lesions information regarding the risk benefit balance of chemopreventive medication, and stress the possibly greater benefit that may accrue to them. The recent data suggesting an evolutionary path of epithelial atypia to low grade and (therefore estrogen receptor positive) malignancy [21, 22] further supports this strategy.

## Surgical Prevention

The most radical preventive measure for high-risk women is bilateral risk-reducing mastectomy (BRRM). Prospective long-term efficacy data on this procedure are scant, and the largest reported experience is a retrospective analysis from the Mayo Clinic [66]. The outcomes of 639 women were reported over a time period of 30 years following BRRM, comparing the women categorized into high and moderate risk of breast cancer to their sisters who did not undergo risk-reducing surgery. An overall 90% relative reduction in breast cancer incidence for women undergoing BRRM was observed, an absolute risk reduction of 16.1% for high-risk patients and 7.9% for moderate-risk patients. With regard to survival, an absolute risk reduction of 2.4–4% was identified. Hamm et al. further investigated the number of women needed to treat to prevent a breast cancer event or death related to breast cancer [67]. Though the findings were analyzed according to the patient's specific risk of breast cancer, overall conclusions were that most women without a documented BRCA mutation, despite increased personal risk of breast cancer, will derive no benefit from prophylactic surgery. Specifically, six high-risk women need to undergo prophylactic surgery to prevent one incident of cancer and 25 high-risk women need to undergo prophylactic surgery to prevent a death related to breast cancer. For women at moderate risk, 13 and 42 women respectively would need to undergo risk-reducing surgery to prevent an incident or death related to breast cancer.

When risk-reducing mastectomy is sought by women with a strong family history who have not undergone genetic testing, the first priority is to provide information and counseling, stressing the benefits of confirming the presence or absence of a mutation in the family. The most suitable family member to undergo testing should be identified (affected with cancer and young age at diagnosis), but if a surviving affected family member is not available, the patient seeking mastectomy may benefit from testing. Among women with high-risk lesions whose affected family members have tested negative, the risk for future breast cancer remains high, and BRRM may be considered if the estimated lifetime breast cancer risk approaches that of a BRCA mutation carrier (40–50%), although chemoprevention should be the first strategy offered. Among premenopausal women with a documented contraindication to tamoxifen (i.e., high risk for thromboembolisms) the rationale for BRRM may be stronger; for postmenopausal women, exemestane is now also an option. The age of the patient should also be considered; the benefit for BRRM is highest for BRCA mutation carriers when it is done at earlier ages [68], and although this has not specifically been addressed for women with high-risk lesions, the relationship of benefit to age is likely to be similar, with marginal if any benefit for women over 60 or so.

## Summary

High-risk lesions of the breast are most commonly detected on breast imaging, and diagnosed by core needle biopsy. The key management decisions relate to (1) need for surgical excision (required in most instances); (2) the need for intense surveillance (not backed by available data); (3) the need for chemoprevention (requires individual assessment, is often justified, but not often accepted); and (4) the need for risk-reducing surgery (not usually necessary or beneficial). Individual counseling and decision-making is the mainstay of rational management of this group of patients, and practitioners need to stay abreast of the rapidly evolving literature in this area.

## References

1. Page DL, Dupont WD, Rogers LW, Rados MS. Atypical hyperplastic lesions of the female breast. A long-term follow-up study. Cancer. 1985;55(11):2698–708.
2. Hartmann LC, Sellers TA, Frost MH, et al. Benign breast disease and the risk of breast cancer. N Engl J Med. 2005;353(3):229–37.
3. Boyd NF, Guo H, Martin LJ, et al. Mammographic density and the risk and detection of breast cancer. N Engl J Med. 2007;356(3):227–36.
4. Dupont WD, Page DL. Risk factors for breast cancer in women with proliferative breast disease. N Engl J Med. 1985;312(3):146–51.
5. Kabat GC, Jones JG, Olson N, et al. A multi-center prospective cohort study of benign breast disease and risk of subsequent breast cancer. Cancer Causes Control. 2010;21(6):821–8.
6. Jackman RJ, Nowels KW, Rodriguez-Soto J, et al. Stereotactic, automated, large-core needle biopsy of nonpalpable breast lesions: false-negative and histologic underestimation rates after long-term follow-up. Radiology. 1999;210(3):799–805.
7. Houssami N, Ciatto S, Bilous M, Vezzosi V, Bianchi S. Borderline breast core needle histology: predictive values for malignancy in lesions of uncertain malignant potential (B3). Br J Cancer. 2007;96(8):1253–7.
8. Eby PR, Ochsner JE, DeMartini WB, et al. Frequency and upgrade rates of atypical ductal hyperplasia diagnosed at stereotactic vacuum-assisted breast biopsy: 9-versus 11-gauge. AJR Am J Roentgenol. 2009;192(1):229–34.
9. Houssami N, Ciatto S, Ellis I, Ambrogetti D. Underestimation of malignancy of breast core-needle biopsy: concepts and precise overall and category-specific estimates. Cancer. 2007;109(3):487–95.

10. Ciatto S, Houssami N, Ambrogetti D, et al. Accuracy and underestimation of malignancy of breast core needle biopsy: the Florence experience of over 4000 consecutive biopsies. Breast Cancer Res Treat. 2007;101(3):291–7.
11. Nagi CS, O'Donnell JE, Tismenetsky M, Bleiweiss IJ, Jaffer SM. Lobular neoplasia on core needle biopsy does not require excision. Cancer. 2008;112(10):2152–8.
12. Kil WH, Cho EY, Kim JH, Nam SJ, Yang JH. Is surgical excision necessary in benign papillary lesions initially diagnosed at core biopsy? Breast. 2008;17(3):258–62.
13. Liberman L, Cohen MA, Dershaw DD, et al. Atypical ductal hyperplasia diagnosed at stereotaxic core biopsy of breast lesions: an indication for surgical biopsy. AJR Am J Roentgenol. 1995;164(5):1111–3.
14. Gadzala DE, Cederbom GJ, Bolton JS, et al. Appropriate management of atypical ductal hyperplasia diagnosed by stereotactic core needle breast biopsy. Ann Surg Oncol. 1997;4(4):283–6.
15. Ely KA, Carter BA, Jensen RA, Simpson JF, Page DL. Core biopsy of the breast with atypical ductal hyperplasia: a probabilistic approach to reporting. Am J Surg Pathol. 2001;25(8):1017–21.
16. Sneige N, Lim SC, Whitman GJ, et al. Atypical ductal hyperplasia diagnosis by directional vacuum-assisted stereotactic biopsy of breast microcalcifications. Considerations for surgical excision. Am J Clin Pathol. 2003;119(2):248–53.
17. Sullivan ME, Khan SA, Sullu Y, Schiller C, Susnik B. Lobular carcinoma in situ variants in breast cores: potential for misdiagnosis, upgrade rates at surgical excision, and practical implications. Arch Pathol Lab Med. 2010;134(7):1024–8.
18. Sohn VY, Causey MW, Steele SR, Keylock JB, Brown TA. The treatment of radial scars in the modern era—surgical excision is not required. Am Surg. 2010;76(5):522–5.
19. Carder PJ, Garvican J, Haigh I, Liston JC. Needle core biopsy can reliably distinguish between benign and malignant papillary lesions of the breast. Histopathology. 2005;46(3):320–7.
20. Marshall LM, Hunter DJ, Connolly JL, et al. Risk of breast cancer associated with atypical hyperplasia of lobular and ductal types. Cancer Epidemiol Biomarkers Prev. 1997;6(5):297–301.
21. Abdel-Fatah TM, Powe DG, Hodi Z, et al. High frequency of coexistence of columnar cell lesions, lobular neoplasia, and low grade ductal carcinoma in situ with invasive tubular carcinoma and invasive lobular carcinoma. Am J Surg Pathol. 2007;31(3):417–26.
22. Lopez-Garcia MA, Geyer FC, Lacroix-Triki M, Marchio C, Reis-Filho JS. Breast cancer precursors revisited: molecular features and progression pathways. Histopathology. 2010;57(2):171–92.
23. Jacobs TW, Byrne C, Colditz G, Connolly JL, Schnitt SJ. Radial scars in benign breast-biopsy specimens and the risk of breast cancer. N Engl J Med. 1999;340(6):430–6.
24. Sanders ME, Page DL, Simpson JF, et al. Interdependence of radial scar and proliferative disease with respect to invasive breast carcinoma risk in patients with benign breast biopsies. Cancer. 2006;106(7):1453–61.
25. Berg JC, Visscher DW, Vierkant RA, et al. Breast cancer risk in women with radial scars in benign breast biopsies. Breast Cancer Res Treat. 2008;108(2):167–74.
26. Ibarra JA. Papillary lesions of the breast. Breast J. 2006;12(3):237–51.
27. Rizzo M, Lund MJ, Oprea G, et al. Surgical follow-up and clinical presentation of 142 breast papillary lesions diagnosed by ultrasound-guided core-needle biopsy. Ann Surg Oncol. 2008;15(4):1040–7.
28. Skandarajah AR, Field L, Yuen Larn MA, et al. Benign papilloma on core biopsy requires surgical excision. Ann Surg Oncol. 2008;15(8):2272–7.
29. Hartman AB, Van De Verg LL, Venkatesan MM. Native and mutant forms of cholera toxin and heat-labile enterotoxin effectively enhance protective efficacy of live attenuated and heat-killed Shigella vaccines. Infect Immun. 1999;67(11):5841–7.
30. Lewis JT, Hartmann LC, Vierkant RA, et al. An analysis of breast cancer risk in women with single, multiple, and atypical papilloma. Am J Surg Pathol. 2006;30(6):665–72.
31. Schnitt SJ. The diagnosis and management of pre-invasive breast disease: flat epithelial atypia—classification, pathologic features and clinical significance. Breast Cancer Res. 2003;5(5):263–8.
32. Brogi E, Tan LK. Findings at excisional biopsy (EBX) performed after identification of columnar cell change (CCC) of ductal epithelium in breast core biopsy (CBX). Mod Pathol. 2002;15(1):29A–30.
33. Kunju LP, Kleer CG. Significance of flat epithelial atypia on mammotome core needle biopsy: should it be excised? Hum Pathol. 2007;38(1):35–41.
34. Piubello Q, Parisi A, Eccher A, et al. Flat epithelial atypia on core needle biopsy: which is the right management? Am J Surg Pathol. 2009;33(7):1078–84.
35. Peres A, Barranger E, Becette V, et al. Rates of upgrade to malignancy for 271 cases of flat epithelial atypia (FEA) diagnosed by breast core biopsy. Breast Cancer Res Treat. 2012;133(2):659–66.
36. Noske A, Pahl S, Fallenberg E, et al. Flat epithelial atypia is a common subtype of B3 breast lesions and is associated with noninvasive cancer but not with invasive cancer in final excision histology. Hum Pathol. 2010;41(4):522–7.
37. Martel M, Barron-Rodriguez P, Tolgay OI, Dotto J, Tavassoli FA. Flat DIN 1 (flat epithelial atypia) on core needle biopsy: 63 cases identified retrospectively among 1,751 core biopsies performed over an 8-year period (1992–1999). Virchows Arch. 2007;451(5):883–91.
38. Forgeard C, Benchaib M, Guerin N, et al. Is surgical biopsy mandatory in case of atypical ductal hyperplasia on 11-gauge core needle biopsy? A retrospective study of 300 patients. Am J Surg. 2008;196(3):339–45.
39. Kohr JR, Eby PR, Allison KH, et al. Risk of upgrade of atypical ductal hyperplasia after stereotactic breast biopsy: effects of number of foci and complete removal of calcifications. Radiology. 2010;255(3):723–30.

40. Dupont WD, Parl FF, Hartmann WH, et al. Breast cancer risk associated with proliferative breast disease and atypical hyperplasia. Cancer. 1993;71(4):1258–65.
41. Dupont WD, Page DL. Breast cancer risk associated with proliferative disease, age at first birth, and a family history of breast cancer. Am J Epidemiol. 1987;125(5):769–79.
42. Haagensen CD, Lane N, Lattes R, Bodian C. Lobular neoplasia (so-called lobular carcinoma in situ) of the breast. Cancer. 1978;42(2):737–69.
43. Koerner F, Maluf H. Uncommon morphologic patterns of lobular neoplasia. Ann Diagn Pathol. 1999;3(4):249–59.
44. Page DL, Kidd Jr TE, Dupont WD, Simpson JF, Rogers LW. Lobular neoplasia of the breast: higher risk for subsequent invasive cancer predicted by more extensive disease. Hum Pathol. 1991;22(12):1232–9.
45. Ibrahim N, Bessissow A, Lalonde L, et al. Surgical outcome of biopsy-proven lobular neoplasia: is there any difference between lobular carcinoma in situ and atypical lobular hyperplasia? AJR Am J Roentgenol. 2012;198(2):288–91.
46. Li CI, Anderson BO, Daling JR, Moe RE. Changing incidence of lobular carcinoma in situ of the breast. Breast Cancer Res Treat. 2002;75(3):259–68.
47. Rendi MH, Dintzis SM, Lehman CD, Calhoun KE, Allison KH. Lobular in-situ neoplasia on breast core needle biopsy: imaging indication and pathologic extent can identify which patients require excisional biopsy. Ann Surg Oncol. 2012;19(3):914–21.
48. Hussain M, Cunnick GH. Management of lobular carcinoma in-situ and atypical lobular hyperplasia of the breast—a review. Eur J Surg Oncol. 2011;37(4):279–89.
49. El-Sayed ME, Rakha EA, Reed J, et al. Predictive value of needle core biopsy diagnoses of lesions of uncertain malignant potential (B3) in abnormalities detected by mammographic screening. Histopathology. 2008;53(6):650–7.
50. Brem RF, Lechner MC, Jackman RJ, et al. Lobular neoplasia at percutaneous breast biopsy: variables associated with carcinoma at surgical excision. AJR Am J Roentgenol. 2008;190(3):637–41.
51. Page DL, Schuyler PA, Dupont WD, et al. Atypical lobular hyperplasia as a unilateral predictor of breast cancer risk: a retrospective cohort study. Lancet. 2003;361(9352):125–9.
52. Muhsen S, Morrogh M, Andrade V, et al. Risk for subsequent breast cancer after lobular carcinoma in situ—do clinical factors matter? J Clin Oncol. 2010;28:(abstr 1593).
53. Bodian CA, Perzin KH, Lattes R. Lobular neoplasia. Long term risk of breast cancer and relation to other factors. Cancer. 1996;78(5):1024–34.
54. Chivukula M, Haynik DM, Brufsky A, Carter G, Dabbs DJ. Pleomorphic lobular carcinoma in situ (PLCIS) on breast core needle biopsies: clinical significance and immunoprofile. Am J Surg Pathol. 2008;32(11):1721–6.
55. Chen YY, Hwang ES, Roy R, et al. Genetic and phenotypic characteristics of pleomorphic lobular carcinoma in situ of the breast. Am J Surg Pathol. 2009;33(11):1683–94.
56. Kauff ND, Brogi E, Scheuer L, et al. Epithelial lesions in prophylactic mastectomy specimens from women with BRCA mutations. Cancer. 2003;97(7):1601–8.
57. Hoogerbrugge N, Bult P, Bonenkamp JJ, et al. Numerous high-risk epithelial lesions in familial breast cancer. Eur J Cancer. 2006;42(15):2492–8.
58. Saslow D, Boetes C, Burke W, et al. American Cancer Society guidelines for breast screening with MRI as an adjunct to mammography. CA Cancer J Clin. 2007;57(2):75–89.
59. Sung JS, Malak SF, Bajaj P, et al. Screening breast MR imaging in women with a history of lobular carcinoma in situ. Radiology. 2011;261(2):414–20.
60. Port ER, Park A, Borgen PI, Morris E, Montgomery LL. Results of MRI screening for breast cancer in high-risk patients with LCIS and atypical hyperplasia. Ann Surg Oncol. 2007;14(3):1051–7.
61. Pisano ED, Gatsonis C, Hendrick E, et al. Diagnostic performance of digital versus film mammography for breast-cancer screening. N Engl J Med. 2005;353(17):1773–83.
62. Fisher B, Costantino JP, Wickerham DL, et al. Tamoxifen for prevention of breast cancer: report of the National Surgical Adjuvant Breast and Bowel Project P-1 study. J Natl Cancer Inst. 1998;90(18):1371–88.
63. Vogel VG, Costantino JP, Wickerham DL, et al. Update of the National Surgical Adjuvant Breast and Bowel Project Study of Tamoxifen and Raloxifene (STAR) P-2 Trial: preventing breast cancer. Cancer Prev Res (Phila). 2010;3(6):696–706.
64. Goss PE, Ingle JN, Ales-Martinez JE, et al. Exemestane for breast-cancer prevention in postmenopausal women. N Engl J Med. 2011;364(25):2381–91.
65. Tchou J, Hou N, Rademaker A, Jordan VC, Morrow M. Acceptance of tamoxifen chemoprevention by physicians and women at risk. Cancer. 2004;100(9):1800–6.
66. Hartmann LC, Schaid DJ, Woods JE, et al. Efficacy of bilateral prophylactic mastectomy in women with a family history of breast cancer. N Engl J Med. 1999;340(2):77–84.
67. Hamm RM, Lawler F, Scheid D. Prophylactic mastectomy in women with a high risk of breast cancer. N Engl J Med. 1999;340(23):1837–8.
68. Grann VR, Jacobson JS, Thomason D, et al. Effect of prevention strategies on survival and quality-adjusted survival of women with BRCA1/2 mutations: an updated decision analysis. J Clin Oncol. 2002;20(10):2520–9.

# Radiological Imaging for the High-Risk Patient

6

Erin Neuschler and Paula Grabler

## Introduction

In this chapter we will discuss the appropriate imaging techniques for women at high risk for breast cancer as well as accepted timelines for imaging. Mammography is the only imaging technique that has been proven to decrease breast cancer mortality as a screening modality. Given the limitations of mammography, other imaging techniques are recommended for the woman at high risk. We will discuss the utility of ultrasound and magnetic resonance imaging (MRI) as additional screening modalities. In addition emerging breast imaging technologies will be reviewed.

## Mammography

The American Cancer Society (ACS), American Medical Association (AMA), and the American College of Radiology (ACR) recommend annual screening mammography for women beginning at the age of 40 [1–3]. Mammography is considered the standard of care in the early detection of breast cancer, before it is symptomatic, with a sensitivity of 77–95% and a specificity of 94–97% [4]. Randomized controlled trials have demonstrated a significant reduction in breast cancer mortality with the widespread use of screening mammography [5–11]. Meta-analyses of the data from multiple, international, randomized controlled trials have reported an approximately 30% reduction in mortality for women between the ages of 50 and 74 [12, 13]. Research conducted in two Swedish counties, comparing deaths from breast cancer diagnosed 20 years before the introduction of screening to deaths during the 20 years after the introduction of screening, demonstrated a significant reduction in breast cancer mortality for women 40 years of age and older [14]. Controversies regarding the benefits of screening for women in their forties have existed for many years with more recent arguments against screening for younger women proposed by the United States Preventive Services Task Force [15]. Given the significant limitations of their analyses, the ACS, AMA, and ACR have stood by their recommendation for annual screening mammography for women beginning at the age of 40.

While research supports these recommendations for women in general, the appropriateness of these recommendations for women who are at higher risk for developing breast cancer have been called into question, especially given that this cohort may develop the disease at a younger age. The ACR recommends beginning screening

E. Neuschler, M.D. (✉)
Department of Breast Imaging, Northwestern Memorial Hospital, 250 East Superior Street, Room 4-2304, Chicago, IL 60611, USA
e-mail: eneuschl@nmff.org

P. Grabler, M.D.
Department of Radiology, Northwestern Memorial Hospital, 250 East Superior Street, Room 4-2304, Chicago, IL 60611, USA
e-mail: Paula.Grabler@nmff.org

N.M. Hansen (ed.), *Management of the Patient at High Risk for Breast Cancer*,
DOI 10.1007/978-1-4614-5891-3_6, © Springer Science+Business Media New York 2013

mammography by the age of 30 but not before the age of 25 for women at highest risk of developing breast cancer [16]. Consequently, the ACS and the National Comprehensive Cancer Network have proposed screening mammography beginning prior to the age of 40 for women at highest risk for breast cancer [17, 18].

This select population of the highest risk patients according to the ACS and NCCN includes: (1) Women who are positive for the BRCA 1 and 2 gene mutation for whom annual screening mammography beginning at the age of 25 is recommended. (2) Women with a strong family history of breast cancer including a mother or sister diagnosed with premenopausal breast cancer or two or more first degree relatives diagnosed with breast or ovarian cancer for whom early mammography beginning 5–10 years prior to the youngest breast cancer case is recommended. (3) Women with a history of mantle field radiation between the ages of 10 and 30 for whom early mammography 8–10 years after radiation treatment, but not before age 25, is recommended. (4) Women with TP53 or PTEN gene mutations (Li-Fraumeni, Cowden, and Bannayan–Riley–Ruvalcaba syndromes) for whom yearly mammography beginning at the age of 30 is recommended. (5) Women between 35 and 40 years of age with a 5-year risk of invasive breast cancer 1.7% or higher for whom annual screening mammography is recommended. (6) Women with an average lifetime risk of invasive breast cancer greater than 20% for whom annual screening mammography beginning at the age of 30 is recommended. (7) Women who have been diagnosed with breast cancer and treated with lumpectomy or mastectomy for whom annual mammography at a minimum, regardless of age, is recommended [17, 18]. Women diagnosed with breast cancer have a 2–15% lifetime risk of developing a metachronous breast cancer and 0.5–1.5% risk for recurrence per year within the first 5 years; in these latter cases, recurrence is typically near the lumpectomy site [19]. Significant differences in the 5-year rates for local recurrence have been reported from 7% for Stage I breast cancer as compared to 13% for Stage III [20].

Regarding breast cancer patients treated with conservation therapy, recommendations for the schedule of mammographic imaging of the treated breast vary. Annual mammography for the contralateral breast is always recommended, regardless of the imaging timeline for the treated breast. Practice guidelines for patients diagnosed with DCIS as well as invasive cancer presenting with calcifications advise a postoperative mammogram to document complete removal of the calcifications, unless complete excision of calcifications is clearly documented on the specimen radiograph. Magnification views with compression in addition to the routine images are used for optimal evaluation of the postoperative lumpectomy site for disease recurrence manifesting as calcifications or new masses [21, 22]. For all breast cancer patients treated with lumpectomy, mammography of the treated breast is recommended 6–12 months following surgery with at least annual mammography thereafter [21–23]. Studies have questioned, however, the need for the postoperative mammography and 6-month follow-up [24–26], especially in light of the fact that the median time to present with a recurrence is greater than 2 years after surgery [27].

Since mammography utilizes X-rays to create images, beginning mammography at an earlier age in women with a genetic or familial predisposition to breast cancer is not without risk [28]. An analysis of 5 studies which examined the effects of low-dose radiation on breast cancer risk was conducted with 4 of the studies focusing on mutation carriers and 1 study focusing on women with family histories of breast cancer. These studies demonstrated an approximately 1.5 times increased risk for radiation-induced breast cancer in both of these groups, suggesting a greater susceptibility to DNA-damaging ionizing radiation in these specific patient populations. Increased risk was especially prevalent in those who began mammography prior to the age of 20 or who underwent five or more exposures at an early age [29]. Consequently, the earliest age that mammography is recommended is 25.

Additional screening modalities other than mammography have been proposed, not only because of the minimum age at which mammography is

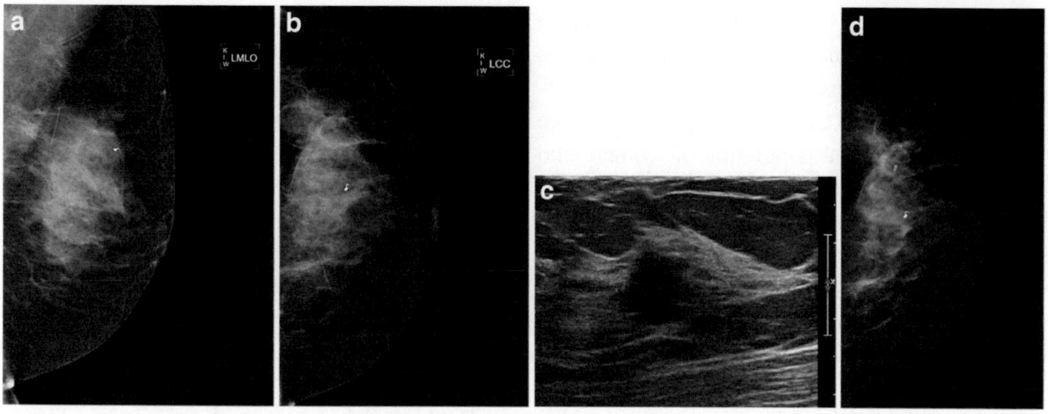

**Fig. 6.1** (**a, b**) Annual left mammogram (MLO and CC views) for a 34-year-old BRCA1 positive woman who has a history of a right mastectomy approximately 2 years prior. Her right breast cancer pathology was invasive ductal carcinoma grade 3 with metastatic involvement of a single right axillary lymph node. The coil-shaped marking clip in the upper central left breast marks the site of a prior benign MR biopsy. The mammogram demonstrates heterogeneously dense breast tissue without a dominant mass or suspicious microcalcifications. (**c**) Ultrasound of the left breast was performed with a 17-5 MHz transducer. There is a 1.3 cm irregular, hypoechoic mass which is located at the 1:30 position, 5 cm from the nipple. This mass is not oriented parallel to the skin surface. (**d**) Ultrasound-guided core needle biopsy was performed of the irregular mass in the left breast. Post-biopsy left mammogram in the CC projection demonstrates the new wing-shaped biopsy marking clip in the outer breast. The pathology demonstrated infiltrating ductal carcinoma grade 2. Given negative MR imaging performed 6 months prior, this represents an interval cancer

recommended and the associated radiation risks, but also because of the inherent limitations of mammography in detecting breast cancer. Reports from screening programs involving women at increased familial risk have indicated a greater number of interval breast cancers (i.e., those diagnosed between screening intervals), cancers which are larger in size, as well as a greater number of cancers which are associated with axillary lymph node involvement. This is especially true in women with dense breasts [30, 31] (Fig. 6.1a–d).

Fifty percent of women less than 50 years of age are considered to have dense breasts. By definition, these breasts are composed of 50% or greater fibroglandular tissue and may obscure detection of small breast lesions, particularly in mammography. Complicating matters further is that dense tissue itself has been shown to increase the risk for breast cancer. Cancers which are clinically detected between screening intervals have a worse prognosis and occur with significantly greater frequency in dense breasts, particularly those with 75% or greater fibroglandular tissue. Extremely dense breasts combined with a non-homogeneous parenchymal pattern are considered the most problematic [32, 33].

In women with dense breasts as well as the overlapping demographic groups of women under the age of 50 and those that are premenopausal, Pisano et al. [34] reported increased effectiveness of digital mammography in detecting breast cancer over analog technology. Overall, the sensitivity of digital mammography in patients with dense breasts is higher than that of film-screen mammography, measuring 70% and 55%, respectively [34].

Specific features of breast cancers have been seen in women with high familial risk [35, 36]. Breast cancers in BRCA1 carriers tend to be high grade, estrogen negative, and invasive cancers which exhibit fast growth rates. The mammographic features are more frequently associated with benign lesions (oval shape with smooth margins which appear to be pushing adjacent parenchymal tissue rather than demonstrating an infiltrative appearance). In addition, these cancers are less frequently associated with calcifications. In contrast, cancers in BRCA2 carriers are more frequently associated with calcifications with many (approximately 1/3) diagnosed as DCIS. In addition, these patients also have cancers presenting as spiculated masses, a finding which is different than their BRCA1 counterparts and more similar to the general population of women who develop breast cancer [37–39].

High-risk women presenting for screening with no clinical complaints obtain a 2 view mammogram of each breast with either digital or film screen technology. Two images of each breast are obtained on routine screening mammography with a mean dose of 6.5 mGy [40]. Images are obtained in the mediolateral oblique projection which enables superior and inferior localization as well as the craniocaudal projection which enables medial and lateral localization of lesions. Analysis of the mammogram includes an assessment of the density of the breasts (almost entirely fat, scattered fibroglandular, heterogeneously dense, and extremely dense) as well as an evaluation for possible lesions (masses, asymmetries, architectural distortion, calcifications, and skin thickening) [41]. Characteristics of the lesions are analyzed to assess the level of suspicion. Having prior mammograms to compare is particularly helpful in evaluating more benign appearing lesions, as the need for additional imaging or biopsy may be obviated if stability over multiple examinations is established. Screening mammograms are typically read in batches following the patient's departure and a letter is sent to the patient with the results within 30 days of the exam, the latter of which is a requirement outlined in the US FDA Mammography Quality Standards Act (MQSA) [42].

Characteristics of benign appearing lesions include masses with circumscribed margins, stable parenchymal asymmetries, and round calcifications. A small percentage of circumscribed masses may represent malignancies that can demonstrate aggressive behavior and high-grade histology. As mentioned previously, this is particularly true for the high-risk patient. Therefore, unless stability is established, biopsy may be required. Characteristics of suspicious lesions include non-circumscribed margins (spiculated, microlobulated, indistinct, obscured) and calcifications which are clustered, pleomorphic, and/or in a linear or segmental in distribution [41]. Architectural distortion is also a suspicious finding unless due to prior surgery or a benign etiology such as a radial scar.

Mammographic interpretation is given a code based upon the ACR Breast Imaging Reporting and Data System, or BI-RADS. The coding is 1: Normal, 2: Benign, 3: Probably benign with short interval follow-up recommended, 4: Suspicious with biopsy recommended, 5: Highly suspicious with appropriate action advised, and 0: Additional imaging required or comparison to prior mammograms [41].

For high-risk women with a clinical finding or who have a history of a prior breast malignancy, diagnostic mammography is typically performed. This may include routine screening images as well as additional diagnostic mammographic views and possible ultrasound as needed. These examinations are supervised by the radiologist.

## Ultrasound

In most breast imaging practices, ultrasound is predominantly used as an adjunct to mammography, primarily for problem-solving after an initial mammogram as well as for the evaluation of palpable findings. In addition, ultrasound is also used as the imaging modality for initial evaluation of palpable abnormalities in women under the age of 30 as well as in women who are pregnant or breastfeeding. Ultrasound is unique in that it uses sound waves to create images, rather than using potentially harmful ionizing radiation. While high frequency transducers are favored for imaging of small, superficial structures, they are limited by their depth of penetration. For this reason, broad bandwidth linear transducers are now available which provide frequencies between 5 and 17 MHz, providing the necessary tools for imaging lesions of varying sizes as well as at a variety of tissue depths [43].

The usefulness of screening ultrasound as a screening methodology has been supported by numerous studies. Berg [44] reviewed six single-center studies which included a total of 42,838 screening ultrasounds. In these studies, 126 women (0.29%) were shown to have 150 cancers which were identified only with supplemental ultrasound. Of these cancers, 141 were invasive and 99 were smaller than 1 cm in size. These studies also demonstrated that the benefit of additional screening sonography was increased with increasing breast density, as 114 of the 126 (90.5%) women with cancers detected on screening sonography had either heterogeneously dense or extremely dense parenchyma [44].

The ACRIN (American College of Radiology Imaging Network) 6666 trial was a multicenter study that compared screening mammography vs. screening mammography plus ultrasound for the detection of breast cancer in high-risk women and those with dense breasts. In this study, radiologists interpreted either the mammographic or sonographic images and were blinded to the results of the other imaging modality. The ACRIN 6666 trial is the largest randomized study of screening ultrasound in which mammography and sonography were performed and interpreted independently. To be eligible for the ACRIN trial, a woman needed to have either heterogeneously dense tissue or extremely dense breast tissue in at least one quadrant. Women with BRCA-1 or BRCA-2 mutations as well as a personal history of breast cancer were included (with the study addressing imaging of the non-affected breast). Women with prior biopsies of lobular carcinoma in situ (LCIS), atypical ductal hyperplasia (ADH), atypical lobular hyperplasia (ALH), or atypical papillary lesion were included if not on chemoprevention. If on chemoprevention, only women with a family history of breast cancer in a relative under 50 were included. Women over 30 years of age treated with prior chest, mediastinal, or axillary irradiation at least 8 years previously also met inclusion criteria. Women with a personal lifetime risk of breast cancer of at least 25%, as defined by either the Gail or Claus models, were included in the study, as were those women with specific 5-year risks based upon the Gail model and density of breast tissue [45].

With 2,705 women recruited for the study, the ACRIN study determined that adding a single screening ultrasound to mammography increased the number of detected cancers from 7.6 to 11.8 per 1,000 women. Of 12 cancers that were detected by screening sonography alone, 11 (92%) were invasive, with a median size of only 10 mm. Eight of nine cancers (89%) had negative lymph nodes. Only 12 out of 136 lesions recommended for biopsy based upon ultrasound review were malignant, equating to a 8.8% positive predictive value. This positive predictive value is low compared with the ACR guidelines of 25–40% for mammography [45].

Berg [46] compiled all of the six single-center studies, the ACRIN trial, and two multicenter Italian studies, and reported that nearly all of the screening ultrasound detected cancers were invasive, but more importantly, most were node negative. The median size of the cancers measured between 9 and 11 mm. In these studies, additional cancers detected with ultrasound alone ranged from 2.7 to 4.6 per 1,000 women [46].

As would be expected, ultrasound is more sensitive for detection of invasive cancers rather than for DCIS, as DCIS is more frequently associated with calcifications and less frequently associated with a soft tissue mass. In the ACRIN study, of the 12 cancers detected only by screening ultrasound, only one cancer was DCIS [45]. In a surveillance study of BRCA carriers with MRI, ultrasound, mammography, and clinical breast examination by Warner et al. [47], a retrospective analysis of the DCIS cases was performed. Zero of 12 DCIS cases were detected by ultrasound. Only two of these cancers were not identified by MRI [47].

In the ACRIN trial, the median time to perform screening breast ultrasound was 19 min for a bilateral ultrasound [45]. The length of time of a typical ultrasound exam is a limitation, particularly in the United States where there is a shortage of breast imaging radiologists. Automated whole breast ultrasound systems (AWBU) have been developed in the hopes of expediting screening breast ultrasound. AWBU uses a computer-guided mechanical arm to acquire images of the breast under the control of a physician or technologist to maintain appropriate orientation and contact of the transducer to the skin. The result is a cine-loop of images simulating real-time imaging which are reviewed at a computer workstation [48]. In a study by Kelly et al., radiologists reviewing screening mammograms, with and without ABWU, were blinded to the diagnosis (whether benign or malignant) in women whose mammograms demonstrated heterogeneously dense or extremely dense parenchyma. This study demonstrated decreased call back rates in dense-breasted women and increased breast cancer detection accuracy [49].

While screening breast ultrasound has been shown to be effective in increasing cancer detection rate when combined with mammography, studies have shown that MRI is superior to ultrasound in cancer detection, particularly in known or suspected BRCA gene mutation carriers [50–53]. In a recent study by Sardenelli et al. [53], 501 high-risk women were screened with all three modalities. In this study, 52 cancers were detected, 49 of which were detected by screening exams and 3 of which were detected clinically in between screening exams. The 91% sensitivity of MRI in this study was much higher than that of mammography or ultrasound, which measured 50% and 52%, respectively [53]. These studies demonstrate that MRI is a critical screening test for high-risk women and should be combined with mammography rather than screening ultrasound and mammography alone. If a high-risk woman chooses not to undergo MRI, then sonography could be utilized as the next screening test of choice. In women with dense breasts, who are at intermediate risk and therefore not typically scheduled for screening MRI examinations, screening sonography could be helpful. As will be discussed in the next section of this chapter, targeted ultrasound can be useful as an adjunct for better characterization and localization of lesions identified on MRI.

The BI-RADS reporting system is used to describe lesions identified by breast ultrasound. The lexicon is based upon a feature analytic approach which emphasizes shape (oval, round, irregular), orientation (parallel or not parallel to the skin), and margin (circumscribed or not circumscribed). Characteristics of typically benign appearing lesions, such as cysts and fibroadenomas, include oval or round masses which are parallel in orientation with circumscribed margins. Characteristics of suspicious lesions are masses which are irregular, not parallel in orientation, and not circumscribed (indistinct, angular, microlobulated, and spiculated) [54].

Ultrasound imaging features may be different in cancers in high-risk patients, similar to that seen with mammography. A prospective study performed by Schrading and Kuhl [39] looked at the imaging phenotypes of breast cancer in high-risk women, BRCA gene mutation carriers, and women at high and moderate risk based upon family history. The imaging phenotypes as well as location of the lesions within the breast were examined. Two-thirds of breast cancers seen in BRCA1 carriers and women deemed to be high risk by family history were found to be in the posterior third of the breast, usually just superficial to the pectoralis muscle. In moderate risk women, cancers were evenly distributed within the anterior, middle, and posterior thirds of the breast. Out of 64 invasive cancers, 15 demonstrated a "fibroadenoma-like" appearance, with oval or round shape as well as smooth or pushing margins. Of the 15 cancers with this appearance, 13 were known or suspected gene mutation carriers [39].

Schrading and Kuhl [39] discuss potential reasons for circumscribed cancers to be present in high-risk women. It has been shown that hereditary breast cancer demonstrates a medullary (or atypical medullar) differentiation, which is associated with pushing margins [35]. In addition, it has been shown that breast cancers in women with familial risk are usually of higher nuclear grade, which may present on mammography and sonography as circumscribed lesions [55]. This is in contrast to intermediate- and low-grade tumors which are more likely to have spiculated borders due to a desmoplastic response which is incited in the surrounding tissue [56]. In the study by Schrading and Kuhl, 13 of the 15 cancers that were high grade demonstrated benign morphologic features. Therefore, when imaging high-risk women, it is important to recognize that malignant lesions can demonstrate benign morphologic features [39] (Fig. 6.2a–e).

## Magnetic Resonance Imaging

As discussed in the "Ultrasound" section, MRI is integral in screening the high-risk patient, both because of the increased sensitivity for detecting cancers as well as because of the lack ionizing

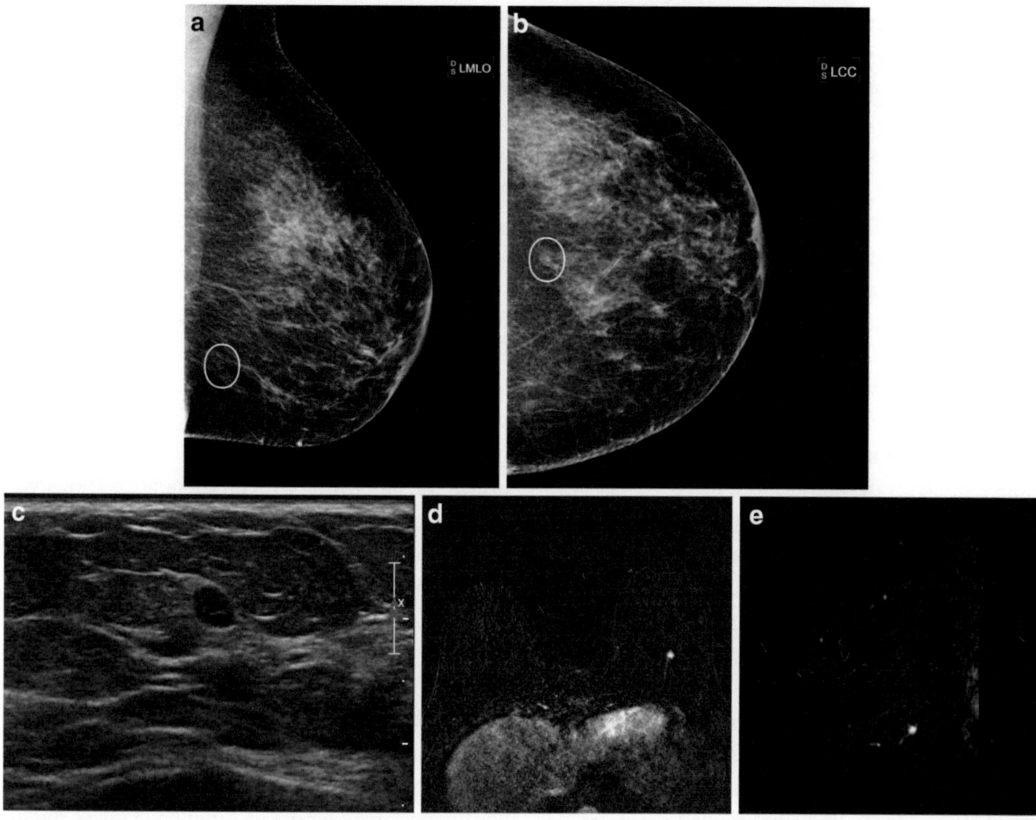


**Fig. 6.2** (**a**, **b**) Annual left mammogram for a 42-year-old woman with a history of a right mastectomy 3 years prior for infiltrating ductal carcinoma grade 3. She has a family history of breast cancer in her sister and grandmother, both premenopausal at diagnosis. MLO and CC views demonstrate a new circumscribed mass in the lower central left breast. (**c**) Targeted left breast ultrasound with a 17-5 MHz transducer demonstrates an oval, circumscribed, and hypoechoic mass which is oriented parallel to the skin surface. The mass is located at the 6 o'clock position, 5 cm from the nipple and measured 0.4 cm. This lesion corresponds to the mammographic mass. (**d**) Bilateral axial contrast-enhanced MR subtraction image and (**e**) sagittal multiplanar reformat subtraction image of the left breast demonstrate an enhancing, circumscribed mass at the 6 o'clock location which corresponds with the mammographic and sonographic findings. Kinetic analysis of the enhancing mass demonstrates washout kinetics. Ultrasound-guided core needle biopsy was performed demonstrating invasive ductal carcinoma grade 3. This is an example of a circumscribed cancer

radiation. MRI is a technology which utilizes a high strength magnet to align the nuclear spins of hydrogen atoms throughout the body. By applying radiofrequency pulses, these aligned spins can be "excited" into higher energy states which will ultimately release radiofrequency energy that is detected by an antenna and is used to create the final images that are interpreted on the PACS viewing station. Since the late 1980s, breast MRI has utilized gadolinium-based intravenous contrast [57, 58]. Detection of breast cancer with gadolinium hinges upon the concept of tumor neovascularity, with the assumption that a neoplastic process will enhance to a greater degree than the surrounding breast parenchyma. Due to hormonal variations in background parenchymal enhancement, breast MRI should be done in the second week of the menstrual cycle [59]. Due to the own inherent risk profile of gadolinium agents, MRI contrast should be avoided in the setting of renal insufficiency as well as pregnancy.

The ACR has issued technical guidelines for MRI. These include a dedicated breast coil and imaging with at least 1.5 T field strength. Some of the other requirements include requirements for slice thickness as well as timing of the post-contrast images. Institutions performing breast MRI should be able to perform MRI-guided biopsies as well as MRI-guided needle localizations. A radiologist interpreting MRI images should have expertise in breast imaging and should work in concert with high-risk clinicians who specialize in risk assessment for breast cancer, to ensure appropriate utilization of the modality [60]. This partnership allows for effective communication of results as well as appropriate follow-up and treatment. It is encouraged that radiologists audit their interpretations so that call-back rates can be assessed as well as biopsy statistics [61].

Similar to mammography and ultrasound, BI-RADS for MRI lesions is based upon a feature analytic approach. The lexicon utilizes categorical descriptors, with the goal being to select the terms from each category which best describes the overarching feature of a particular lesion. The lesion types include focus/foci (area of enhancement less than 5 mm), mass, and nonmasslike enhancement (area of enhancement that does not fit criteria for a mass). For a mass, the important descriptors are shape (oval, round, lobulated), margin (smooth, irregular, spiculated), and the internal enhancement of the mass (homogeneous, heterogeneous, rim-enhancement, dark internal septations, enhanced internal septations, and central enhancement). For non-masslike enhancement the descriptors are based upon the distribution of the enhancement [62].

In addition to morphology, evaluation of MRI lesions is based upon kinetic analysis. This is determined by the perfusion and diffusion of intravenous contrast from vessels into the extracellular space over time. The BI-RADS for MRI describes these kinetic curves and their importance in differentiating benign from malignant lesions was shown by Kuhl et al. in 1999 [62, 63]. The initial portion of the kinetic curve describes percentage of wash-in of contrast into the lesion which is characterized as slow, medium, or rapid. The delayed phase of enhancement is characterized as either persistent, plateau, or washout. A Type 1, or persistent curve, is seen when there is continued increase in contrast signal over time. These kinetics are usually associated with benign lesions. A Type II, plateau curve, is seen when there is no increase in signal over time after initial wash-in. Lastly, a Type III, washout curve, is seen when there is a decrease in signal after an initial wash-in. Type 1 curves are typically associated with benign processes. Type II and III curves have been shown to have a high positive predictive value for malignancy, measuring 77% [63]. Tumor neovascularity results in rapid uptake of contrast, and, in many cancers, results in early washout of contrast. These findings create a type III enhancement curve [64].

Assessment of lesions is based upon a combination of morphology and kinetics, with morphology being the most important factor. Kinetics are useful for supporting a recommendation; however, morphology should be the basis of the recommendation. As with mammography and ultrasound, a mass with a spiculated margin is suspicious regardless of its kinetic curve. Similarly, an oval mass is more likely to be benign. If a mass has an oval shape, circumscribed margin, is bright on T2 weighted sequence (a fluid sensitive sequence), and has a low-signal non-enhancing internal septation, this lesion may be considered benign. with confidence irrespective of kinetics. This is due to the high negative predictive value of a low-signal, non-enhancing septation [65]. The assessment of whether an enhancing focus is felt to be benign or suspicious depends upon the background enhancement within both breasts. In the high-risk patient, a solitary asymmetric focus with suspicious kinetics would be suspicious for a tiny cancer. For non-mass enhancement the descriptors are based upon the distribution of the enhancement, it is the distribution that is the most important feature, with kinetics playing little if any role in the recommendation for biopsy. A focal area of enhancement, which is an area of enhancement less than 25% of a quadrant, is the least suspicious, followed by linear enhancement, which is enhancement which is not in a ductal distribution. Ductal and segmental enhancement are more likely to be associated with ductal carcinoma in situ or invasive cancer. Regional and diffuse enhancement are larger areas of enhancement with the latter usually seen in the setting of background parenchymal enhancement and felt to be benign [64].

The ACS is specific in their recommendations regarding breast MRI, which are based upon clinical trials assessing breast MRI in high-risk women [66]. The ACR endorses these recommendations. The first of these published trials was by Kuhl et al. [67] in 2000 and included 192 asymptomatic women who were proven or suspected to carry a breast cancer susceptibility gene. These patients underwent a regular clinical breast exam, yearly mammogram, and breast MRI as well as twice yearly ultrasound. Nine cancers were identified in two screening rounds, and all were detected by breast MRI. Only four of the malignancies in the asymptomatic group were identified by both mammography and ultrasound. The positive predictive values of mammography, ultrasound, and MRI were 30%, 12%, and 64%, respectively [67].

Eight early clinical trials assessing breast MRI effectiveness in high-risk women were reviewed by Lehman in 2006 [61]. Out of 4,271 total women included in these eight studies, 144 malignancies were detected, yielding a 3% cancer detection rate. Depending on the woman's risk status and age, approximately 31 out of every 1,000 women screened would have an otherwise occult cancer detected by MRI. The sensitivities ranged between 71 and 100% and the specificities ranged between 81 and 97%. In 8–17% of cases the patients had to be recalled for additional evaluation.

The ACS recommends annual MRI screening in women who are BRCA1 or BRCA2 gene mutation carriers, have a first-degree relative who is a BRCA carrier but has not been screened themselves, or a lifetime risk of breast cancer of at least 20–25% based upon the BRCAPRO model or other models dependent on family history. The second group for which annual MRI screening is recommended is in women who have had chest radiation between the ages of 10 and 30 for Hodgkin's disease and women who have or their first degree relatives have the Li-Fraumeni, Cowden, and Bannayan–Riley–Ruvalcaba genetic syndromes [66].

For women with a lifetime risk of breast cancer between 15 and 20%, history of LCIS, ALH or ADH, heterogeneously or extremely dense parenchyma on mammography, or a personal history of breast cancer, the ACS has found insufficient evidence to recommend for or against MRI screening [66]. The National Comprehensive Cancer Network differs from the ACS in its recommendations regarding women with a history of LCIS and atypical hyperplasias, stating that MRI should be considered in these women, in addition to mammography, clinical breast exam, and risk reduction strategies [18]. In a study by Friedlander et al. malignancy was found in 3.8% of women with a history of LCIS screened by MRI [68].

The scheduling of imaging in the high-risk patient is important. It has been advocated alternating screening mammography and breast MRI, one every 6 months. Le-Petross et al. [69] investigated the use of alternating screening mammography and breast MRI every 6 months in women at high risk for breast cancer based upon a retrospective chart review. All of the women had BRCA mutations. Thirteen cancers were identified, 12 of which were identified on MR, and were not identified on the mammogram 6 months prior. One of the cancers was found by prophylactic mastectomy specimen and not by imaging [69].

There have been no randomized controlled trials to assess the effect of screening MRI on mortality, although other markers of mortality can be assessed. These include the size of the tumor and nodal involvement, both of which are important prognostic indicators. Kriege et al. [70] used age-matched control groups to look at the incidence of nodal disease and tumor size in women screened with MRI vs. those that were not. Tumors which were 10 mm or less comprised 43.2% of the group screened by MRI, vs. 14.0 and 12.5% in the control groups not screened by MRI. Lymph node involvement was 21.4% in the group screened with MRI vs. 52.4 and 56.4% in the group not screened with MRI [70].

In a study by Tilanus-Linthorst et al. [71], woman at high risk were shown to benefit from MRI screening with regard to stage of malignancy and nodal disease. Early T1NO cancers were identified in only 46% of women not screened vs. 81% of women screened with MRI. Women not screened with breast MRI had a 42% chance of nodal disease vs. 19% of women screened with breast MRI [71].

There has been a more recent prospective study by Warner et al. [72] which compares the incidence of breast cancer in BRCA mutation carriers who were screened with MRI vs. those that were not. In this study, 445 BRCA gene mutation carriers underwent annual MRI screening. The incidence of breast cancer in this MRI screened cohort was compared with the incidence of breast cancer in BRCA gene mutation carriers who did not undergo MRI screening (830 total women). This MRI screening paradigm was performed for an average of 3.2 years. The purpose of the study was to compare the incidence of noninvasive cancers, stage I cancers, and stage II to IV cancers between the two cohorts. The hypothesis was that if MRI screening could reduce mortality in BRCA gene mutation carriers, then higher stage cancers and positive nodes would occur more frequently in women who were not screened with MRI. The cumulative incidence of malignancy was assessed at 6 years. The percentage of cancers detected for each group was 9.2%. This study demonstrated a decreased incidence of advanced-stage breast cancer in the screened cohort. The incidence of DCIS and stage I breast cancers was 13.8% in the MRI screened group and 7.2% in the group not screened with MRI. In contrast, the incidence of stage II to IV breast cancers was 1.9% in the MRI screened group and 6.6% in the group not screened with MRI [72].

Schrading and Kuhl [39] investigated the MRI phenotypes of breast cancer in women at high risk. The "fibroadenoma-like" (or so-called benign appearing) malignancies which can be misleading on mammography and ultrasound are less common in MRI. On MRI, fibroadenomas typically demonstrate dark, non-enhancing septations. None of the 15 cancers which had a "fibroadenoma-like" appearance on mammography or ultrasound demonstrated this feature on MRI. Rather, these 15 cancers instead demonstrated suspicious MRI features, including rim enhancement or Type III kinetics with rapid washout. These features are not usually associated with fibroadenomas. A limitation of MRI in evaluation of familial breast cancers is that benign kinetic features can be seen in cancers and that cancers can present as nonmasslike enhancement, rather than a discrete mass [39].

Targeted ultrasound is frequently employed to evaluate abnormalities seen on MRI, often referred to as a second look ultrasound. If there is a suspicious finding identified on the second-look ultrasound, then an ultrasound-guided core needle biopsy could be performed, rather than performing a more expensive, more time-consuming MRI-guided biopsy. In a review article by Leung [73], a meta-analysis of 13 studies on second-look ultrasound demonstrated that lesion type on MRI is the most important feature in determining whether the lesion would be identified at second-look ultrasound. Enhancing masses are more likely to have sonographic correlates than nonmasslike enhancement. Additional features which were predictive of being found on second-look ultrasound were larger size and malignant histology, with invasive cancer being more commonly found than DCIS. The probability of an MRI lesion being malignant is greater if there is a sonographic correlate. Based upon the recommendations proposed by Leung, if no sonographic correlate is identified, MRI biopsy should be performed [73].

Lesions identified at second-look ultrasound are often understated, as reported by Abe et al. [74]. Malignant lesions identified at second-look ultrasound were oval or round in greater than 60% of cancers and greater than 30% were isoechoic or similar sonographic appearance to fat. They also demonstrated that typically malignant features were often not identified, with no suspicious features identified in 11 of 33 malignant lesions [74].

## Emerging Breast Imaging Modalities

Early stage cancers are more often associated with longer term survival rates, the ability to perform lumpectomy rather than mastectomy, as well as less need for chemotherapy [75]. In an attempt to improve on the benefits of mammography, ultrasound, and MRI, additional technologies have been introduced to further improve breast cancer detection.

The FDA-approved technique, tomosynthesis, involves movement of an X-ray tube in an arc around the compressed breast and creates multiple low dose projection images [76, 77]. 2D and 3D images are acquired with the latter resulting in a series of high-resolution thin slice images. When MLO and CC 2D and 3D images are obtained, the radiation exposure is approximately twice that of a typical digital mammogram [78]. Poplak demonstrated comparable or better image quality for breast tomosynthesis over digital mammography, with a major benefit being the elimination of overlapping structures in dense breast tissue [79]. Mass margins may be more precisely characterized and the number and distribution of findings better seen. Research by Andersson et al. [80] demonstrated improved cancer visibility with tomosynthesis compared to digital mammography. This may be due to superior delineation of masses and architectural distortion [80]. Thus, tomosynthesis may have a higher sensitivity for breast cancer detection. Tomosynthesis has been shown to be superior to digital mammography in the assessment of tumor size and stage [81]. Tomosynthesis may also be helpful in evaluating women with dense breasts, particularly in high-risk young women with dense breasts, given the ability to eliminate overlapping breast tissue and improve visibility of subtle cancers. This modality, however, should be used cautiously in this patient population due to the increased radiation dose. Therefore, tomosynthesis is not currently recommended to be used as a screening modality in high-risk women at this time.

Dedicated cone-beam breast CT is currently under investigation as an adjunct to mammography and an alternative to tomosynthesis, given its potential to identify lesions obscured by overlapping breast tissue on conventional imaging. A major feature of breast CT compared to tomosynthesis and mammography is that it does not require compression, thus eliminating patient discomfort. Additionally, lack of compression utilized by this modality does not alter blood flow to the breast if contrast is utilized [82]. In dedicated cone-beam breast CT, the patient lies prone with the breast hanging through an opening in the table. A detector and X-ray tube rotate 360° around the breast over a period of approximately 10s, obtaining cross-sectional slices with the ability to reformat in any 3D plane. Studies have demonstrated imaging of the breast from the chest wall to the nipple with sufficient spatial and contrast resolution to detect and characterize masses and their margins as well as calcifications. A benefit of this technique is that the lack of compression does not distort the spatial relationships within the breast. The radiation dose for this technique is lower than that of tomosynthesis and not much more than that of conventional mammography (mean glandular dose of 8.2 mGy for CT vs. 6.5 mGy for conventional mammography). Imaging of the axilla and axillary tail region, however, is less inclusive compared to that of mammography [40]. Preliminary research suggests that calcifications are better depicted on mammography [83].

Further attempts to improve breast cancer detection have involved nuclear medicine imaging. Breast-specific gamma imaging (BSGI) and positron emission mammography (PEM) are FDA-approved adjuncts to mammography. BSGI utilizes the radiotracer technetium-99m sestimibi with high-resolution breast-specific gamma cameras to detect both DCIS and invasive carcinoma with sensitivities greater than 90%, regardless of breast density [84]. It is based on cell function and is particularly sensitive to malignant cells which have increased metabolic activity and thus localize and emit more gamma radiation.

PEM provides images of biochemical activity in the breast, utilizing the glucose-based radiotracer 18F-FDG. It is able to detect invasive and in situ cancers with sensitivities of approximately 90%. Image creation in this modality is also based on the higher metabolic activity of cancer cells with preferential localization of the glucose analog radiotracer [85].

The major limitation of both BSGI and PEM for high-risk patients is that they have higher radiation exposure, with mean doses greater than that of conventional mammography and with the

**Table 6.1** Breast imaging recommendations for screening women based upon risk

| | Screening mammography | Screening MRI | Screening breast ultrasound |
|---|---|---|---|
| Highest risk | Per the ACR: Yearly starting by age 30 (but not before age 25) or 10 years earlier than the age of diagnosis of the youngest affected relative, whichever is later<br>Per the NCCN: Yearly starting by age 25 for hereditary breast and ovarian cancer patients. 5–10 years earlier than age of diagnosis of youngest affective relative for strong family history or other genetic predisposition | Alternate MRI with mammography every 6 months | Not indicated unless there is a contraindication to MRI |
| Intermediate risk | 10 years earlier than the age of diagnosis of the youngest affected relative, but not before 30 | Consider MRI if history of LCIS (per NCCN). If performed, alternate MRI with mammography every 6 months | Consider in women with dense breasts |
| Average risk | Age 40 | Not indicated | Insufficient evidence to support screening at this time |

radiation-induced cancer risks at least 20 times greater than digital mammography [86].

## Conclusion

Mammography remains the mainstay of breast imaging as it is the only imaging modality that has been shown to reduce breast cancer mortality. It unfortunately has limited sensitivity in dense breasts, which are found in many young women at high risk. Ultrasound has been shown to find additional cancers in dense breasts and is used in the everyday breast imaging practice. However, it suffers from a lack of specificity, and therefore is not suitable for a screening modality. Women at high risk benefit most from adding MRI to the screening regimen. Newer technologies such as tomosynthesis, breast CT, BSGI, and PEM may be helpful in imaging the woman at high risk; however, they are not screening modalities because of their higher radiation dose. In summary, screening recommendations exist for those women at the highest risk of developing breast cancer, those with intermediate risk, and those of average risk and these recommendations are outlined in Table 6.1.

## References


1. Smith RA, Cokkinides V, Brooks D, Saslow D, Brawley OW. Cancer screening in the United States, 2010: a review of current American Cancer Society guidelines and issues in cancer screening. CA Cancer J Clin. 2010;60(2):99–119.
2. American Medical Association. Mammography screening in asymptomatic women forty years and older (AMA Policy H-525.993). Washington, DC: American Medical Association; 1999.
3. ACR Practice Guidelines for the Performance of Screening and Diagnostic Mammography. 2008. Available at: http://www.acr.org/~/media/ACR/Documents/PGTS/guidelines/Screening_Mammography.pdf. Accessed 1 Feb 2012.
4. Humphrey LL, Helfand M, Chan BK, Woolf SH. Breast cancer screening: a summary of the evidence for the U.S. Preventive Services Task Force. Ann Intern Med. 2002;137(5 Pt 1):347–60.
5. Verbeek ALM, Hendricks JHCL, Holland R, Mravunac M, Sturmans F. Screening and breast cancer mortality, age specific effects in Nijmegen project, 1975–82. Lancet. 1985;1(8433):865–6.
6. Shapiro S, Venet W, Strax P, Venet L. Periodic screening for breast cancer: the Health Insurance Plan Project and its sequelae, 1963–1986. Baltimore, MD: Johns Hopkins University Press; 1988.
7. Nystrom L, Rutqvist LE, Wall S, et al. Breast cancer screening with mammography: overview of Swedish randomized trials. Lancet. 1993;341(8851):973–8.

8. Roberts MM, Alexander FE, Anderson TJ, et al. Edinburgh trial of screening for breast cancer: mortality at seven years. Lancet. 1990;335(8684):241–6.
9. Miller AB, Baines CJ, To T, et al. Canadian national breast screening study: 1. Breast cancer detection and death rates among women aged 40 to 49 years. CMAJ. 1992;147:1459–76.
10. Moss SM, Summerley ME, Thomas BT, Ellman R, Chamberlain JOP. A case-control evaluation of the effect of breast cancer screening in the United Kingdom trial of early detection of breast cancer. J Epidemiol Community Health. 1992;46(10):362–4.
11. Otto SJ, Fracheboud J, Looman CWN, et al. National Evaluation Team for breast cancer screening initiation of population-based mammography screening in Dutch municipalities and effect on breast-cancer mortality: a systematic review. Lancet. 2003;361(9367): 411–7.
12. Kerlikowske K, Grady D, Rubin SM, Sandrock C, Ernster VL. Efficacy of screening mammography. A meta-analysis. JAMA. 1995;273(2):149–54.
13. Elwood JM, Cox B, Richardson AK. The effectiveness of breast cancer screening by mammography in younger women. Online J Curr Clin Trials. 1993; Doc No. 32.
14. Tabar L, Yen MF, Vitak B, Chen HH, Smith RA, Duffy SW. Mammography service screening and mortality in breast cancer patients: 20-year follow-up before and after introduction of screening. Lancet. 2003;361(9367):1405–10.
15. U.S. Preventive Services Task Force. Screening for breast cancer: U.S. Preventive Services Task Force recommendation statement. Ann Intern Med. 2009;151(10):716–26.
16. Lee CH, Dershaw DD, Kopans D, et al. Breast cancer screening with imaging: recommendations from the Society of Breast Imaging and the ACR on the use of mammography, breast MRI, breast ultrasound, and other technologies for the detection of clinically occult breast cancer. J Am Coll Radiol. 2010;7(1):18–27.
17. American Cancer Society. Breast cancer: early detection. 2011. Available at: http://www.cancer.org/acs/groups/cid/documents/webcontent/003165-pdf.pdf. Accessed 1 Feb 2012.
18. National Comprehensive Cancer Network. NCCN clinical practice guidelines in oncology: NCCN guidelines TM. Breast cancer screening and diagnosis, version 1.2011. NCCN.org.
19. Brewster AM, Hortobagyi GN, Broglio KR, Kau S, Santa-Maria CA. Residual risk of breast cancer recurrence 5 years after adjuvant therapy. J Natl Cancer Inst. 2008;100(16):1179–83.
20. Hartman M, Czene K, Reilly M, Adolfsson J, Bergh J, Adami HO, et al. Incidence and prognosis of synchronous and metachronous bilateral breast cancer. J Clin Oncol. 2007;25(27):4210–6.
21. ACR-ACS-CAP-SSO practice guideline for the management of ductal carcinoma in-situ of the breast (DCIS). Revised 2006 (Resolution 21). Available at: http://www.acr.org/~/media/ACR/Documents/PGTS/guidelines/DCIS.pdf. Accessed 1 Feb 2012.
22. ACR-ACS-CAP-SSO practice guideline for breast conservation therapy in the management of invasive breast carcinoma. Revised 2006 (Resolution 20). Available at: http://www.acr.org/~/media/ACR/Documents/PGTS/guidelines/Invasive_Breast_Carcinoma.pdf. Accessed 1 Feb 2012.
23. Khatcheressian JL, Wolff AC, Smith TJ, Grunfeld E. American Society of Clinical Oncology 2006 update of the breast cancer follow-up and management guideline in the adjuvant setting. J Clin Oncol. 2006;24(31):5091–7.
24. Grann A, Abdou JC, Dragman N, Goodman R. The value of postexcision preradiation mammography in patients with early-stage breast cancer. Am J Clin Oncol. 2004;27(3):285–8.
25. Link K, Eradat J, Mehta NH, Bent C. Is a short-interval postradiation mammogram necessary after conservative surgery and radiation in breast cancer? Int J Radiat Oncol Biol Phys. 2008;72(4):1041–7.
26. Hymas RV, Gaffney DK, Parkinson BT, Belnap T. Is short interval mammogram necessary after breast-conservation surgery and radiation treatment in breast cancer patients? J Clin Oncol. 2010;28(15 Suppl):603.
27. Elder EE, Kennedy CW, Gluch L, Carmalt HL. Patterns of breast cancer relapse. Eur J Surg Oncol. 2006;32(9):922–7.
28. MacLachlan TK, Somasundaram K, Sgagias M, et al. BRCA1 effects on the cell cycle and the DNA damage response are linked to altered gene expression. J Biol Chem. 2000;275(4):2777–85.
29. Jansen-van der Weide MC, Greuter MJ, Jansen L, Oosterwijk JC, Pijnappel RM, de Bock GH. Exposure to low-dose radiation and the risk of breast cancer among women with a familial or genetic predisposition: a meta-analysis. Eur Radiol. 2010;20(11):2547–56.
30. Brekelmans CT, Seynaeve C, Bartels CC, et al. Effectiveness of breast cancer surveillance in BRCA ½ gene mutation carriers and women with high familial risk. J Clin Oncol. 2001;19(4):924–30.
31. Komenaka IK, Ditkoff BA, Joseph KA, et al. The development of interval breast malignancies in patients with BRCA mutations. Cancer. 2004;100(10):2079–83.
32. Harvey JA, Bovbjerg VE. Quantitative assessment of mammographic breast density: relationship with breast cancer risk. Radiology. 2004;230(1):29–41.
33. Boyd NF, Guo H, Martin LJ, Sun L. Mammographic density and the risk and detection of breast cancer. N Engl J Med. 2007;356(3):227–36.
34. Pisano ED, Gatsonis C, Hendrick E, Yaffe M. Diagnostic performance of digital versus film mammography for breast-cancer screening. N Engl J Med. 2005;356(17):1773–83.
35. Lakhani SR, Jacquemier J, Sloane JP, et al. Multifactorial analysis of differences between sporadic breast cancers and cancers involving BRCA1 and BRCA2 mutations. J Natl Cancer Inst. 1998;90(15):1138–45.
36. Breast Cancer Linkage Consortium. Pathology of familial breast cancer: differences between breast can-

cers in carriers of BRCA1 or BRCA2 mutations and sporadic cases. Lancet. 1997;349(9064):1505–10.
37. Tilanus-Linthorst M, Verhoog L, Obdeign IM, et al. A BRCA ½ mutation, high breast density and prominent pushing margins of a tumor independently contribute to a frequent false-negative mammography. Int J Cancer. 2002;102(1):91–5.
38. Hamilton LJ, Evans AJ, et al. Breast imaging findings in women with BRCA1 and BRCA2 associated breast carcinoma. Clin Radiol. 2004;59(10):895–902.
39. Schrading S, Kuhl C. Mammographic, US, and MR imaging phenotypes of familial breast cancer. Radiology. 2008;246(1):58–70.
40. O'Connell A, Conover DL, Zhang Y. Cone-beam CT for breast imaging: radiation dose, breast coverage, and image quality. AJR Am J Roentgenol. 2010;195(2):496–509.
41. ACR. BI-RADS mammography. In: American College of Radiology Breast Imaging Reporting and Data System Atlas. 4th ed. Reston, VA: American College of Radiology; 2003.
42. Mammography Quality Standards Act. Available at: http://www.fda.gov/Radiation-EmittingProducts/MammographyQualityStandardsActandProgram/default.htm. Accessed 1 Feb 2012.
43. Madjar H, Mendelson EB. The practice of breast ultrasound. 2nd ed. Stuttgart, Germany: Thieme; 2008.
44. Berg WA. Supplemental screening sonography in dense breasts. Radiol Clin North Am. 2004;42(5):845–51.
45. Berg WA, Blume JD, Cormack JB, et al.; ACRIN 6666 Investigators. Combined screening with ultrasound and mammography vs mammography alone in women at elevated risk of breast cancer. JAMA. 2008;299(18):2151–63.
46. Berg WA. Tailored supplemental screening for breast cancer: what now and what next? AJR Am J Roentgenol. 2009;192(2):390–9.
47. Warner E, Causer PA, Wong JW, et al. Improvement in DCIS detection rates by MRI over time in a high-risk breast screening study. Breast J. 2011;17(1):9–17.
48. Kelly KM, Dean J, Comulada WS, Lee SJ. Breast cancer detection using automated whole breast ultrasound and mammography in radiographically dense breasts. Eur Radiol. 2010;20(3):734–42.
49. Kelly KM, Dean J, Lee SJ, Comulada WS. Breast cancer detection: radiologists' performance using mammography with and without automated whole-breast ultrasound. Eur Radiol. 2010;20(11):2557–64.
50. Lehman CD, Isaacs C, Schnall MD, et al. Cancer yield of mammography, MR, and US in high-risk women: prospective multi-institution breast cancer screening study. Radiology. 2007;244(2):381–8.
51. Warner E, Plewes DB, Hill KA, et al. Surveillance of BRCA1 and BRCA2 mutation carriers with magnetic resonance imaging, ultrasound, mammography, and clinical breast examination. JAMA. 2004;292(11):1317–25.
52. Kuhl CK, Schrading S, Leutner CC, et al. Mammography, breast ultrasound, and magnetic resonance imaging for surveillance of women at high familial risk for breast cancer. J Clin Oncol. 2005;23(33):8469–76.
53. Sardanelli F, Podo F, Santoro F, et al.; High Breast Cancer Risk Italian 1 (HIBCRIT-1) Study. Multicenter surveillance of women at high genetic breast cancer risk using mammography, ultrasonography, and contrast-enhanced magnetic resonance imaging (the high breast cancer risk Italian 1 study): final results. Invest Radiol. 2011;46(2):94–105.
54. Mendelson EB, Baum JK, Berg WA, Merritt CRB, Rubin E. Breast imaging reporting and data system, BI-RADS: ultrasound. Reston, VA: American College of Radiology; 2003.
55. Marcus JN, Watson P, Page DL, et al. Hereditary breast cancer: pathobiology, prognosis, and BRCA1 and BRCA2 gene linkage. Cancer. 1996;77(4):697–709.
56. Lamb PM, Perry NM, Vinnicombe SJ, Wells CA. Correlation between ultrasound characteristics, mammographic findings and histological grade in patients with invasive ductal carcinoma of the breast. Clin Radiol. 2000;55(1):40–4.
57. Kaiser WA, Zeitler E. MR imaging of the breast: fast imaging sequences with and without Gd-DTPA. Preliminary observations. Radiology. 1989;170(3 Pt 1):681–6.
58. Heywang SH, Wolf A, Pruss E, et al. MR imaging of the breast with Gd-DTPA: use and limitations. Radiology. 1989;171(1):95–103.
59. Kuhl CK, Bieling HB, Gieseke J, et al. Healthy premenopausal breast parenchyma in dynamic contrast-enhanced MR imaging of the breast: normal contrast medium enhancement and cyclical-phase dependency. Radiology. 1997;203(1):137–44.
60. ACR MRI accreditation program requirements. Available at: http://www.acr.org/~/media/ACR/Documents/PGTS/guidelines/MRI_Breast.pdf. Accessed 1 Feb 2012.
61. Lehman CD. Role of MRI in screening women at high risk for breast cancer. J Magn Reson Imaging. 2006;24(5):964–70.
62. American College of Radiology. ACR BI-RADS: magnetic resonance imaging, in ACR Breast Imaging Reporting and Data System: Breast Imaging Atlas. Reston, VA: American College of Radiology; 2003.
63. Kuhl CK, Mielcareck P, Klaschik S, et al. Dynamic breast MR imaging: are signal intensity time course data useful for differential diagnosis of enhancing lesions? Radiology. 1999;211(1):101–10.
64. Weinstein S, Rosen M. Breast MR imaging: current indications and advanced imaging techniques. Radiol Clin North Am. 2010;48(5):1013–42.
65. Kuhl C. Dynamic breast magnetic resonance imaging. In: Morris EA, Liberman L, editors. Breast MRI: diagnosis and intervention. New York, NY: Springer; 2005. p. 79–139.
66. Saslow D, Boetes C, Burke W, et al. American Cancer Society guidelines for breast screening with MRI as an adjunct to mammography. CA Cancer J Clin. 2007;57(2):75–89.

67. Kuhl CK, Schmutzler RK, Leutner CC, et al. Breast MR imaging screening in 192 women proved or suspected to be carriers of a breast cancer susceptibility gene: preliminary results. Radiology. 2000;215(1):267–79.
68. Friedlander LC, Roth SO, Gavenonis SC. Results of MR imaging screening for breast cancer in high-risk patients with lobular carcinoma in situ. Radiology. 2011;261(2):421–7.
69. Le-Petross HT, Whitman GJ, Atchley DP, et al. Effectiveness of alternating mammography and magnetic resonance imaging for screening women with deleterious BRCA mutations at high risk of breast cancer. Cancer. 2011;117(17):3900–7.
70. Kriege M, Brekelmans CT, Boetes C, et al. Magnetic Resonance Imaging Screening Study Group. Efficacy of MRI and mammography for breast-cancer screening in women with a familial or genetic predisposition. N Engl J Med. 2004;351(5):427–37.
71. Tilanus-Linthorst MM, Bartels CC, Obdeijn AI, Oudkerk M. Earlier detection of breast cancer by surveillance of women at familial risk. Eur J Cancer. 2000;36(4):514–9.
72. Warner E, Hill K, Causer P, et al. Prospective study of breast cancer incidence in women with a *BRCA1* or *BRCA2* mutation under surveillance with and without magnetic resonance imaging. J Clin Oncol. 2011;29(13):1664–9.
73. Leung JW. Utility of second-look ultrasound in the evaluation of MRI-detected breast lesions. Semin Roentgenol. 2011;46(4):260–74.
74. Abe H, Schmidt RA, Shah RN, et al. MR-directed ("second-look") ultrasound examination for breast lesions detected initially on MRI: MR and sonographic findings. AJR Am J Roentgenol. 2010;194(2):370–7.
75. Tabár L, Vitak B, Chen HH, et al. The Swedish two-county trial twenty years later. Updated mortality results and new insights from long-term follow-up. Radiol Clin North Am. 2000;38(4):625–51.
76. Baldwin P. Digital breast tomosynthesis. Radiol Technol. 2009;81(1):57M–74.
77. Sarkar A, Shi C, Rassiah-Szegedi P, Diaz A, Eng T, Papanikolaou N. The effect of a limited number of projections and reconstruction algorithms on the image quality of megavoltage digital tomosynthesis. J Appl Clin Med Phys. 2009;10(3):2970.
78. Hologic Selenia Dimensions 3D System, Sponsor executive summary. 2010;40–1. Available at: http://www.fda.gov/downloads/AdvisoryCommittees/Committees-MeetingMaterials/MedicalDevices/Medical-DevicesAdvisoryCommittee/Radiological DevicesPanel/UCM226662.pdf. Accessed 14 March 2011.
79. Poplack SP, Tosteson TD, Kogel CA, Nagy HM. Digital breast tomosynthesis: initial experience in 98 women with abnormal digital screening mammography. AJR Am J Roentgenol. 2007;189(3):616–23.
80. Andersson I, Ikeda DM, Zackrisson S, et al. Breast tomosynthesis and digital mammography: a comparison of breast cancer visibility and BIRADS classification in a population of cancers with subtle mammographic findings. Eur Radiol. 2008;18(12):2817–25.
81. Förnvik D, Zackrisson S, Ljungberg O, et al. Breast tomosynthesis: accuracy of tumor measurement compared with digital mammography and ultrasonography. Eur Radiol. 2008;18(3):2817–25.
82. Boone JM, Kwan AL, Yang K, Burkett GW, Lindfors KK, Nelson TR. Computed tomography for imaging the breast. J Mammary Gland Biol Neoplasia. 2006;11(2):103–11.
83. Lindfors KK, Boone JM, Nelson TR. Dedicated breast CT: initial clinical experience. Radiology. 2008;246(3):725–33.
84. Brem RF, Floerke AC, Rapelyea JA, Teal C, Kelly T, Mathur V. Breast-specific gamma imaging as an adjunct imaging modality for the diagnosis of breast cancer. Radiology. 2008;247(3):651–7.
85. Berg WA, Weinberg IN, Narayanan D, et al. High-resolution fluorodeoxyglucose positron emission tomography with compression ("positron emission mammography") is highly accurate in depicting primary breast cancer. Breast J. 2006;12(4):309–23.
86. Hendrick RE. Radiation doses and cancer risks from breast imaging studies. Radiology. 2010;257(1):246–53.

# Risk Reduction Strategies: Medical Oncology

7

Virginia Kaklamani

## Introduction

In the United States it is estimated that in 2012 more than 40,000 women will die of breast cancer and 229,060 women will be diagnosed with the disease [1]. Although early detection strategies, such as mammograms, have been successfully implemented, 10 (of women will be diagnosed with four or more lymph nodes involved [2]. It has long been thought that the steps leading to cancer development in the breast take place during a long period of time. Support of this notion comes from data in women exposed to radiation. Among patients who received chest radiation for Hodgkin's disease, a cancer of the lymph nodes, as well as the survivors of the atomic bombing, it has been found that the greatest risk of developing breast cancer is when the radiation exposure took place during the early teen years [3]. However breast cancer in those individuals occurred at least 10–15 years later. Additional data come from infants undergoing radiation to the thymic gland, a gland located in the chest, [4] and girls in puberty who received radiation during a procedure for the diagnosis of tuberculosis [5].

Owing to the long natural history of cancer initiation, and the high incidence and severity of the disease, breast cancer is a unique model for successful prevention [6]. Lifestyle modification has been suggested but so far such strategies have been implemented in clinical trials for too short a period to prove successful in preventing breast cancer. Most of the focus has been on developing medications for prevention (chemoprevention). To date three medications have been extensively studied and approved as chemopreventive agents for breast cancer: tamoxifen, raloxifene, and exemestane. However several other agents are currently undergoing clinical testing.

## Selective Estrogen Receptor Modulators

These agents change the effect of estrogen in tissues. The word selective is used because in some tissues they promote the effect of estrogens and in other tissues they inhibit its effect. Therefore these agents can have estrogenic effects in some tissues but antiestrogenic effects in others.

### Tamoxifen

Tamoxifen was initially developed in the 1960s to be used as a contraceptive pill. It was found however to have strong antiestrogenic properties

V. Kaklamani, M.D., D.Sc. (✉)
Division Hematology/Oncology,
Northwestern University, 676 North St. Clair Street,
Suite 850, Chicago, IL 60611, USA
e-mail: v-kaklamani@northwestern.edu

N.M. Hansen (ed.), *Management of the Patient at High Risk for Breast Cancer*,
DOI 10.1007/978-1-4614-5891-3_7, 

and to prevent the growth of breast tumors in rats [7, 8]. Tamoxifen, like other selective estrogen receptor modulators (SERMs), is unique and acts as an estrogen in some tissues and as an antiestrogen in others [9]. It has long been the hormone drug of choice for all stages of hormone responsive breast cancer and has been shown to decrease the risk of recurrence as well as mortality in early stage breast cancer [10].

Tamoxifen was considered for breast cancer chemoprevention for three reasons. Primarily tamoxifen has an excellent safety profile [6]. This is important since any agent used for chemoprevention would have to be used for a long period of time, in healthy individuals. Secondly, tamoxifen has been found to prevent breast cancer in mice and rats [7, 8]. Finally, studies showed that when giving tamoxifen to treat breast cancer, there was a decreased risk of developing breast cancer in the other breast [10].

## NSABP P-1

The NSABP P-1 trial was the first large preventive trial in breast cancer and enrolled 13,388 patients between June 1992 and September 1997 [11]. Women were eligible to participate in the trial if they were over the age of 60 or between 35 and 59 years of age with a high risk for breast cancer. Women with lobular carcinoma in situ (LCIS), a high-risk factor for breast cancer, were also eligible for the study. After a median follow-up of 7 years tamoxifen was found to reduce the incidence of breast cancer by 43( and that of precancerous lesions by 37 (, in all age groups [12]. The benefit was found to be only in hormone receptor-positive breast cancers where the overall risk was reduced by 69(. The rate of hormone receptor-negative tumors did not significantly differ from the placebo group. Tamoxifen led to a 32( reduction in bone fractures due to osteoporosis and increased the risk of uterine cancer, stroke, blood clots, and cataracts whereas there was no difference in the risk of heart attacks and death in the two arms [12].

Overall the NSABP P-1 trial was able to demonstrate a 43( reduction of the incidence of breast cancer among healthy but high risk for breast cancer women who took tamoxifen for 5 years. So far it hasn't been shown that women who will take tamoxifen for 5 years will live longer although they will have a significantly lower risk of being diagnosed with breast cancer. It has been suggested, however, that a longer follow-up is needed to demonstrate that women at high risk for developing breast cancer will live longer if they take tamoxifen for 5 years.

## IBIS-I

A total of 7,145 women aged 35–70 and at high risk for breast cancer were randomly assigned to take either tamoxifen or a sugar pill (placebo) for a 5 years [13]. After a median follow-up of 96 months women in the tamoxifen arm had a 27% reduced risk for breast cancer compared with placebo. This reduction in risk was again seen only in hormone receptor positive tumors whereas there was no difference in the risk for hormone receptor negative tumors. Side effects associated with tamoxifen therapy were similar to those observed in the NSABP P-1 trial.

## Royal Marsden and Italian Trial

Two other trials failed to show an advantage to the use of tamoxifen as a chemopreventive agent. The Royal Marsden trial [14] enrolled 2,494 healthy women aged 30–70 years with a family history of breast cancer. The trial accrued patients between October of 1986 and April of 1996. Unlike the NSABP trial, 40( of women in this trial were on hormone replacement therapy (HRT). After a median follow-up of 70 months, the overall incidence of breast cancer was similar between the two arms. It has been suggested that the reason for not finding a benefit for tamoxifen in this trial is because of the relatively small number of patients as well as the unknown effect of HRT in combination with tamoxifen.

An Italian trial randomized 5,408 women, unselected for breast cancer risk, who had undergone hysterectomy followed by tamoxifen versus placebo [15]. However, only 149 of those participating in the trial completed 5 years of tamoxifen. Furthermore 47( of the participants had had their ovaries removed at that time of their hysterectomy which decreased their risk of subsequent breast cancer. The study did not show any difference between the two groups as far as breast cancer development. This study has been criticized for the small number of participants completing 5 years of therapy, as well as the fact that the high rate of ovarian removal would place these women in a low-risk group for developing breast cancer. Despite these drawbacks the Italian study showed a trend toward a significant benefit of tamoxifen among the patients who took it for 1 year.

Based on the NSABP P-1 trial tamoxifen at a dose of 20 mg/day was approved by the FDA for use as a chemopreventive agent in high-risk individuals for developing breast cancer. It is unclear, however, if tamoxifen is preventing breast cancer or treating early stage breast cancer present at the initiation of therapy.

## Raloxifene

Raloxifene is an SERM that like tamoxifen acts as an antiestrogen in the breast tissue and prevents breast cancer in mice and rats [16, 17]. Furthermore it has an estrogenic-like effect on the bones and therefore prevents and treats osteoporosis and appears to be less estrogenic than tamoxifen in the human uterus and therefore does not seem to increase the risk of uterine cancer [16, 18]. It is approved for the prevention of osteoporosis in postmenopausal women at a dose of 60 mg/day. Early data on raloxifene suggested that like tamoxifen it may be a useful chemopreventive agent for breast cancer. Furthermore the potential advantage of raloxifene is the fact that it is less estrogenic on the uterus and may therefore not cause an increased incidence of uterine cancer [18]. The Multiple Outcomes of Raloxifene Evaluation (MORE) trial in which 7,704 postmenopausal women were randomized to receive two different doses of raloxifene or placebo [19] found that there was a 70( reduction in breast cancer incidence in the raloxifene treated arms.

### STAR Trial

Based on these findings, the Study of Tamoxifen and Raloxifene (STAR) trial was initiated in postmenopausal women at high risk for breast cancer [20]. The STAR trial randomized 19,747 eligible postmenopausal women to tamoxifen 20 mg/day or raloxifene 60 mg/day for 5 years. With a median follow-up of 81 months tamoxifen was found to be a better chemopreventive agent compared with raloxifene, indicating that the rate in the raloxifene group was about 24( higher than the rate in the tamoxifen group. There was no difference in the two treatment groups in precancerous lesions. The incidence of uterine cancer was significantly lower in the raloxifene group as was the incidence of blood clots and cataracts [20]. Overall this study demonstrated that both tamoxifen and raloxifene are effective chemopreventive medications with tamoxifen potentially being the better chemopreventive agent and raloxifene being the less toxic agent. However since raloxifene has only been studied in postmenopausal women, tamoxifen is still the only medication used for breast cancer prevention in premenopausal women. Both agents have only been found to prevent hormone receptor positive breast cancer [20].

## Other SERMs

Due to the toxicity profile of tamoxifen several other SERMs are currently being developed with the potential of being more potent chemopreventive agents with less toxicity. In a recent trial of 8,556 postmenopausal women lasofoxifene at a dose of 0.5 mg per day was found to significantly decrease hormone receptor positive breast cancer risk, coronary heart disease, stroke, and spinal fractures, whereas it increased blood clots and had no effect on uterine cancer [21]. In 9,354 postmenopausal women, arzoxifene at 20 mg/day was compared to placebo and found at 48 months to significantly reduce the risk of invasive breast cancer and spinal fractures. It was also found to significantly increase uterine polyps, blood clots, and muscle cramps but not heart attacks [22].

## Aromatase Inhibitors

Aromatase inhibitors are a newer class of breast cancer drugs which block the production of estrogens. These agents work on an enzyme, called aromatase, which is responsible for the production of estrogens in postmenopausal women. They are currently used to treat breast cancer and have been shown to be more efficacious than tamoxifen in breast cancer treatment. However unlike tamoxifen they can only be used in postmenopausal women.

### Exemestane

Exemestane is one of the three aromatase inhibitors which is currently being used for the treatment of breast cancer. Given data in invasive breast cancer where aromatase inhibitors (AIs) have been shown to decrease the incidence of a second breast cancer more so than tamoxifen, exemestane was studied in women at high risk for developing breast cancer. The NCIC CTG MAP3 [23] randomized 4,560 women at high risk for breast cancer to exemestane or placebo. Women received the medications for 5 years. At a median follow-up of 35 months women who received exemestane had a 65( decreased incidence of breast cancer. There were no significant differences in side effects between the two groups although women on placebo felt better than the women on exemestane. Furthermore, exemestane has been shown to increase the risk of bone fractures and the follow-up period in this trial may not have been enough to show this. The results of this trial lead to the approval of exemestane in the prevention of breast cancer in postmenopausal women.

#### Ongoing Trials with AIs

The IBIS-II trial [24] planned to randomize 6,000 women at high risk for breast cancer to anastrozole or placebo. As of January 2012, 6,844 women had already been randomized and the study was not accruing any more volunteers. Results should be expected in the next few years.

## Future Strategies for Chemoprevention

### Other Agents

Recent data has suggested that bisphosphonates, medications that are widely being used for the treatment and prevention of osteoporosis, can help prevent breast cancer. In women who participated in the Women's Health Initiative (WHI) oral bisphosphonate use was associated with a 30( decreased risk of hormone receptor positive breast cancer and a nonsignificant 44( decrease in the risk of hormone receptor negative breast cancer [25].

Other agents such as COX-2 inhibitors [26], statins [27], PARP inhibitors [28], metformin [29], and retinoids [30] are also being considered as chemopreventive agents although data are still preliminary.

## Conclusions

Currently three agents have been approved for breast cancer chemoprevention, tamoxifen in pre- and postmenopausal women and raloxifene and exemestane only in postmenopausal women. Emerging agents such as bisphosphonates and COX-2 inhibitors show promise although their side effect profile may limit their use. However most of the agents to date show activity in preventing mostly hormone receptor positive breast cancers and the lack of any survival benefit in the prevention trials suggests that these agents may prevent breast cancers that would have been cured with our current treatments without having any effect in preventing aggressive, life-threatening breast cancers. It is our hope that future research will build on our current chemopreventive strategies finding novel agents to prevent all subtypes of breast cancers.

## References


1. Siegel R, Naishadham D, Jemal A. Cancer statistics, 2012. CA Cancer J Clin. 2012;62:10–29.
2. Jemal A, Siegel R, Ward E, Hao Y, Xu J, Thun MJ. Cancer statistics, 2009. CA Cancer J Clin. 2009;59:225–49.
3. Tokunaga M, Land CE, Yamamoto T, et al. Incidence of female breast cancer among atomic bomb survivors, Hiroshima and Nagasaki, 1950–1980. Radiat Res. 1987;112:243–72.
4. Hildreth NG, Shore RE, Dvoretsky PM. The risk of breast cancer after irradiation of the thymus in infancy. N Engl J Med. 1989;321:1281–4.
5. Miller AB, Howe GR, Sherman GJ, et al. Mortality from breast cancer after irradiation during fluoroscopic examinations in patients being treated for tuberculosis. N Engl J Med. 1989;321:1285–9.
6. Jordan VC, Costa AF. Chemoprevention. In: Harris JR, editor. Diseases of the breast. 2nd ed. Philadelphia: Lippincott Williams & Wilkins; 2000.
7. Jordan VC, Lababidi MK, Mirecki DM. Anti-oestrogenic and anti-tumour properties of prolonged tamoxifen therapy in C3H/OUJ mice. Eur J Cancer. 1990;26:718–21.
8. Jordan VC, Lababidi MK, Langan-Fahey S. Suppression of mouse mammary tumorigenesis by long-term tamoxifen therapy. J Natl Cancer Inst. 1991;83:492–6.
9. O'Regan RM, Jordan VC. Tamoxifen to raloxifene and beyond. Semin Oncol. 2001;28:260–73.
10. Anonymous. Tamoxifen for early breast cancer: an overview of the randomised trials. Early Breast Cancer Trialists' Collaborative Group. Lancet. 1998;351:1451–67.
11. Fisher B, Costantino JP, Wickerham DL, et al. Tamoxifen for prevention of breast cancer: report of the National Surgical Adjuvant Breast and Bowel Project P-1 Study. J Natl Cancer Inst. 1998;90:1371–88.
12. Fisher B, Costantino JP, Wickerham DL, et al. Tamoxifen for the prevention of breast cancer: current status of the National Surgical Adjuvant Breast and Bowel Project P-1 study. J Natl Cancer Inst. 2005;97:1652–62.
13. Cuzick J, Forbes JF, Sestak I, et al. Long-term results of tamoxifen prophylaxis for breast cancer—96-month follow-up of the randomized IBIS-I trial. J Natl Cancer Inst. 2007;99:272–82.
14. Powles T, Eeles R, Ashley S, et al. Interim analysis of the incidence of breast cancer in the Royal Marsden Hospital tamoxifen randomised chemoprevention trial. Lancet. 1998;352:98–101.
15. Veronesi U, Maisonneuve P, Costa A, et al. Prevention of breast cancer with tamoxifen: preliminary findings from the Italian randomised trial among hysterectomised women. Italian tamoxifen prevention study. Lancet. 1998;352:93–7.
16. Anzano MA, Peer CW, Smith JM, et al. Chemoprevention of mammary carcinogenesis in the rat: combined use of raloxifene and 9-cis-retinoic acid. J Natl Cancer Inst. 1996;88:123–5.
17. Gottardis MM, Jordan VC. Antitumor actions of keoxifene and tamoxifen in the N-nitrosomethylurea-induced rat mammary carcinoma model. Cancer Res. 1987;47:4020–4.
18. Delmas PD, Bjarnason NH, Mitlak BH, et al. Effects of raloxifene on bone mineral density, serum cholesterol concentrations, and uterine endometrium in postmenopausal women. N Engl J Med. 1997;337:1641–7.
19. Cummings SR, Eckert S, Krueger KA, et al. The effect of raloxifene on risk of breast cancer in postmenopausal women: results from the more randomized trial. Multiple outcomes of raloxifene evaluation. JAMA. 1999;281:2189–97.
20. Vogel VG, Costantino JP, Wickerham DL, et al. Update of the National Surgical Adjuvant Breast and Bowel Project Study of Tamoxifen and Raloxifene (STAR) P-2 Trial: Preventing Breast Cancer. Cancer Prev Res (Phila). 2010;3(6):696–706.
21. Cummings SR, Ensrud K, Delmas PD, et al. Lasofoxifene in postmenopausal women with osteoporosis. N Engl J Med. 2010;362:686–96.
22. Powles T, Diem S, Wickerham DL, et al. Effects of arzoxifene on breast cancer incidence in postmenopausal women with osteoporosis or with low bone mass. Cancer Res. 2009;69:499s.
23. Goss PE, Ingle JN, Ales-Martinez JE, et al. Exemestane for breast-cancer prevention in postmenopausal women. N Engl J Med. 2011;364:2381–91.
24. Anonymous. IBIS-II. International Breast Cancer Intervention Study. 2010
25. Chlebowski RT, Chen Z, Cauley JA, et al. Oral bisphosphonate and breast cancer: prospective results from the Women's Health Initiative (WHI). Cancer Res. 2009;69:489s.
26. Li Y, Brown PH. Prevention of ER-negative breast cancer. Recent Results Cancer Res. 2009;181:121–34.
27. Boudreau DM, Yu O, Johnson J. Statin use and cancer risk: a comprehensive review. Expert Opin Drug Saf. 2010;9(4):603–21.
28. Lord CJ, Ashworth A. Targeted therapy for cancer using PARP inhibitors. Curr Opin Pharmacol. 2008;8:363–9.
29. Larsson SC, Mantzoros CS, Wolk A. Diabetes mellitus and risk of breast cancer: a meta-analysis. Int J Cancer. 2007;121:856–62.
30. Liby K, Rendi M, Suh N, et al. The combination of the rexinoid, LG100268, and a selective estrogen receptor modulator, either arzoxifene or acolbifene, synergizes in the prevention and treatment of mammary tumors in an estrogen receptor-negative model of breast cancer. Clin Cancer Res. 2006;12:5902–9.

# Risk Reduction Strategies: Surgical Perspective

# 8

Lisa Renee-Palko Spiguel and Nora Hansen

## Introduction

Breast cancer is estimated to affect over 200,000 women in the United States in 2012, accounting for up to 40,000 deaths [1]. Based on SEER database rates from 2006 to 2008, the cumulative lifetime risk of breast cancer for an average woman in the general US population is 12.29%, with the greatest risk occurring in the sixth decade of life [1]. Although the majority of these breast cancers are sporadic, approximately 25% of breast cancers are secondary to some inherited predisposition, commonly related to identifiable mutations in inherited genes such as BRCA1, BRCA2, *CHEK2*, and PTEN. Women born with these gene mutations are at a significantly higher risk of developing breast cancer over the general population, as well as other associated cancers, and do so typically at a younger age.

Mutations in the tumor suppressor genes, BRCA1 and BRCA2, account for the majority of known familial breast cancer risk. Studies demonstrate that women with germ line mutations in BRCA1 gene have an estimated lifetime risk of breast cancer ranging from 65–87%, with the average lifetime risk of 45–55% in BRCA2 carriers. The greatest risk occurs in women younger than the age of 40. These women are also at an increased risk of ovarian cancer with a lifetime risk in BRCA1 carriers of 39–51%, and 11–35% for BRCA2 mutation carriers. The greatest risk of ovarian cancer occurs in women over the age of 60 [2]. Although studies looking specifically at breast cancer-specific survival in women with germ line BRCA mutations have not demonstrated a decrease in overall or disease-free survival, they have demonstrated that in addition to an increase in lifetime risk of breast cancer, there is an increase in the incidence of metachronous breast cancers as compared to the general population, with up to 20% of BRCA1 carriers and over 10% of BRCA2 carriers diagnosed with a new cancer at 5 years, as compared to 2–5% for the general population diagnosed with sporadic cancer [3, 4].

Although evidence of known genetic mutations confirms a women's predilection for cancer, not all inherited conditions are known. Furthermore other factors such as a personal history of breast cancer, as well as personal history of high risk lesions such as LCIS and atypical hyperplasia, increase a woman's risk above the general population. Due to the increased risk of cancer in these patients, various options exist to either increase the detection of cancer at an earlier stage or decrease the overall risk of cancer from occurring. Options include increased surveillance which is discussed in depth in chapter 6 as well as chemoprevention strategies through the use of selective estrogen receptor modulators, such as tamoxifen, which have demonstrated a

L.R.-P. Spiguel (✉) • N. Hansen
Lynn Sage Comprehensive Breast Center,
250 East Superior Street, Prentice 4-420,
Chicago, IL 60611, USA
e-mail: lisa.spiguel@gmail.com; nhansen@nmh.org

N.M. Hansen (ed.), *Management of the Patient at High Risk for Breast Cancer*,
DOI 10.1007/978-1-4614-5891-3_8, © Springer Science+Business Media New York 2013

49% decrease in the risk of invasive cancer in healthy high risk patients with a median follow-up of 55 months. In subset analysis of BRCA mutation carriers, the use of tamoxifen demonstrated an equivalent reduction in breast cancer incidence among BRCA2 carriers; however, tamoxifen beginning at the age of 35 in healthy BRCA1 mutation carriers did not significantly reduce breast cancer risk. These results are likely related to the overall low incidence (6.6%) of BRCA carriers in the Breast Cancer Prevention trial, as well as the majority of BRCA1 cancers being ER- and PR- negative [5].

Additional options to reduce risk are surgical, consisting of prophylactic bilateral mastectomy (PBM) and prophylactic bilateral salpingo-oophorectomy (PBSO) in high risk women, as well as contralateral prophylactic mastectomy (CPM) in women with a personal history of breast cancer diagnosis. This chapter will discuss these surgical options for cancer risk reduction, focusing on the ability of surgery not only to reduce the occurrence of a primary breast cancer, but also to reduce the occurrence of subsequent metachronous cancers and associated mortality. Furthermore it will discuss safety of nipple sparing mastectomy (NSM) on risk reduction and cancer treatment in high risk women, as well as the role for sentinel lymph node biopsy (SLNB) in prophylactic surgery.

## Surgical Strategies

### Prophylactic Bilateral Mastectomy

Several prospective and retrospective studies have investigated the utility of PBM for the prevention of breast cancer (Table 8.1). All of these studies demonstrate a 85–100% breast cancer risk reduction following PBM with up to a 14-year median follow-up.

One of the first studies that investigated the efficacy of PBM in cancer prevention was a study looking specifically at moderate and high risk women based on family history. Hartmann and colleagues conducted this retrospective review of all women with a family history of breast cancer who underwent PBM for risk reduction—10% of which underwent total mastectomy, while 90% underwent subcutaneous mastectomy. Women were divided into two groups, high risk and moderate risk on the basis of family history. A total of 639 women were identified, 214 at high risk and 425 at moderate risk. Following a median follow-up of 14 years, a 89.5% reduction in breast cancer risk in the moderate risk group was demonstrated as compared to the predicted incidence based on the Gail risk model, and a 90–94% breast cancer risk reduction occurred in the high risk group based on incidence of breast cancer in related sisters. They also concluded a reduction in the risk of death from breast cancer in both groups up to 94% [6]. On subset analysis of 26 BRCA1 and BRCA2 mutation carriers, with a median follow-up of 13.4 years, no patients developed subsequent breast cancer following PBM, translating into a breast cancer risk reduction of up to 100% [7].

A second study investigating the role of PBM in breast cancer risk reduction specifically in BRCA patients was a prospective study conducted on 139 BRCA1 and BRCA2 carriers, 76 of which underwent PBM with 63 electing for surveillance alone [8]. Following a mean follow-up of 2.9 years, no women developed breast cancer following PBM, whereas 8 (17.7%) women developed breast cancer in the surveillance group, demonstrating a substantial breast cancer risk reduction in BRCA mutation carriers.

**Table 8.1** Prophylactic bilateral mastectomy

| Study | Year | Study design | F/U (years) | Patients (*n*) | Breast cancer risk reduction (%) |
|---|---|---|---|---|---|
| Hartmann et al. | 1999 | Retrospective | 14 | 639 | 90–94 |
| Hartmann et al. | 2001 | Retrospective | 13.4 | 26 | 85–100 |
| Meijers-Heijboer et al. | 2001 | Prospective | 2.9 | 139 | 100 |
| Rebbeck et al. | 2004 | Prospective | 6.4 | 483 | 90–95 |

A larger prospective cohort study of 483 BRCA carriers with a longer mean follow-up of 6.4 years compared 105 BRCA mutation carriers who underwent PBM to 378 matched controls who underwent routine surveillance [9]. Four different statistical analyses were performed to determine breast cancer risk reduction associated with PBM, as well as the effects of concomitant PBSO on overall risk reduction. Women either underwent subcutaneous, total, or modified radical mastectomy (MRM). Following 6.4 years follow-up, 2 (1.9%) women who underwent PBM were diagnosed with breast cancer compared with 184 (48.7%) of the 378 matched controls, demonstrating up to a 95% breast cancer risk reduction in BRCA mutation carriers who undergo PBM.

A more recent study by Heemskerek-Gerritsen investigated the role of both PBM and CPM in high risk women with either known BRCA status or 50% risk carriers from a hereditary breast/ovarian cancer (HB(O)C) family [10]. Their study comprised 358 women, 65.9% of which were known BRCA mutation carriers, while the other 34.1% were from HB(O)C families. Fifty-one percent of which were affected women with a history of breast cancer, and 49% had no prior history of breast cancer. All patients underwent skin sparing mastectomies. A considerable portion of BRCA mutation carriers also opted for PBSO, with 57% of unaffected BRCA carriers and 67% of affected BRCA carriers. Following a 4.5-year median follow-up, no primary breast cancers occurred after CPM. One BRCA1 mutation carrier who underwent PBM was found to have metastatic cancer in an axillary node, as well as bone and liver metastases 3.5 years following PBM, suggesting a missed occult primary at the time of her PBM. No additional patients undergoing PBM developed subsequent breast cancer.

Although none of the studies investigating the role of PBM on breast cancer risk reduction are randomized prospective trials, they all demonstrate at least a 90% reduction in breast cancer risk following prophylactic mastectomy. Based on such provocative risk reduction, one would infer a survival benefit directly from PBM in these high risk patients; however, there has been no strong evidence to date. One of the first studies investigating PBM in high risk patients by Hartman and colleagues did confer up to a 94% reduction in the risk of death from breast cancer in both moderate and high risk groups; however, this was calculated based on the probability of breast cancer for each year of follow-up with the breast cancer-relative survival rates from the SEER database [6].

Schrag and colleagues also suggested a gain in life expectancy following prophylactic surgery among women who carry mutations in either BRCA1 or BRCA2; however, their data was calculated based on a Markov decision analysis model. They used available data on the incidence of cancer, prognosis of women with various cancer types, and the efficacy of PBM and PBSO in preventing breast and ovarian cancer to estimate the effects of prophylactic surgery on life expectancy among women with different levels of cancer risk [11]. They compared nine case scenarios based on whether patients underwent immediate prophylactic surgery, delayed prophylactic surgery, or surveillance alone. They assumed all women undergoing PBSO would continue to receive hormone replacement therapy until the age of natural menopause, hypothetically abating any effect PBSO would have on breast cancer prevention. Their results demonstrated, on average, that 30-year-old women who carry BRCA mutations would gain approximately 2.9–5.3 years of life expectancy from PBM and 0.3–1.7 years of life expectancy from PBSO depending on their cumulative risk of cancer, and that the gain in life expectancy from undergoing both prophylactic surgeries was greater than the sum of each procedure alone. In regards to optimal timing for surgery, PBSO could be delayed up to the age of 40 years with little loss of life expectancy. However the overall gain in life expectancy did decline with age, with minimal benefits for women 60 years and older.

Based on the above studies, it is evident that PBM confers over a 90% reduction in breast cancer risk in high risk women; however, there is only a suggested mortality reduction, with the overall gain being greater for younger women, and little benefit on survival for women over the age of 60.

## Prophylactic Bilateral Salpingo-Oophorectomy

The impact of PBSO in regards to breast cancer and ovarian cancer risk reduction has also been well studied (Table 8.2). These studies demonstrate an approximate 50% risk reduction of breast cancer risk following PBSO and up to a 96% risk reduction of gynecologic malignancies following PBSO. The greatest effect of PBSO on both breast and gynecologic malignancies occurs in women less than the age of 50, supporting the use of PBSO as a prophylactic surgery for women soon after childbearing ages.

Rebbeck and colleagues performed one of the first retrospective case–control cohort studies investigating the reduction of breast cancer risk following PBSO in BRCA1 mutation carriers [12]. They included women with BRCA1 mutations who underwent PBSO but had no prior history of breast or ovarian cancer and had not undergone PBM. These women were matched with a control group comprising BRCA1 mutation carriers that had not undergone either PBSO or PBM, had similar date of birth, and were from the same collaborative institution from which the case cohort was ascertained. Following 9 years of postsurgical follow-up, PBSO demonstrated a 47% reduction in the risk of developing breast cancer, which persisted for greater than 10 years after surgery and was not negated by the use of postsurgical hormone replacement therapy. When further analyzing risk reduction based on age, women older than the age of 50 demonstrated little benefit, indicating that the therapeutic benefit of PBSO occurs at earlier ages.

In a later publication, Rebbeck and colleagues investigated the benefit of PBSO for both breast and ovarian cancer risk reduction in both BRCA1 and BRCA2 mutation carriers as compared to matched controls [13]. In the subgroup of 259 women studied for ovarian cancer risk reduction, only 2 (0.8%) cases of papillary serous peritoneal cancer were diagnosed 3.8 and 8.6 years after surgery, as compared to 58 (19.9%) cases in 292 matched controls, leading to an overall ovarian cancer risk reduction of 96%. The mean age of ovarian cancer diagnosis was 50 years of age supporting the role of PBSO as soon as possible after childbearing is completed. In the subgroup of 241 women studied for breast cancer risk reduction, 21 (21.2%) of the 99 patients who underwent PBSO subsequently developed breast cancer, as compared to 60 (42.3%) of the controls, constituting a 53% breast cancer risk reduction.

A prospective study by Kauff and colleagues investigated the prevention of breast and ovarian cancer in women 35 years of age or older with BRCA1 or BRCA2 mutations who underwent PBSO as compared to women who underwent surveillance [14]. With a mean follow-up of 24.2 months, 5 (6.9%) ovarian or primary peritoneal cancers developed in women who elected to undergo surveillance, compared to 1 (1.0%) woman who underwent PBSO. Eight (12.9%) women with breast tissue in the surveillance group developed breast cancer, as compared to 3 (4.3%) women who underwent PBSO. When both breast cancer and ovarian cancer occurrences were analyzed together, a 75% risk reduction of BRCA-related breast or ovarian cancer was found. When analyzed separately, a reduction in both BRCA-related breast and ovarian cancer occurred; however the risk reduction was not statistically significant.

In a more recent prospective study by Kauff and colleagues, the efficacy of PBSO for the prevention of BRCA-associated breast and gynecologic cancer was investigated in women with BRCA1 and BRCA2 mutations independently [15]. Following 33 months of follow-up, 28 (9.5%) women who underwent surveillance developed breast cancer, as compared to 19 (6.3%) women who underwent PBSO, leading to a 47% risk reduction in BRCA-related breast cancer. In BRCA1 mutation carriers, 19 (10.6%) developed a new breast cancer, as compared to 15 (7.9%) women who underwent PBSO, representing a 39% risk reduction in BRCA1 patients. In BRCA2 carriers, 9 (7.8%) patients developed breast cancer in the surveillance group, as compared to 4 (3.5%) breast cancers in the PBSO group, leading to an overall 72% risk reduction in BRCA2 carriers. The larger reduction in breast cancer risk in BRCA2 carriers following PBSO

**Table 8.2** Prophylactic bilateral salpingo-oophorectomy

| | | | | BRCA1 | | BRCA2 | | Risk reduction | |
|---|---|---|---|---|---|---|---|---|---|
| Study | Year | F/U (years) | Patients (*n*) | BSO (%) | Control (%) | BSO (%) | Control (%) | Breast cancer | Gynecologic cancer |
| Rebbeck et al. | 1999 | 9 | 122 | 100 | – | – | – | HR 0.53 (CI, 0.33–0.84) | – |
| Rebbeck et al. | 2002 | 8 | 551 | 84.6 | 82.2 | 16.2 | 18.2 | – | HR 0.04 (CI, 0.01–0.16) |
| Rebbeck et al. | 2002 | 10 | 241 | 83.8 | 85.2 | 18.2 | 14.8 | HR 0.47 (CI, 0.29–0.77) | – |
| Kauff et al. | 2002 | 2 | 170 | 57 | 67 | 43 | 33 | HR 0.32 (CI, 0.08–1.20) | HR 0.15 (CI, 0.02–1.31) |
| Eisen et al. | 2005 | – | 3,295 | 73.6 | 73.6 | 26.4 | 26.4 | OR 0.46 (CI, 0.35–0.62) | – |
| Finch et al. | 2006 | 3.5 | 1,828 | 79 | 70 | 20 | 30 | – | HR 0.20 (CI, 0.07–0.58) |
| Kauff et al. | 2008 | 3 | 1,079 | 63 | 61 | 37 | 39 | HR 0.53 (CI, 0.29–0.96) | HR 0.12 (CI, 0.03–0.41) |

was thought to be related to the higher proportion of ER-positive breast cancers occurring in BRCA2 mutation carriers as compared to BRCA1 carriers.

In regards to BRCA-associated gynecologic cancers, 12 (4.2%) women who underwent surveillance, as compared to 3 (0.6%) women who underwent PBSO developed gynecologic cancers, leading to an 88% risk reduction of BRCA-associated gynecologic cancers following PBSO. When their analysis was limited to BRCA1 carriers, 10 (5.8%) women developed gynecologic cancers in the surveillance group, as compared to 3 (0.9%) in the PBSO group, leading to an 85% overall risk reduction. In BRCA2 carriers, only 2 (1.8%) women developed gynecologic cancer in the surveillance group, with no patients developing cancer in the PBSO group. Risk reduction in BRCA2 carriers did not reach statistical significance related to the low incidence of BRCA2-associated gynecologic cancers. PBSO therefore appears to confer a larger risk reduction in BRCA-associated breast cancer in BRCA2 mutation carriers and a larger risk reduction in BRCA-associated gynecologic cancers in BRCA1 mutation carriers.

Eisen and colleagues performed an international case–control study also investigating the extent of protection offered against BRCA-associated breast cancer following PBSO in BRCA1 and BRCA2 mutation carriers, as well as the affect of age at PBSO [16]. They identified 1,439 matched sets in 3,295 patients, 74% were BRCA1 carriers, 26% were BRCA2 carriers. As compared to the surveillance group, PBSO was associated with a 57% reduction in breast cancer risk in BRCA1 carriers, and a 46% reduction in risk in BRCA2 patients. This protective effect was evident up to 15 years following PBSO. When investigating the effect of age at PBSO, a statistically significant reduction was seen only up to the age of 50 in BRCA1 carriers. There was no clear trend associated with timing of PBSO for BRCA2 carriers likely related to the lower number of BRCA2 carriers in their study, as well as an older age of breast cancer onset in BRCA2 carriers.

In a subsequent prospective case–control cohort study investing the effect of PBSO on BRCA-associated gynecologic malignancies, Finch and colleagues demonstrated an 80% reduction in gynecologic cancer risk in patients undergoing PBSO as compared to surveillance alone [17]. One thousand eight hundred and twenty-eight women were enrolled, with 75.5% BRCA1 mutation carriers, and 24.1% BRCA2 mutation carriers. Eight patients carried both BRCA1 and BRCA2 mutations. Thirty two (4.1%) gynecologic cancers were observed in the surveillance group, 29 (5.3%) in BRCA1 carriers and 3 (1.3%) in BRCA2 mutation carriers, as compared to 7 (1.3%) in women undergoing PBSO, 6 (1.3%) in BRCA1 carriers and 1 (1.0%) in BRCA2 carriers. After adjustment for covariates, there was an 80% reduction in risk of gynecologic cancers associated with PBSO in BRCA carriers.

As demonstrated in the above studies, there is an approximate 50% risk reduction for breast cancer and up to a 96% risk reduction for gynecologic-associated cancer in BRCA mutation carriers who undergo PBSO as compared to surveillance. In subset analysis, it appears that PBSO may confer a larger breast cancer risk reduction in BRCA2 carriers as compared to BRCA1 carriers. This greater risk reduction is likely related to the increased prevalence of ER-positive cancers in BRCA2 mutation carriers as compared to BRCA 1 carriers. On the other hand, it appears from various studies that PBSO may confer a larger gynecologic cancer risk reduction in BRCA1 carriers, which is likely related to an increased prevalence of gynecologic cancers at younger ages in BRCA1 carriers. The greatest reduction in both breast and gynecologic cancers following PBSO is shown to occur at ages less than 50, supporting the use of PBSO for prophylactic surgery soon after a woman's childbearing years.

Does breast and gynecologic cancer risk reduction following PBSO equate to a mortality benefit in these high risk women? Domcheck and colleagues performed a large prospective analysis of over 600 BRCA1 or BRCA2 mutation carriers, with the primary intent to determine whether PBSO improves overall mortality and cancer-specific mortality in these high risk patients [18].

In their matched cohort analysis, results demonstrated a 7% incidence of breast cancer in BRCA carriers following PBSO, as compared to 13% in women undergoing surveillance, leading to a breast cancer risk reduction of 64% following PBSO in BRCA patients. Subsequent mortality analysis demonstrated a statistically significant reduction in overall mortality (HR 0.24), breast cancer-specific mortality (HR 0.10), and gynecologic-specific mortality (HR 0.05) in BRCA carriers. When investigating the association between PBSO and mortality reduction in BRCA1 independent of BRCA2 mutation carriers, a statistically significant reduction in overall, breast cancer-specific, and ovarian cancer-specific mortality reduction was demonstrated in BRCA1 carriers only, likely related to the lack of cancer-specific deaths in BRCA2 mutation carriers who underwent PBSO.

In a more recent multicenter prospective cohort study by Domcheck and colleagues, the relationship of both PBSO and PBM in cancer-specific and overall mortality reduction was investigated in BRCA carriers [19]. Both PBSO and PBM resulted in breast cancer risk reduction. After 3 years follow-up, none of the women undergoing PBM developed breast cancer, while 7% of the surveillance women did. PBSO in both BRCA1 and BRCA2 mutation carriers led to a statistically significant breast cancer risk reduction, with a 37% reduction in BRCA1 carriers and 64% reduction in BRCA2 carriers. Breast cancer risk reduction was only significant in women who underwent PBSO prior to the age of 50. In regards to gynecologic cancer risk reduction, PBSO was associated with risk reduction in BRCA1 mutation carriers only, with a risk reduction of 85% in women with a prior diagnosis of breast cancer, and 69% in women with no prior history of breast cancer. No cases of gynecologic cancer following PBSO were detected in BRCA2 carriers. Furthermore, PBSO was associated with significantly lower all-cause mortality and cancer-specific mortality when all BRCA mutation carriers were combined, with the greatest gain in women younger than the age of 50. However when analyzed independently based on mutation status, all-cause mortality reduction and cancer-specific mortality remained significant only in BRCA1 mutation carriers. This is likely related to the limited number of BRCA2 mutation carriers, as well as fewer events that occurred in BRCA2 mutation carriers.

The above studies demonstrate a significant breast and gynecologic cancer risk reduction, as well as a significant lower cancer-specific mortality and increased overall survival in women who undergo PBSO as compared to women who elect to undergo increased surveillance. Importantly this overall survival benefit and lower cancer-specific mortality was found to occur in women younger than the age of 50, supporting the notion that women who elect to undergo PBSO should do so soon after childbearing years [12, 16, 19]. As mentioned above, when BRCA mutation carriers were independently evaluated based on BRCA1 vs. BRCA2 mutation status, the survival benefit was more significant in BRCA1 carriers. This is most likely related to the lower number of BRCA2 carriers enrolled in the above studies, as well as the overall lower incidence of BRCA-associated cancers occurring at younger ages in BRCA mutation carriers.

When discussing PBSO as a prophylactic option for BRCA mutation carriers, it is important to address concerns regarding premature menopause in premenopausal women. Premature menopause may lead to increased risk of osteoporosis and cardiovascular disease, as well as early symptoms of hot flashes, vaginal dryness, sexual dysfunction, and cognitive dysfunction [16]. It is important to counsel women that the use of short-term hormone replacement therapy appears safe in such women, with studies demonstrating no significant difference in breast risk cancer reduction in women who took short-term HRT following PBSO, as compared to those who did not [20, 21]. Although the data on duration of HRT is not concrete, it appears that women who undergo PBSO in their premenopausal years are safe to take short-term HRT until the age when they would have experienced natural menopause, typically at the age of 50. This allows physicians the ability to prescribe HRT until the natural age of menopause to abate premature menopausal symptoms in women following PBSO.

## Contralateral Prophylactic Mastectomy

In addition to women with strong family histories or known inherited mutations, women with a history of primary breast cancer are also at higher risk of developing a subsequent primary cancer, approximating 1% per year, with some studies demonstrating a risk of contralateral breast cancer (CBC) up to 35% by 16 years after the first breast cancer diagnosis [22]. This risk is higher in women with known BRCA1 or BRCA2 germ line mutations, with up to a 27% risk at 5 years and 43% risk at 10 years depending on the specific mutation and history of endocrine therapy [23]. Due to this increased risk of metachronous cancer, more women are electing to undergo CPM for breast cancer risk reduction. Recent SEER data demonstrates that the use of CPM in the United States has more than doubled from 1998 to 2003, with up to 11% of women undergoing mastectomy for their index cancer electing to undergo concomitant CPM [24].

One of the first studies investigating CBC risk reduction following CPM, was a study by McDonnell and colleagues who retrospectively evaluated women with a family history of breast and/or ovarian cancer who underwent CPM at the time of their therapeutic mastectomy. To determine CBC risk reduction they used the Anderson statistical model calculating risk reduction based on family history and menopausal status [22]. Following a median follow-up of 10 years, only 8 (1.1%) women developed CBC post CPM. Through use of their statistical model, breast cancer risk reduction was up to 96% following CPM which varied slightly based on menopausal status, with a 94.8% reduction in premenopausal women and 96.3% risk reduction in postmenopausal women. The risk reduction was similar regardless of whether adjuvant therapy was used for the woman's primary cancer.

Metcalfe and colleagues looked specifically at CBC risk reduction in BRCA mutation-detected families. Based on their analysis, they determined a 5-year actuarial risk of CBC following the diagnosis of a first breast cancer to be 16.9% in women who saved their contralateral unaffected breast, and a 10-year risk of 29.5%. The 10-year actuarial risk of CBC was shown to be slightly higher for BRCA1 patients, 32%, as compared to BRCA2 patients, 24.5%. With a mean follow-up of 9.2 years, only 1 (0.7%) patient following CPM developed a CBC, as compared to 97 (28.9%) in women who saved their contralateral breast, leading to a 97% overall CBC risk reduction following CPM [23]. They also demonstrated a 59% CBC risk reduction in their patients who underwent PBSO, which was greater for women younger than the age of 50 at time of diagnosis.

Van Sprundel and colleagues also demonstrated a significant CBC risk reduction following CPM in BRCA mutation carriers [25]. After a mean follow-up of 3.4 years, only 1 (1.3%) patient following CPM developed a CBC, whereas 6 (14%) patients undergoing surveillance developed CBC, leading to an overall 91% CBC risk reduction following CPM, independent of the impact of PBSO. A significant overall survival was observed in the CPM groups as compared to the surveillance group; however, this was related to the effect of concomitant PBSO. Women who underwent both CPM and PBSO did demonstrate a better overall and breast cancer-specific survival than either prophylactic surgery alone.

Herrinton and colleagues also demonstrated a protective benefit of CPM on the incidence of CBC, as well as an associated decrease in breast cancer-specific mortality and all-cause mortality [26]. After a median follow-up of 5.7 years, CPM was associated with a 97% reduction in CBC risk. Furthermore, 8.1% of women who underwent CPM died of breast cancer as compared to 11.7% of women who did not, representing a 43% risk reduction in breast cancer-specific death. On further analysis, the CPM cohort did have a lower all-cause mortality suggesting a possible of selection bias for overall healthier patients undergoing CPM. CPM was also less effective against preventing subsequent distant metastasis, leading to a larger effect of CBC risk reduction than expected mortality reduction.

Boughey and colleagues also investigated the effect of CPM on recurrence and survival in high risk women with Stage I and II breast cancer [27]. High risk women were defined as any woman with history of either first- or second-degree relative. Their control cohort was matched on age of breast cancer diagnosis, year of diagnosis, tumor stage, and nodal status. After a median follow-up of 17.3 years, 2 (0.5%) patients developed a CBC in the CPM cohort as compared to 31 (8.1%) patients who did not undergo CPM, representing a 95% risk reduction of CBC. Reduction in CBC risk remained statistically significant after adjustment for age, stage, nodal status, and first-degree family history. Ten-year overall survival estimates for CPM vs. Patients undergoing only therapeutic mastectomy were 83% vs. 74%, with a 22% overall survival benefit for patients undergoing CPM. A disease-free survival benefit of 34% was also seen in women who underwent CPM. There was also a trend towards improved breast cancer-specific survival in women undergoing CPM.

In a recent large population-based study on data from the SEER registry, Bedrosian and colleagues investigated the utility of CPM on breast cancer-specific survival, with further analyses based on age, disease stage, and ER status [28]. Of 311,643 cases of breast cancer diagnosed in the 6-year study period, 107,106 women underwent mastectomy for the treatment of unilateral breast cancer. Eight thousand nine hundred and two (8.3%) underwent CPM. As compared to non-CPM patients, CPM patients were significantly younger and had earlier-stage disease. In a univariate analysis, CPM was associated with improved disease-specific survival for women with stages I-III, with an overall 47% improvement in disease-specific survival. Additional variables associated with disease-specific survival were disease stage, lymph node status, tumor grade, ER status, race, histology, and age, all of which remained statistically significant following multivariate analysis. To determine the role of selection bias for healthier women, they found that cancer-specific survival associated with CPM declined with age, with women older than 60 years having no risk reduction from CPM, which was likely related to a strong association between CPM and non-cancer causes of death in women older than 60. Among younger women, there was no association between CPM and non-cancer causes of death.

In a subset analysis investigating age, disease stage, and ER status, they demonstrated that patients diagnosed before the age of 50 years with stage I or II ER-negative breast cancer had a significant reduction in the risk of disease-specific mortality, with a risk reduction of 47%, accounting for a 4.8% increase in 5-year adjusted breast cancer-specific survival favoring CPM. This was not seen in early-stage ER-positive breast cancers in young women. Among women between the ages of 50 and 59, CPM was associated with improved breast cancer-specific survival for women who had early-stage ER-negative disease and those with later-stage ER-positive disease. No reduction in breast cancer-specific death was associated with CPM in women older than 60 years of age. As illustrated by Bedrosian and colleagues, these results may be related to the larger absolute lifetime risk of metachronous CBC combined with the low probability of competing causes of death in younger women. Furthermore the role of endocrine therapy in reducing subsequent breast cancer may have a role in the decreased effects of CPM in younger women with ER+ disease. In addition, no survival benefit was seen amongst women who underwent CPM for DCIS, pure lobular cancers, or locally advanced (stage III) disease.

Overall, the above studies demonstrate up to a 97% risk reduction of CBC in women who undergo CPM as compared to women who save their unaffected breast. This risk reduction has been shown to confer a survival benefit that seems to be affected by selection bias of healthier women who undergo for CPM. However, based on the SEER database study by Bedrosian and colleagues there may be a subset of women for which CPM would provide the greatest survival benefit, consisting of young women with early stage ER-negative disease (Table 8.3).

**Table 8.3** Surgical strategies for risk reduction

| Surgical strategies for risk reduction |
|---|
| Prophylactic bilateral mastectomy (PBM)<br>• PBM has been shown to confer over a 90% breast cancer risk reduction in women at moderate to high risk based on family history alone<br>• Subset analysis of BRCA mutation carriers continues to demonstrate a 85–100% breast cancer risk reduction following PBM<br>• No strong evidence exists to date regarding an associated mortality benefit from breast cancer risk reduction following PBM; however, analytic decision models do suggest a gain of 2.9–5.3 years of life in BRCA mutation carriers |
| Prophylactic bilateral salpingo-oophorectomy (PBSO)<br>• A 47–68% breast cancer risk reduction is demonstrated following PBSO, with a 80–96% gynecologic cancer risk reduction in BRCA mutation carriers<br>• The greatest breast cancer and gynecologic cancer risk reduction occurred in BRCA women younger than the age of 50 years, supporting the use of PBSO soon after childbearing years<br>• A significant reduction in overall mortality, breast cancer-specific mortality, and gynecologic cancer-specific mortality is demonstrated following PBSO alone or in combination with PBM in BRCA mutation carriers<br>• In subset analysis investigating BRCA 1 and BRCA 2 mutation carriers independently, survival benefit was only statistically significant in BRCA 1 carriers, likely related to the limited number of BRCA 2 carriers in the studies, as well as the fewer cancer events that occurred in BRCA 2 mutation carriers as compared to BRCA1 carriers<br>• Similar to cancer-specific risk reduction, mortality benefit following PBSO was found to be significant only in women younger than the age of 50 years |
| Contralateral prophylactic mastectomy (CPM)<br>• A 91–97% contralateral breast cancer (CBC) risk reduction has been shown to occur in women undergoing CPM during the treatment of their index cancer<br>• Several studies suggest an overall and breast cancer-specific survival benefit following CPM; however, concern exists for selection bias for younger healthier women electing to undergo CPM<br>• In subset analysis of a large SEER registry study, young women with ER-negative tumors may demonstrate the greatest survival benefit due to the inability of the use of endocrine agents<br>• No survival benefit following CPM is demonstrated in women undergoing CPM for DCIS, pure lobular cancers, locally advanced disease, as well as women over the age of 60 |

## Nipple Sparing Mastectomy for Risk Reduction and Cancer Treatment

Based on the above studies, both PBM as well as CPM provide significant breast cancer risk reduction in patients undergoing both prophylactic and therapeutic surgery. However, what surgery is the best oncologic option for these patients? Over the past few years, NSM has resurfaced as a surgical option due to tighter selection criteria and advanced reconstructive options. NSM is a mastectomy technique similar to skin sparing mastectomy (SSM), however unlike SSM, NSM preserves the nipple areola complex with a small amount of retroareolar tissue. From an aesthetic standpoint, nipple areola complex preservation is thought to maintain the aesthetic integrity of the women's breast, by preserving the most symbolic component—the nipple and areola. However from an oncologic standpoint, preserving the nipple areola complex leaves the theoretical potential for occult cancer in a clinically negative nipple as well as the potential for future cancer to occur. This risk is thought to be heightened in high risk women undergoing prophylactic surgery due to their predilection for cancer, which is emphasized by Hartmann and Rebbeck's earlier studies demonstrating in-breast recurrences to only occur in women who underwent NSM as compared to total mastectomy [6, 9].

### Occult Nipple Involvement

Numerous studies supporting the safety of NSM for both therapeutic and prophylactic mastectomy arise from studies investigating the incidence of occult nipple involvement in mastectomy specimens. In a recent study, Reynolds and colleagues investigated both the presence of terminal duct lobular units (TDLUs) in the nipple as well as the incidence of premalignant and malignant lesions within the NACs of BRCA carriers [29]. Sixty-two therapeutic and prophylactic mastectomy specimens from 33 BRCA mutation carriers were sectioned and microscopically examined. Seventy-six percent of women were BRCA1 mutation carriers, while 24% were BRCA2 carriers. Twenty-eight women (85%) underwent therapeutic mastectomy, and 82% underwent concomitant CPM. Five women (15%) underwent PBM for risk reduction. Interestingly only 24% of mastectomy specimens demonstrated TDLUs in the NAC, the majority of which were in the retroareolar tissue, with only 5 (8%) specimens demonstrating TDLUs in the nipple papilla alone. There was no evidence of premalignant or invasive cancer found in the 33 NACs of prophylactic mastectomies, including both CPM and PBM specimens. Of the 29 therapeutic mastectomies, only 1 (3.5%) NAC demonstrated invasive cancer, 1 (3.5%) demonstrated DCIS, and 1 (3.5%) demonstrated atypical lobular hyperplasia.

Brachtel and colleagues then investigated clinicopathologic characteristics predictive of NAC involvement [30]. Three hundred and sixteen mastectomy specimens, 232 therapeutic and 84 prophylactic, were sectioned and analyzed. Thirty-eight percent of patients were known BRCA mutation carriers. None of the prophylactic mastectomy specimens contained invasive carcinoma or DCIS, although 5% were positive for LCIS. Twenty-one percent of the 232 therapeutic mastectomy specimens contained pathologic findings of DCIS (62%), IDC (<10%), ILC (<10%), and lymphovascular invasion (<20%). On multivariate analysis, tumor size, tumor-nipple distance, and HER2-Neu amplification were predictive of NAC involvement. No statistical correlation was found with BRCA mutation status. Furthermore they demonstrated an 80% sensitivity and 96% negative predictive value of retroareolar biopsy in determining nipple involvement.

One of the most recent and largest studies by Li and colleagues examined 2,323 mastectomy specimens to determine the frequency of occult NAC involvement as well as to identify clinicopathologic features predictive of occult NAC involvement [31]. Two hundred and forty-eight (10.7%) mastectomy specimens demonstrated occult nipple involvement, with more than half of the involved nipples occurring only at the base of the nipple margin. Only 5% of all involved nipples had a negative base with involved papillae or skin. Of the 248 involved nipples, 56.5% were DCIS only, 29.4% were invasive cancer, 3.2% LVI only, and 1.6% LCIS. Seventy-eight percent of the index cancers with occult nipple involvement were IDC or IDC accompanied with DCIS. On multivariate analysis, tumor size, tumor-to-nipple distance, central tumor location, multicentricity or multifocality, as well as lymph node involvement, LVI, and HER2-Neu amplification were statistical predictors of occult nipple involvement.

The above studies demonstrate a higher likelihood of NAC involvement in therapeutic mastectomy specimens as compared to prophylactic specimens, with both Reynolds and Brachtel demonstrating a 0% incidence of malignant or premalignant pathology involving the nipple base in prophylactic mastectomy specimens [29, 30]. In regards to therapeutic mastectomies, the likelihood of NAC involvement was as high as 21%, which was affected by factors such as tumor size, tumor-to-nipple distance, multicentricity, higher stage cancers, LVI, and the presence of HER2-Neu amplification, demonstrating the importance of patient selection in nipple areola preservation [31].

## Oncologic Safety of Nipple Sparing Mastectomy

On a clinical note, numerous single-institution studies with at least 5 years of follow-up have demonstrated oncologic safety in terms of acceptable local, regional, and distant recurrence rates, as well as favorable 5-year overall survival in patients undergoing NSM [32–37] (Table 8.4). One of the largest studies with longest follow-up was published by Benediktsson and colleagues, with a median follow-up of 13.4 years [33]. Although they demonstrated one of the highest overall locoregional recurrence rates of 24.1%, 0% of their recurrences occurred at the NAC. High local recurrence rates were likely related to their patient population, in which over 50% of their patients had Stage II or Stage III disease with up to 40% having axillary node involvement. Furthermore, following subgroup analysis of patients who received adjuvant radiotherapy, the locoregional recurrence rate was decreased to 8.5% after 13 years.

**Table 8.4** Nipple sparing mastectomy (NSM)

| Study | Year | Patients (*n*) | F/U (years) | NAC recurrence (%) | Locoregional recurrence (%) | Distant recurrence (%) | Post-op XRT (%) | Stage II/III (%) | Five-year overall survival (%) |
|---|---|---|---|---|---|---|---|---|---|
| Caruso et al. | 2006 | 56 | 5.5 | 2 | 2 | 10 | 0 | 38 | 92 |
| Benediktsson et al. | 2008 | 216 | 13 | 0 | 24.1 | 20.3 | 21.8 | 53.2 | 76.4 |
| Gerber et al. | 2009 | 238 | 8.4 | 1.6 | 13.4 | 23.3 | 27 | 81 | 76.6 |
| Kim et al. | 2010 | 520 | 5.5 | 1.3 | 2.0 | – | 5.3 | 41.5 | 97.1 |
| Lim et al. | 2010 | 897 | 5.2 | – | 4.6 | – | 56.3 | 100 | 79.4 |
| Jensen et al. | 2011 | 99 | 5 | 0 | 0 | 0 | 16 | 36.4 | 100 |

**Table 8.5** Oncologic safety of nipple sparing mastectomy

- A 10–20% incidence of occult nipple areola complex (NAC) involvement has been demonstrated in women undergoing therapeutic mastectomy, with a 0% incidence of occult nipple involvement in women undergoing prophylactic mastectomy for risk reduction
- Clinicopathologic factors related to increased NAC involvement are larger tumor size, shorter tumor-to-nipple distance, central tumor location, tumor multicentricity or multifocality, presence of lymph node involvement, as well as HER2-neu amplification
- Clinical studies demonstrate locoregional recurrences to occur in 0–24% of women undergoing NSM for breast cancer treatment, with NAC recurrences only as high as 1.6%
- Intra-operative retroareolar tissue biopsy is recommended with studies demonstrating a 80% sensitivity and 96% negative predictive value of retroareolar biopsy in determining NAC involvement

A second series published by Gerber and colleagues compared 246 patients who underwent MRM, SSM, or NSM, with an average follow-up of 8.4 years [34]. Each surgical group was statistically equivalent in terms of multicentricity, AJCC staging, axillary involvement, tumor grade, as well as pre- and postoperative systemic and radiotherapy. Their results demonstrated no significant differences in locoregional recurrences, isolated distant metastases, or breast cancer-specific death. Their locoregional recurrence rates for MRM, SSM, and NSM were 14.6, 12.5, and 13.4%, respectively, with only a 1.6% incidence of NAC recurrence in their NSM patients. Of more recent studies with a minimum 5-year median follow-up, local recurrence rates ranged from 0 to 5%, with NAC recurrence rates ranging from 0 to 1.3% [35–37].

A recent study by Filho and colleagues investigated the use of NSM for both prophylactic and oncologic purposes in high risk women [38]. Fifty six percent were for breast cancer risk reduction, as compared to 44% for therapeutic mastectomies. NSM was offered as a therapeutic option to patients with clinically negative axillas, tumors less than 3 cm, and a tumor-to-nipple distance of at least 1 cm. Approximately 20% of their patients were known BRCA mutation carriers, with 70% of their patients having a positive family history. Although with a limited median follow-up of 10.4 months, there were no reported local or NAC recurrences.

Based on the above studies, NSM for prophylactic surgery appears to be oncologically safe in regards to the low probability of occult nipple involvement, as well as the acceptable recurrence rate and overall survival. Additional long-term follow-up in high risk patients would be helpful in fully elucidating the clinical outcomes in such patients. NSM for therapeutic surgery also appears safe; however, appropriate patient selection appears to be paramount and the use of intra-operative frozen section of retroareolar tissue is recommended (Table 8.5).

## Role of Sentinel Lymph Node Biopsy in Prophylactic Mastectomy

SLNB in the setting of prophylactic mastectomy currently is not standard of care, although the use of SLNB has been demonstrated to occur in up to 85% of patients undergoing CPM based solely on surgeon preference [39]. Many surgeons fear the need to perform staging axillary lymph node dissection (ALND) in patients found to have occult invasive malignancies in their prophylactic specimens, when an axillary dissection potentially could have been prevented with a negative SLNB. Although some institutions do report the utility of SLNB following mastectomy, the overall accuracy is unknown [40]. Although postsurgical complications following ALND are reported in up to 70% of patients, SLNB is also not without risk, with recent data from prospective randomized trials demonstrating up to a 25% postoperative complication rate following SLNB alone, which includes up to an 8% risk of lymphedema at 6 months [41]. Furthermore the incidence of an occult invasive cancer in prophylactic specimens is reportedly low. Both Hartmann and colleagues, as well as Heemskerk-Gerritsen and colleagues demonstrated a <1% incidence of occult invasive cancer in their prophylactic mastectomy specimens of high risk women undergoing PBM [6, 10].

Since then numerous retrospective studies have investigated the role of SLNB for prophylactic surgery [42–48] (Table 8.6). The incidence

**Table 8.6** Sentinel lymph node biopsy

| | | | | | | Mastectomy specimen | | Contralateral SLNB |
|---|---|---|---|---|---|---|---|---|
| Study | Year | Study design | Patients ($n$) | BRCA (%) | Family history + (%) | Invasive cancer (%) | DCIS (%) | Positive (%) |
| Dupont et al. | 2000 | Prospective | 57 | – | – | 3.5 | 0 | 3.5 |
| Boughey et al. | 2006 | Retrospective | 409 | 5.6 | 57 | 1.8 | 3.2 | 1.9 |
| Black et al. | 2007 | Retrospective | 173 | 17.0 | 52.6 | 2.6 | 7.3 | 3.6 |
| Soran et al. | 2007 | Retrospective | 155 | 7 | 52.3 | 1.3 | 1.9 | 1.3 |
| McLaughlin et al. | 2008 | Retrospective | 529 | 9.3 | 59 | 1.6 | 3.8 | 2 |
| Laronga et al. | 2009 | Retrospective | 449 | – | 53.2 | 1.4 | 2.9 | 2 |
| Nasser et al. | 2010 | Retrospective | 99 | – | 48.5 | 2 | 6 | 2 |
| Czyszczon et al. | 2011 | Retrospective | 184 | 6 | 6 | 1 | 5 | 1.3 |

**Table 8.7** Role of sentinel lymph node biopsy (SLNB) in risk reducing surgery

- The incidence of occult invasive carcinoma found in prophylactic mastectomy is low, occurring in less than 3.5% of women undergoing PBM
- When calculating the total benefit rate of sentinel lymph node biopsy based on the number of negative sentinel lymph nodes when occult cancer is found and the number of positive sentinel lymph nodes when no cancer is found, the benefit rate is only 2.8%—in turn not supporting the use of routine SLNB during prophylactic surgery
- Some studies investigating sentinel lymph node biopsy in CPM also demonstrate an increased risk of cross metastasis to contralateral sentinel nodes, questioning the utility of routine SLNB in this subset of patients

of occult invasive carcinoma in prophylactic specimens has been shown to occur between 1 and 3.5% of the time. Furthermore the majority of occult disease if found, is typically in situ disease. In a recent meta-analysis incorporating 1,251 patients undergoing routine SLNB in 1,343 prophylactic mastectomies from 6 retrospective studies, occult invasive cancer was found in 21 specimens, representing an occult invasive cancer rate of only 1.7% [49]. Of these 21 cases, only 4 cases had positive SLNs, therefore only 17 patients of 1,343 pooled prophylactic mastectomies were able to avoid potential ALND. Eighteen cases demonstrated positive SLNs where no occult cancer was identified. A total benefit rate of SLNB was calculated, which was defined as the number of negative SLNs at the time of prophylactic mastectomy in cases with occult cancer plus the number of positive SLNs at the time of prophylactic mastectomy in cases where no invasive cancer was identified divided by the number of prophylactic mastectomies. The overall benefit rate was 2.8%.

Although Zhou and colleagues demonstrated only an overall 2.8% benefit rate, is there a patient population that would benefit from routine SLNB? Of the studies reviewed, the majority demonstrate a higher incidence of occult cancer in CPM specimens for known index cancers as compared to PBM for risk reduction. Therefore patients undergoing PBM for risk reduction may not be suitable candidates for routine SLNB. However in CPM patients, clinicopathologic factors have been identified as predictive in both contralateral occult disease as well as contralateral sentinel lymph node involvement. Boughey and colleagues demonstrated postmenopausal status, age over 60 years, or history of either ILC or LCIS to be predictive of contralateral occult disease. They did not demonstrate BRCA mutation status to be a predictive variable [43]. Laronga and colleagues found that larger index cancer size, ipsilateral nodal metastases, higher index tumor grade, skin and nipple involvement, and LVI did play independent roles in contralateral nodal involvement in the absence of contralateral occult disease [46]. This was true in 6 of the 8 studies and likely represented cross metastasis from locally advanced or inflammatory index cancers, as well as patients undergoing delayed CPM in the face of an ipsilateral recurrence with prior axillary dissection. Such clinicopathologic characteristics may be helpful in patient selection for SLNB in patients undergoing CPM [39, 43, 44, 46–48] (Table 8.7).

## Conclusion

The decision to undergo prophylactic surgery for risk reduction remains complex. Although prospective randomized clinical trials would be ideal to truly evaluate the efficacy of prophylactic surgeries on risk reduction and survival, these studies would be difficult for accrual and would take years of follow-up. Based on numerous prospective and retrospective studies, PBM, PBSO, as well as CPM demonstrate significant cancer-specific risk reduction. Although only analytical models demonstrate expected survival benefit for patients undergoing PBM, stronger retrospective and prospective studies demonstrate an overall survival and cancer-specific survival in younger women undergoing PBSO. Furthermore, a recent population-based analysis demonstrates a potential survival benefit in younger patients with

ER-negative tumors undergoing CPM. In regards to type of prophylactic surgery, total mastectomy, SSM, and NSM all appear to be safe options for prophylactic surgery. Patient selection remains imperative for NSM decision in patients undergoing NSM for therapeutic mastectomy, with tumor characteristics and anatomical factors of clinical importance. Whereas the routine use of SLNB is not fully supported based on the available literature, the use of SLNB in selected patients undergoing CPM may appear clinically appropriate, such as patient with locally advanced index cancers.

## References


1. Howlader N, Noone AM, Krapcho M, et al. SEER Cancer Statistics Review, 1975–2008. Bethesda, MD: National Cancer Institute. http://seer.cancer.gov/csr/1975_2008/, based on November 2010 SEER data submission, posted to the SEER web site, 2011.
2. Antoniou A, Pharoah PDP, Arod S, et al. Average risks of breast and ovarian cancer associated with BRCA1 or BRCA2 mutations detected in case series unselected for family history: a combined analysis of 22 studies. Am J Hum Genet. 2003;72:1117.
3. Verhoog LC, Brekelmans CTM, Seynaeve C, et al. Survival and tumour characteristics of breast-cancer patients with germline mutations of BRCA1. Lancet. 1998;351:316–21.
4. Verhoog LC, Brekelmans CTM, Seynaeve C. Survival in hereditary breast cancer associated with germline mutations of BRCA2. J Clin Oncol. 1999;17: 3396–402.
5. King MC, Wieand S, Hale K, et al. Tamoxifen and breast cancer incidence among women with inherited mutations in BRCA1 and BRCA2: National Surgical Adjuvant Breast and Bowel Project (NSABP-P1) Breast Cancer Prevention Trial. JAMA. 2001;286:2251–6.
6. Hartmann LC, Schaid DJ, Woods JE, et al. Efficacy of bilateral prophylactic mastectomy in women with a family history of breast cancer. N Engl J Med. 1999;340:77–84.
7. Hartmann LC, Sellers TA, Schaid DJ, et al. Efficacy of bilateral prophylactic mastectomy in BRCA1 and BRCA2 gene mutation carriers. J Natl Cancer Inst. 2001;93:1633–7.
8. Meijers-Heijboer H, van Geel B, van Putten WLJ, et al. Breast cancer after prophylactic bilateral mastectomy in women with a BRCA1 or BRCA2 mutation. N Engl J Med. 2001;345:159–64.
9. Rebbeck TR, Friebel T, Lynch H, et al. Bilateral prophylactic mastectomy reduces breast cancer risk in BRCA1 and BRCA2 mutation carriers: the PROSE study group. J Clin Oncol. 2004;22:1055–62.
10. Heemskerek-Gerritsen BAM, Brekelmans CTM, Menke-Pluymers MBE, et al. Prophylactic mastectomy in BRCA1/2 mutation carriers and women at risk of Hereditary Breast Cancer: long-term experiences at the Rotterdam Family Cancer Center. Ann Surg Oncol. 2007;14:3335–44.
11. Schrag D, Kuntz KM, Garber JE, et al. Decision analysis-effects of prophylactic mastectomy and oophorectomy on life expectancy among women with BRCA1 or BRCA2 mutations. N Eng J Med. 1997;336:1465–71.
12. Rebbeck TR, Levin AM, Eisen A, et al. Breast cancer risk after bilateral prophylactic oophorectomy in BRCA1 mutation carriers. J Natl Cancer Inst. 1999;91:1475–9.
13. Rebbeck TR, Lynch HT, Neuhausen SL, et al. Prophylactic oophorectomy in carriers of BRCA1 or BRCA2 mutation. N Engl J Med. 2002;346:1616–22.
14. Kauff ND, Satagopan JM, Robson ME, et al. Risk-reducing salpingo-oophorectomy in women with BRCA1 or BRCA2 mutation. N Engl J Med. 2002;346:1609–15.
15. Kauff ND, Domcheck SM, Friebel TM, et al. Risk-reducing salpingo-oophorectomy for the prevention of BRCA1- and BRCA2- associated breast and gynecologic cancer: a multicenter, prospective study. J Clin Oncol. 2008;26:1331–7.
16. Eisen A, Lubinski J, Klijn J, et al. Breast cancer risk following bilateral oophorectomy in BRCA1 and BRCA2 mutation carriers: an international case–control study. J Clin Oncol. 2005;23:7491–6.
17. Finch A, Beiner M, Lubinski J, et al. Salpingo-oophorectomy and the risk of ovarian, fallopian tube, and peritoneal cancers in women with a BRCA1 or BRCA2 mutation. JAMA. 2006;296:185–92.
18. Domcheck SM, Friebel TM, Neuhausen SL, et al. Mortality after bilateral salpingo-oophorectomy in BRCA1 and BRCA2 mutation carriers: a prospective cohort study. Lancet Oncol. 2006;7:223–9.
19. Domcheck SM, Friebel TM, Singer CF, et al. Association of risk-reducing surgery in BRCA1 or BRCA2 mutation carriers with cancer risk and mortality. JAMA. 2010;304:967–75.
20. Rossouw JE, Prentice RL, Manson JE, et al. Postmenopausal hormone therapy and risk of cardiovascular disease by age and years since menopause. JAMA. 2007;297:1465–77.
21. Rebbeck TR, Friebel T, Wagner T, et al. Effect of short-term hormone replacement therapy on breast cancer risk reduction after bilateral prophylactic oophorectomy in BRCA1 and BRCA2 mutation carriers: the PROSE study group. J Clin Oncol. 2005;23:7804–10.
22. McDonnell SK, Schaid DJ, Myers JL, et al. Efficacy of contralateral prophylactic mastectomy in women with a personal and family history of breast cancer. J Clin Oncol. 2001;19:3938–43.
23. Metcalfe K, Lynch HT, Ghadirian P, et al. Contralateral breast cancer in BRCA1 and BRCA2 mutation carriers. J Clin Oncol. 2004;22:2328–35.
24. Tuttle TM, Habermann EB, Grund EH, et al. Increasing use of contralateral prophylactic mastectomy for breast cancer patients: a trend toward more aggressive surgical treatment. J Clin Oncol. 2007;25:5203–8.

25. Van Sprundel TC, Schmidt MK, Rookus MA, et al. Risk reduction of contralateral breast cancer and survival after contralateral prophylactic mastectomy in BRCA1 or BRCA2 mutation carriers. Br J Cancer. 2005;93:287–92.
26. Herrinton LJ, Barlow WE, Yu O, et al. Efficacy of prophylactic mastectomy in women with unilateral breast cancer: a cancer research network project. J Clin Oncol. 2005;23:4275–86.
27. Boughey JC, Hoskin TL, Degnim AC, et al. Contralateral prophylactic mastectomy is associated with a survival advantage in high-risk women with a personal history of breast cancer. Ann Surg Oncol. 2010;17:2702–9.
28. Bedrosian I, Hu CY, Chang GJ. Population-based study of contralateral prophylactic mastectomy and survival outcomes of breast cancer patients. J Natl Cancer Inst. 2010;102:401–9.
29. Reynolds C, Davidson JA, Lindor NM, et al. Prophylactic and therapeutic mastectomy in BRCA mutation carriers: can the nipple be preserved? Ann Surg Oncol. 2011;18:3102–9.
30. Brachtel EF, Rusby JE, Michaelson JS, et al. Occult nipple involvement in breast cancer: clinicopathologic findings in 316 consecutive mastectomy specimens. J Clin Oncol. 2009;27:4948–54.
31. Li W, Wang S, Guo X, et al. Nipple involvement in breast cancer: retrospective analysis of 2323 consecutive mastectomy specimens. Int J Surg Pathol. 2011;19:328–34.
32. Caruso F, Ferrara M, Castiglione G, et al. Nipple sparing subcutaneous mastectomy: sixty-six months follow-up. Eur J Surg Oncol. 2006;32:937–40.
33. Benediktsson KP, Perbeck L. Survival in breast cancer after nipple sparing subcutaneous mastectomy in immediate reconstruction with implants: a prospective trial with 13 years median follow-up in 216 patients. Eur J Surg Oncol. 2008;34:143–8.
34. Gerber B, Krause A, Dieterich M, et al. The oncological safety of skin paring mastectomy with conservation of the nipple-aerola complex and autologous reconstruction: an extended follow-up study. Ann Surg. 2009;249:461–8.
35. Kim HJ, Park EH, Lim WS, et al. Nipple areola skin-sparing mastectomy with immediate transverse rectus abdominis musculocutaenous flap reconstruction is an oncologically safe procedure: a single center study. Ann Surg. 2010;251(3):493–8.
36. Lim W, Ko BS, Kim HJ, et al. Oncological safety of skin sparing mastectomy followed by immediate reconstruction for locally advanced breast cancer. J Surg Oncol. 2010;102:39–42.
37. Jensen JA, Orringer JS, Guiliano AE. Nipple-sparing mastectomy in 99 patients with a mean follow-up of 5 years. Ann Surg Oncol. 2011;18:1665–70.
38. Filho PA, Capko D, Barry J, et al. Nipple-sparing mastectomy for breast cancer risk-reducing surgery: The Memorial Sloan-Kettering Cancer Center experience. Ann Surg Oncol. 2011;18:3117–22.
39. Soran A, Falk J, Bonaventura M, et al. Is routine sentinel lymph node biopsy indicated in women undergoing contralateral prophylactic mastectomy: Magee-Womens hospital experience. Ann Surg Oncol. 2007;14:646–51.
40. Karam A, Stempel M, Cody HS, et al. Reoperative sentinel lymph node biopsy after previous mastectomy. J Am Coll Surg. 2008;207:543–8.
41. Lucci A, McCall LM, Beitsch PD, et al. Surgical complications associated with sentinel lymph node dissection (SLND) plus axillary lymph node dissection compared with SLND alone in the American College of Surgeons Oncology Group Trial Z0011. J Clin Oncol. 2007;25:3657–63.
42. Dupont EL, Kuhn MA, Mcann C, et al. The role of sentinel lymph node biopsy in women undergoing prophylactic mastectomy. Am J Surg. 2000;180:274–7.
43. Boughey JC, Khakpour N, Meric-Bernstam F, et al. Selective use of sentinel lymph node surgery during prophylactic mastectomy. Cancer. 2006;107:1440–7.
44. Black D, Specht M, Lee JM. Detecting occult malignancy in prophylactic mastectomy: preoperative MRI versus sentinel lymph node biopsy. Ann Surg Oncol. 2007;14:2477–84.
45. McLaughlin SA, Stempel M, Morris EA, et al. Can magnetic resonance imaging be used to select patients for sentinel lymph node biopsy in prophylactic mastectomy? Cancer. 2008;112:1214–21.
46. Laronga C, Lee MC, McGuire KP. Indications for sentinel lymph node biopsy in the setting of prophylactic mastectomy. J Am Coll Surg. 2009;209:746–52.
47. Nasser SM, Smith SG, Chagpar AB. The role of sentinel node biopsy in women undergoing prophylactic mastectomy. J Surg Res. 2010;164:188–92.
48. Czyszczon IA, Roland L, Sahoo S. Routine prophylactic sentinel lymph node biopsy is not indicated in women undergoing prophylactic mastectomy. J Surg Oncol. 2012;105:650–4.
49. Zhou WB, Liu XA, Dai JC, et al. Meta-analysis of sentinel lymph node biopsy at the time of prophylactic mastectomy of the breast. Can J Surg. 2011;54:300–6.

# 9 Options and Advances in Breast Reconstruction

John Y.S. Kim, Vinay Rawlani, and Jennifer E. Cheesborough

## Introduction

Women at high risk for developing breast cancer are increasingly turning to risk reduction surgery, and the majority of these women will pursue breast reconstruction. Therefore, to fully understand the surgical management of high-risk women, one must be aware of the reconstructive options available including prosthetic and autologous modalities. Each of these procedures has distinct advantages and disadvantages, which are discussed in the following chapter. The key aspects of these procedures and their outcomes are also reviewed.

## Introduction to the High-Risk Patient

For women in the United States, the lifetime risk for developing breast cancer is 12.2% [1]. There are also women who carry a heightened risk of developing cancer. These include women with a strong family history of breast cancer, a BRCA1 or BRCA2 mutation, in situ breast cancer, and atypia. Approximately 5–19% of women have a strong family history of breast cancer [2]. Additionally, 1 in 400 women in the general population are carriers of the BRCA mutation, 1 in 40 women of Ashkenazi Jewish decent are carriers of the BRCA mutation, and 0.4% of women have known breast cancer in situ [3]. Prophylactic risk reduction mastectomy serves to reduce the chance of developing breast cancer in these "high-risk" patients. Data shows that the risk of breast cancer can be reduced by 90% with bilateral prophylactic mastectomy (BPM) and up to 95% when combined with prophylactic oophorectomy [4, 5].

While breast reconstruction rates after BPM vary from 60 to 92%, the increasing incidence of risk reduction breast surgery will ultimately lead to a heightened utilization of reconstructive techniques [6, 7]. These patients comprise a unique, typically younger group of women undergoing breast reconstruction. Although satisfaction rates for BPM and subsequent reconstruction fall between 70 [8] and 100% [9], these patients have greater reconstructive expectations than their counterparts undergoing therapeutic mastectomy [10]. Nearly all high-risk patients will have questions prior to surgery; however, 69% of these concerns are related to reconstruction rather than oncologic issues [10]. Therefore, understanding of the approach to the high-risk patient cannot be complete without knowledge of the reconstructive options available for these patients.

J.Y.S. Kim, M.D. (✉) • V. Rawlani, M.D. • J.E. Cheesborough, M.D.
Division of Plastic and Reconstructive Surgery, Northwestern Memorial Hospital, 675 North St Clair, Suite 19-250, Chicago, IL, USA
e-mail: jokim@nmh.org

N.M. Hansen (ed.), *Management of the Patient at High Risk for Breast Cancer*,
DOI 10.1007/978-1-4614-5891-3_9, 

## Reconstructive Goals and Limitations

For all breast reconstruction patients, the goal of surgery is to restore *reasonable* shape, volume, and symmetry of the breasts. These factors have been associated with improved self-image and self-confidence in women undergoing mastectomy reconstruction [11–15]. Traditionally, the ability to restore breast volume, shape, and symmetry relies on suitable preservation and rearrangement of skin and appropriate substitution of volume. Whether the volume replacement is in the form of an implant or autologous tissue rearrangement, the key is to provide sufficient bulk and position the volume in an aesthetic fashion. In the high-risk population, there is one additional factor that has a dramatic effect on reconstructive outcomes: *whether or not the nipple can be spared*. Preserving the nipple can significantly impact overall aesthetic outcomes [16, 17].

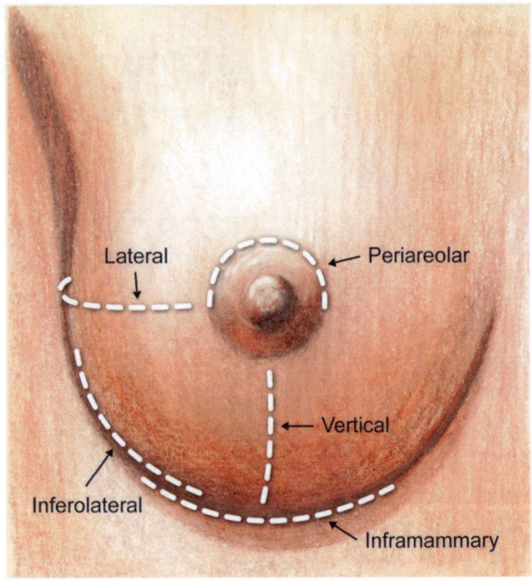


**Fig. 9.1** Schematic drawing of common nipple sparing mastectomy (NSM) incisions. Several incision patterns have been proposed for the NSM. The periareolar, lateral, and inframammary incisions are the most common. Incision designs require balancing effects on exposure vs. nipple viability. Note that the periareolar incision alone directly limits radial blood flow to the nipple and therefore is not recommended. The inferolateral incision is a modification of the inframammary incision and allows better access to the upper outer quadrant

## Reconstructive Planning: Nipple Sparing Mastectomy

The oncologic indications for nipple sparing mastectomy (NSM) are broadening. In general, NSM is considered for all high-risk patients and most cancer patients with T0 to T2 tumors smaller than 4.5 cm in size, further than 2.5 cm from the areola edge and 4 cm from the nipple center, with no clinical involvement of the nipple areola complex (NAC) or skin [18, 19]. In these circumstances, the incidence of local recurrence appears to be equivalent to skin sparing mastectomies [19–23].

Following a NSM, the blood supply to the NAC is based solely upon the subdermal plexus of the mastectomy skin flap. Several surgical techniques have been described for NSM that focus on increasing NAC viability. The most common incisions used in NSM are periareolar, lateral, transareolar, vertical, or inframammary [24–26] (Fig. 9.1). Each incision has advantages and disadvantages (Table 9.1). Periareolar incisions enable central access to all quadrants of the breast during the mastectomy while maintaining a well-hidden scar within the periphery of the NAC. However, the radial blood supply to the nipple is disrupted along the length of the incision, such that incisions that cover a greater percentage of the radial circumference of the NAC increase the risk of nipple necrosis (Fig. 9.2a–c). Lateral incisions also allow for easy access to all quadrants of the breast, but do not directly disrupt the radial blood supply to the nipple. While the scar lies on the breast mound, it is often well-hidden in a bra or bathing suit (Fig. 9.3a, b). The transareolar incision placed horizontally directly across the NAC provides a similar amount of exposure as the periareolar and lateral incisions; however, scar contracture may cause nipple distortion. The vertical incision preserves blood supply to the NAC similar to a lateral incision, improves visibility near the inframammary fold (IMF), but the scar remains on the breast mound and reduces access to the axillary tail. Inframammary incisions allow the scar to be well-concealed in the IMF with minimal disruption of the dermal blood supply to the NAC (Fig. 9.4a, b). The inframammary incision may be modified by shifting the incision to the inferolateral portion of the IMF (inferolateral

**Table 9.1** Nipple sparing mastectomy incision: advantages and disadvantages

| | Pro | Con |
|---|---|---|
| Periareolar | Good central access for mastectomy, reasonable scar aesthetics | Increased nipple necrosis/loss |
| Lateral | Good central access for mastectomy, good blood supply | More visible scar, possible nipple malposition |
| Transareolar | Good central access for mastectomy, good blood supply | More visible scar, possible loss of nipple projection or retraction |
| Vertical | Good blood supply, allow removal of excess skin in horizontal dimension | Technically difficult to reach upper outer quadrant |
| Inframammary | Good scar aesthetics | Questionable vascularity in larger breasts, poor access for larger volume mastectomies |
| Inferolateral | Good scar aesthetics, improved access to upper outer quadrant | Poor access for larger volume mastectomies |

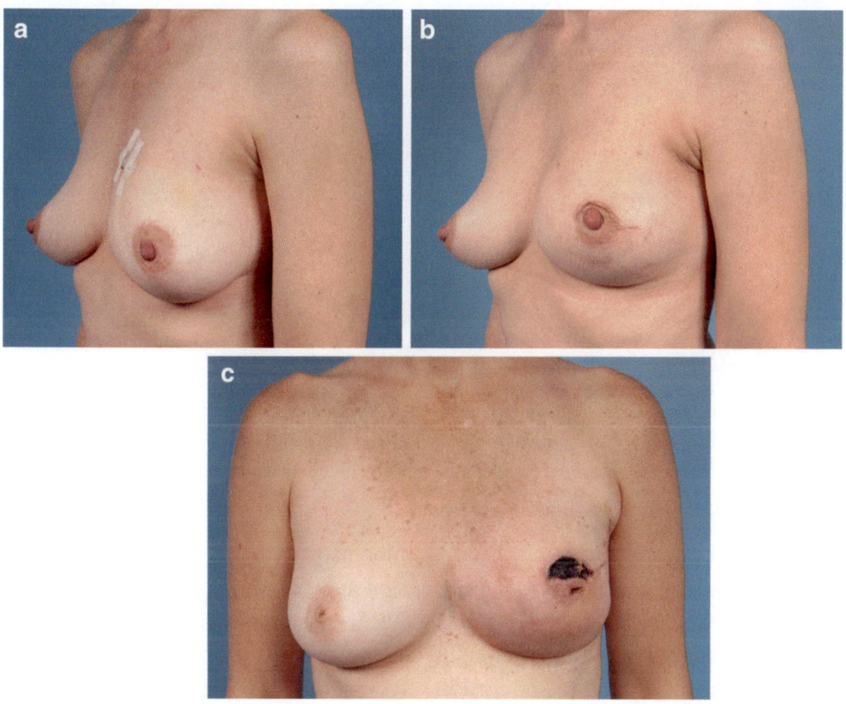

**Fig. 9.2** Nipple necrosis following a unilateral nipple sparing mastectomy (NSM) using a periareolar incision. (**a**) Preoperative photograph. (**b**) Postoperative result demonstrating the aesthetic benefits of a nipple sparing approach to mastectomy with a periareolar incision. (**c**) (Different patient) the periareolar incision is more likely to result in nipple necrosis. With a periareolar incision, the radial blood supply to the nipple areolar complex is disrupted along the length of the incision. The greater the circumference covered by the incision, the greater the risk of necrosis

incision). This potentially allows for better preservation of inferior perforating vessels and provides better access to the upper outer quadrant, which is often difficult with a traditional inframammary incision.

The reported incidence of nipple necrosis rates varies from 0 to 68%, with a propensity towards higher rates of necrosis with periareolar incisions [24, 25, 27–30]. Several other patient and technical factors may affect the risk for nipple necrosis.

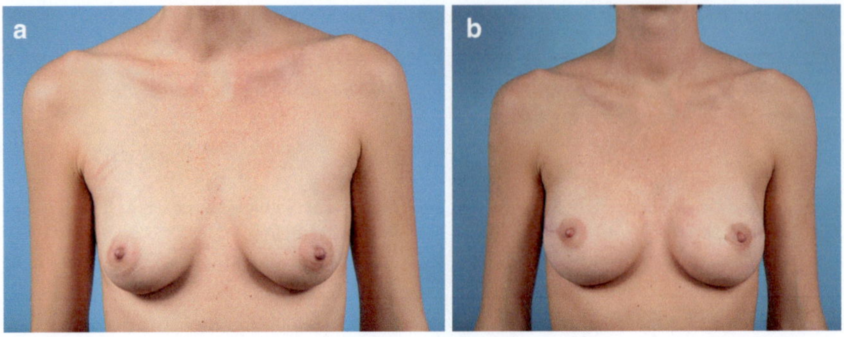

**Fig. 9.3** Bilateral tissue expander-implant reconstruction following nipple sparing mastectomy via lateral incision. (**a**) Preoperative photograph. (**b**) Postoperative result demonstrating the aesthetic benefits of a nipple sparing approach to mastectomy with a lateral incision

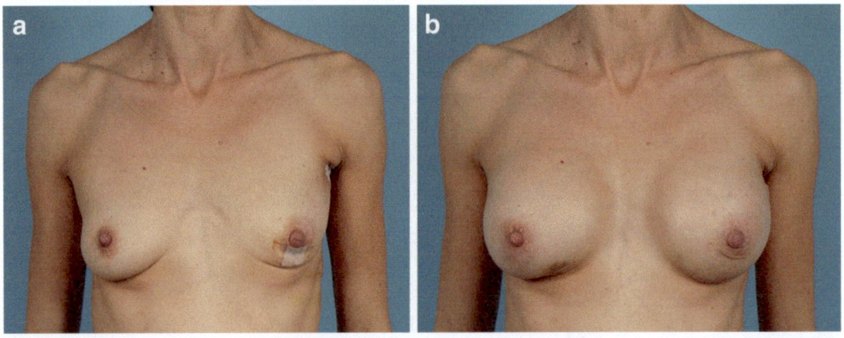

**Fig. 9.4** Unilateral tissue expander-implant reconstruction following nipple sparing mastectomy via inframammary incision. (**a**) Preoperative photograph of a patient with atypical lobular hyperplasia of left breast who underwent a small infra-areolar biopsy. (**b**) Postoperative result demonstrating the aesthetic benefits of an inframammary nipple sparing approach to mastectomy. This patient with moderate-sized breasts and minimal ptosis is the ideal candidate for an inframammary approach to nipple sparing mastectomy. She had a contralateral breast augmentation

Patients with larger or ptotic breasts will have a longer NAC to chest wall distance and attenuated blood supply to the NAC [31]. In general, patients who are diabetic and actively smoking are thought to have poorer perfusion of mastectomy skin flaps and may not be the best candidates for a nipple sparing procedure [32, 33]. Thinner mastectomy skin flaps and the use of tumescent solution with epinephrine are thought to potentially increase risk of wound complications, but the use of tumescent solution may facilitate the generation of the mastectomy flaps for the surgical oncologist/breast surgeon [31].

Reconstructive techniques may also have an effect on nipple viability [34]. With any type of reconstruction, one must limit the amount of pressure placed on skin flaps as this may decrease the blood supply to the NAC. Autologous reconstruction may provide a secondary source of blood supply to the nipple via an underlying vascularized tissue bed. In prosthetic reconstruction, various techniques have been described to increase nipple viability. In two-stage expander-based reconstruction, the expanders may be initially underinflated to reduce tension on the skin flaps. With single-stage prosthetic reconstruction, there is impetus to restore all or part of the breast volume immediately following the mastectomy, but consideration must be given to the viability of the NAC at the time of surgery. If an adjustable implant is utilized, the implant may be underfilled if the flaps appear threatened and fully inflated at a later clinic visit.

At our institution, we have adopted a patient-specific, multidisciplinary approach to nipple sparing mastectomies. The decision to pursue a NSM is determined by the breast surgeon and patient. Prior to the mastectomy, the breast and reconstructive surgeons discuss the incision design, taking into consideration the patient's risk factors and anticipated techniques for mastectomy and reconstruction. For patients with small breasts without lesions in the upper outer breast quadrant, an inferolateral incision is used. In cases not meeting these criteria, a lateral incision is preferred. We rarely utilize a periareolar incision, except in the outlier cases of preexisting periareolar scars, as the minimal benefit it provides is outweighed by the risk of nipple necrosis. During the reconstructive procedure, the mastectomy skin flaps and nipple viability are assessed. If the NAC or surrounding skin is not thought to be viable, the mastectomy is converted into a skin sparing mastectomy (SSM). If there is any doubt of complete flap viability, the reconstruction may be delayed and the mastectomy skin flaps monitored.

## Reconstructive Planning: Skin Sparing Mastectomy

Although NSM allows for complete preservation of the skin envelope, the technique is not suitable for all patients [19, 35]. Such patients are candidates for a SSM (Fig. 9.5a). Although the NAC and some skin are removed during an SSM, the similar principle of optimizing mastectomy skin flap preservation is utilized to enhance the outcomes of SSM (Fig. 9.5b). Most breast surgeons use an elliptical or fusiform skin excision with a length to width ratio of 3:1, which is thought to permit a tension-free closure without relative excess at the apices. While this incision design may be appropriate for patients with excess skin, a significant amount of skin is removed and can affect reconstructive outcomes. Therefore, planning of the SSM incision warrants discussion.

From the oncologic surgeon's perspective, a mastectomy incision is designed to achieve two goals: to adequately excise skin to aid in tumor control and to provide access for the mastectomy procedure. From the reconstructive surgeon's perspective, the incision is designed to optimize the outcome of the reconstruction. Mathematical modeling has shown the amount of skin removed in the vertical dimension has greater negative effects on breast volume and shape than skin removed in the horizontal dimension [36]. The relationship between the vertical dimension of the mastectomy incision and breast volume is quadratic in nature. Additionally, the volume loss caused by loss of vertical skin height occurs in areas that impact breast projection and ptosis, which are two very important components of an aesthetically acceptable result (Fig. 9.6). Fortunately for the breast surgeon, horizontal extension of the incision provides excellent visual access to the breast [36]. Therefore, the ideal SSM

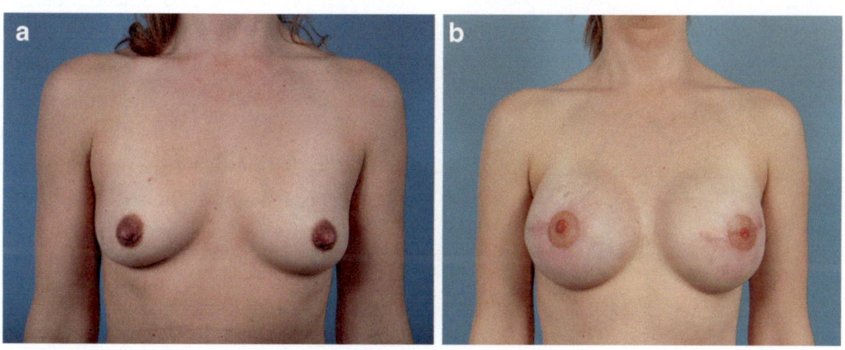

**Fig. 9.5** Bilateral tissue expander-implant and nipple areolar complex reconstruction following skin sparing mastectomy (SSM). (**a**) Preoperative photograph. (**b**) Postoperative result demonstrating a reasonable appearance of the breast after reconstruction is completed. Note how the reconstruction of the nipple areolar complex visually improves the outcome

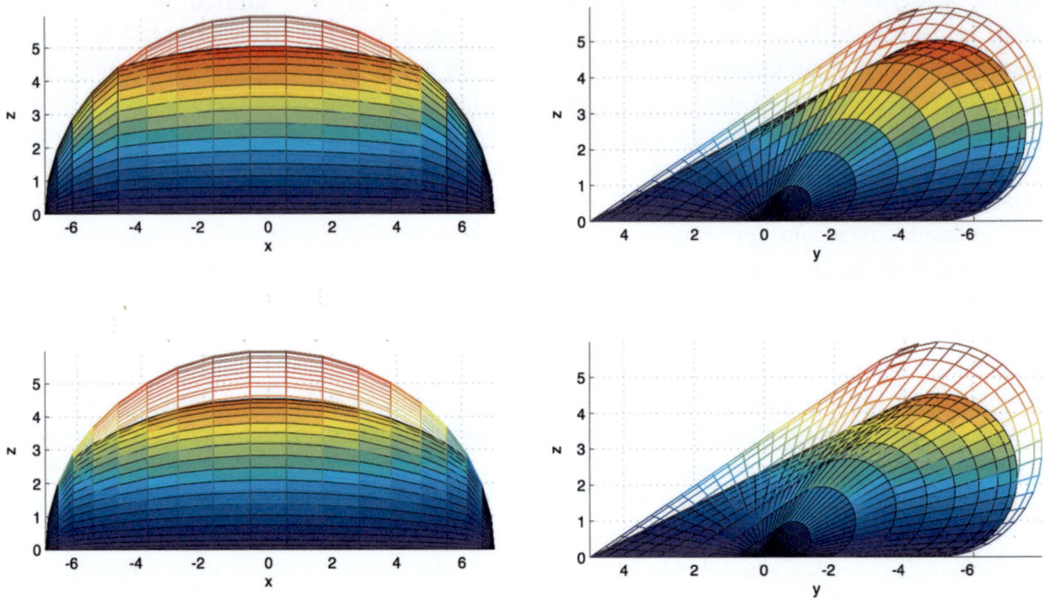


**Fig. 9.6** Mathematical modeling demonstrating the effect vertical incision dimensions on breast volume. *Top*: effect of an elliptical skin excision with vertical dimension measuring 40 mm on breast volume. *Bottom*: effect of an elliptical skin excision with vertical dimension measuring 60 mm on breast volume. Note the significant reduction in breast volume compared to the 40 mm ellipse, and the greater effect of volume loss on projection and ptosis. There is a quadratic relationship between the vertical dimension of an elliptical mastectomy incision and breast volume

would involve a complete periareolar incision with a horizontal extension in the lateral or superolateral direction. Alternatively, a fusiform incision in the same vector may be used with minimal additional effect on reconstructed breast volume (Fig. 9.7). Planning of the incision is important for both prosthetic and autologous-based reconstructions. In prosthetic breast reconstruction, preservation of the native mastectomy flap minimizes the need for serial expansions. In autologous reconstruction, aesthetic outcomes are better when the visible flap skin paddle is minimized to the size and shape of the reconstructed NAC.

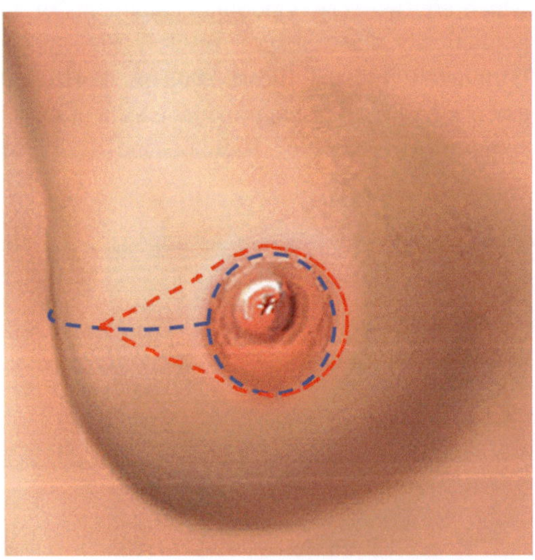

**Fig. 9.7** Schematic drawing of the preferred SSM incisions. Optimal skin preservation is an important aspect of achieving good aesthetic outcomes after SSM. The vertical dimension of an incision has greater effect on breast volume loss than the horizontal component and therefore

**Fig. 9.7** (continued) should be minimized. Secondly, medial extension of the incision into the breast cleavage area should be avoided. Therefore, the preferred design of an SSM incision is a circum-areolar incision at a minimal, yet oncologically safe, distance from the areolar with a lateral extension. Alternatively, a fusiform incision with the apex pointing in the same vector may be used with minimal effect on breast volume loss

## Breast Reconstruction: Techniques

As alluded to above, the best reconstructive outcomes begin with an appropriately planned mastectomy. The second focus of breast reconstruction is replacement of the excised parenchymal volume to achieve reasonable size, shape, and symmetry. In selecting the appropriate method of reconstruction, one must consider the advantages and disadvantages of each technique and evaluate the patient's goals and expectations.

There are two methods of breast reconstruction: prosthetic (i.e., tissue expander-implant reconstruction) and autologous (pedicled or free flap tissue transfer). The advantages and disadvantages of each technique are summarized in Table 9.2. In general, prosthetic reconstruction is a less invasive procedure, with a shorter immediate recovery period than autologous reconstruction. However, this method carries an overall greater incidence of long-term complications, requires that a prosthetic device be permanently implanted in the body and has greater limitation in achieving a natural appearance. Alternatively, autologous reconstruction is highly effective in producing a natural breast appearance and texture. However, autologous reconstruction is more invasive and requires a longer recovery time. While the overall incidence of complications is lower, the possibility of complete flap failure and complications at the flap donor site is always present [37].

While reconstructive options may be discussed preoperatively with the patient, one must remember that the definitive method of reconstruction cannot be determined until intraoperative evaluation of the skin flaps and the mastectomy defect is completed. In prosthetic reconstruction, the viability of skin flaps has a significant impact on whether the reconstructive surgeon can perform a one or two-stage prosthetic reconstruction. In cases of autologous reconstruction, the perfusion of the reconstructive flaps must be assessed as well as the patency of recipient vessels.

## Unilateral vs. Bilateral Reconstruction

The majority of high-risk patients will undergo BPM and reconstruction [38]. In general, the outcomes of bilateral prosthetic-based reconstruction are better compared to unilateral cases because such reconstruction gives the surgeon more control over achieving symmetry [17]. However, women undergoing bilateral reconstruction may not have sufficient tissue to undergo bilateral breast reconstruction with autologous tissue alone.

**Table 9.2** Prosthetic vs. autologous reconstruction: advantages and disadvantages

| | Tissue expander/implant | Latissimus flap ± implant | Abdominal tissue transfer (TRAM, DIEP, SIEA) |
|---|---|---|---|
| Initial surgery impact | Minimal | Moderate | Greatest |
| Secondary surgery (excluding nipple reconstruction) | Always, unless candidate for one-stage reconstruction | Occasional | Infrequent |
| Hospital stay | 1–2 days | 2–3 days | 3–7 days |
| Shape and feel | No ptosis, firm, little motion, no change with body weight changes | Moderate to natural ptosis, less firm, more motion, little change with weight fluctuation | Natural ptosis, soft, normal motion, changes proportionate to weight fluctuation |
| Potential for abdominal weakness | None | None | Risk even with muscle sparing techniques (except SIEA) |
| Return to work | 2 weeks | 4 weeks | 6–8 weeks |
| Procedure-specific risks | Skin flap loss, delayed healing, expander exposure/infection | Donor site seroma, flap loss | Flap loss, partial flap loss, abdominal weakness, fat necrosis |

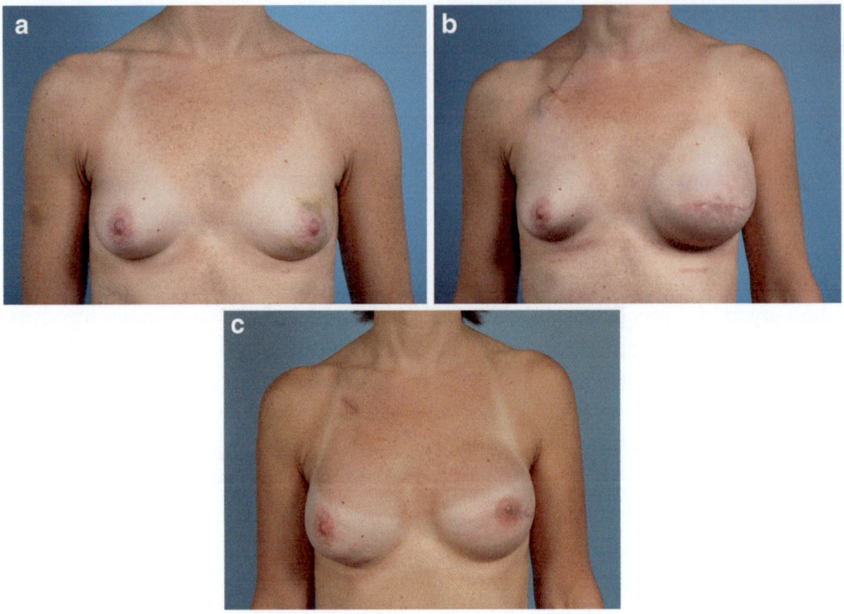

**Fig. 9.8** Unilateral tissue expander-implant-based reconstruction following SSM. (**a**) Preoperative photograph of a patient who desired an increase in breast size following unilateral SSM. (**b**) Postoperative result demonstrating the aesthetic benefits of tissue expander-implant. In general, serial tissue expansion allows the surgeon to increase the breast size to that desired by the patient. (**c**) Postoperative result following nipple areolar complex reconstruction and contralateral augmentation for symmetry

There are high-risk patients with atypia and in situ lesions who will decide to undergo a unilateral mastectomy and reconstruction. Inherently, it is more difficult to achieve symmetry in unilateral reconstruction since the surgeon must try and match the appearance of a natural breast. It is especially difficult to attain symmetry in women with larger and/or ptotic breasts. In these cases, one may consider a contralateral procedure for symmetry or autologous-based reconstruction (Fig. 9.8a–c).

## Timing

Most high-risk patients who desire breast reconstruction will undergo immediate reconstruction following their mastectomy [38]. The advantages of immediate reconstruction include fewer surgeries, more pliable tissues unhindered by soft tissue contracture, superior breast shape and symmetry, lower cost, and positive psychological outcomes [39]. The disadvantages include longer initial surgery times and possible mastectomy skin flap necrosis. A few high-risk patients will delay reconstruction in consideration of the risk of occult cancer diagnosis in the mastectomy specimen. Data suggest that the detection rate of occult cancer (DCIS or invasive carcinoma) in a prophylactic mastectomy specimen for a high-risk patient is 5–15% [40]. In this incidence, one must consider whether the patient requires radiation and whether there is adequate skin to reestablish the breast envelope. These factors may lead a surgeon to recommend autologous reconstruction.

# Prosthetic-Based Reconstruction

Prosthetic-based breast reconstruction accounts for nearly 80% of breast reconstruction procedures across the United States [41]. The procedure involves replacing the breast parenchyma with a breast implant. While the majority of high-risk patients are candidates for prosthetic reconstruction, it may not be suitable for all patients. Important factors to consider prior to prosthetic reconstruction include the patient's body habitus and breast size, whether the reconstruction is unilateral or bilateral, the patient's expectations for symmetry, and ability to tolerate the possibility of a second operative procedure and serial expansions. The ideal candidates for prosthetic reconstruction are women with small- to medium-sized breasts, minimal breast ptosis, and planned bilateral reconstruction. In patients undergoing unilateral prosthetic reconstruction, symmetry is increasingly difficult to achieve with increasing size and ptosis of the contralateral native breast.

Obese patients pose an additional challenge in prosthetic breast reconstruction. In addition to often having large, ptotic breasts, this patient population often demonstrates a broader chest with excess lateral chest wall tissue. Given the limitation of tissue expander and implant sizes, prosthetic reconstruction may not restore the breast volume to that of the original breasts or provide the appropriate relationship between the body habitus and reconstructed breasts. In this situation, the addition of autologous tissue to an implant-based reconstruction, or the use of autologous tissue alone, may achieve a more pleasing result.

On the other hand, there are circumstances in which prosthetic reconstruction may be highly favored over autologous reconstruction. In active women with minimal excess body tissue, there may not be sufficient tissue to perform autologous breast reconstruction. Active patients may also not tolerate the possibility of donor site morbidity, such as abdominal weakness. For patients with multiple medical problems, prosthetic-based reconstruction offers a less invasive, simpler operation with faster recovery.

## Two-Stage (Tissue Expander-Implant) Reconstruction: Technical Considerations

The majority of prosthetic-based reconstructions are performed in two stages. The first stage involves placement of a tissue expander in a subpectoral pocket following mastectomy. Postoperatively, serial inflations of the tissue expander are performed until the desired breast size is achieved. During the second stage, the tissue expander is exchanged for an implant. In general, two-stage reconstruction maximizes the reconstructive surgeon's control over the size, shape, and pocket position by allowing for revision during the tissue expander to implant exchange. This differs from one-stage implant-based reconstruction in which the permanent implant is placed during the primary procedure.

There are several aspects of prosthetic-based breast reconstruction that are influenced by the mastectomy technique and merit discussion. To begin, the IMF determines the inferior position of the tissue expander during the first stage operation. Therefore, care should be taken to avoid disturbing the IMF during the mastectomy. Its desired position should be marked on the patient preoperatively in case it is disrupted during the mastectomy.

Next, the preferred placement of the tissue expander is in a submuscular or subfasical pocket. There are two main methods of creating the pocket. A subpectoral–subfascial pocket may be developed by elevating the pectoralis major muscle and fascia of the serratus anterior and rectus abdominis muscles. With this technique, the pectoralis major is elevated off the chest wall and pectoralis minor. As the dissection is carried laterally, the pocket is elevated in continuity with the subfascial plane of the serratus anterior. As dissection is carried inferiorly to the IMF, the tissues above the rectus muscles are elevated in continuity with the subpectoral space. This creates a complete subpectoral/subfascial space for placement of the tissue expander. Therefore, during the mastectomy, care should be taken not to violate the fascia above the rectus abdominus or serratus anterior muscles. In a separate technique, a subpectoral–subdermal pocket may be created by completely disoriginating the pectoralis major from the chest wall. In this scenario, only the superior portion of the expander is covered by the pectoralis. While a healthy inferior mastectomy skin flap can support the inferior portion of the expander, a thin or compromised skin flap may provide inadequate soft-tissue coverage of the inferior pole of the expander thereby increasing the risk for implant exposure. To address this, a piece of acellular dermal matrix (ADM) is often used to cover the inferior portion of the tissue expander and augment implant coverage. There are many potential benefits and pitfalls to this technique, which are discussed in the section on ADM.

Once the pocket is created, the appropriate tissue expander is selected and placed into the pocket. Selection of the appropriate expander is based on several factors including: desired breast volume, breast dimensions (height, width, and projection), and the patient's body habitus. The extent of intraoperative inflation of the tissue expander is highly dependent on the status of the mastectomy skin flaps. The tissue expander is filled to a volume that optimally eliminates dead space, but does not impart excessive pressure on the mastectomy skin flaps. Greater intraoperative expansion allows for improved outcomes by preserving native mastectomy skin; however, the viability of mastectomy skin will determine how much expansion can safely be performed intraoperatively. Tissue expansion is continued postoperatively until the desired breast size is achieved. The amount of skin removed during SSM will inherently influence the amount of expansion that needs to be performed postoperatively to reestablish the breast envelope.

The second stage involves exchange of the tissue expander for a permanent implant. The selection of a saline or silicone implant largely depends on patient preference. All patients undergoing breast reconstruction are candidates for use of a silicone gel implant as long as they meet the inclusion criteria determined by the manufacturer. During the second stage, the capsule that develops around the expander can be modified via a capsulotomy and/or a partial capulectomy to gain control over the final implant and IMF position.

In unilateral reconstructions, a procedure may be performed on the contralateral breast to improve symmetry. Contralateral symmetry procedures include augmentation mammaplasty, mastopexy, or reduction mammaplasty. These procedures are most often undertaken during the second stage once the reconstruction is complete to maximize the surgeon's control of overall symmetry.

## One-Stage (Implant) Reconstruction: Technical Considerations

In select cases, prosthetic-based breast reconstruction can be completed in one operation. The procedure is performed in the same manner as the primary operation for the two-stage prosthetic reconstruction, except that a permanent implant is inserted instead of a tissue expander. In the ideal case, implants are selected to fill the mastectomy defect and act to preserve the native mastectomy skin flaps in their entirety. This technique is particularly beneficial for patients undergoing NSM, where all of the breast skin is preserved.

Not all patients are candidates for one-stage implant reconstruction and both the anatomical and patient factors that influence whether this procedure is appropriate must be considered. Anatomically, the patient should have small- to moderate-sized breasts with minimal ptosis. Following the mastectomy, the skin flaps must demonstrate excellent viability with adequate tissue to fulfill the patient's desired final breast size. If there is not enough skin, undue tension will be placed on the flap by a permanent implant, thereby increasing the risk of skin flap necrosis. In cases where there is adequate skin, the use of an adjustable permanent saline implant can aid in one-stage reconstruction. In these cases, the permanent implant has a remote access port that is used for minor volume modification postoperatively until the desired size is achieved. While there are advantages to this method, breast projection and final implant position may be more difficult to finesse than in two-stage reconstruction.

In addition to anatomic considerations, there are patient factors to consider in one-stage prosthetic reconstruction. First, the patient must demonstrate tolerance for a potentially smaller breast size with a one-stage approach. Second, patients should be prepared to undergo revision surgery in order to achieve their desired aesthetic outcome. This may prove difficult when the expectation is for a single procedure.

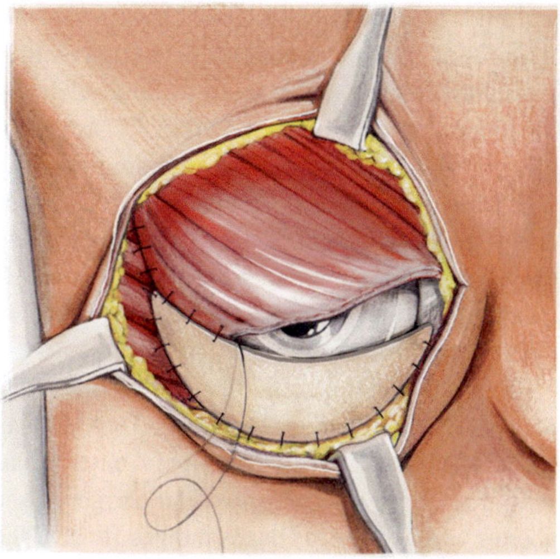

**Fig. 9.9** Schematic representation of acellular dermal matrix-assisted tissue expander-implant breast reconstruction. During the reconstructive procedure, ADM is sutured to the chest wall to re-establish the IMF and the inferior border of the dis-inserted pectoralis muscle to create a dermal sling

## Acellular Dermal Matrix

Today, nearly one-half of prosthetic breast reconstructions are being performed with ADM [42]. The benefits of this procedure have been alluded to above and include: (1) enhanced positioning of the prosthesis, (2) more precise definition of the IMF, (3) faster expansion curve (with concomitant reduction in clinic visits and time to exchange), (4) improved cosmesis resulting from better expansion of the lower pole, (5) decreased dissection of serratus anterior and rectus fascia (with possible reduction in postoperative pain), and (6) dissipation of pressure placed on skin flaps by the tissue expander or implant. There are also potential benefits of reducing long-term capsular contracture. In general, the ADM is inserted as an inferior pole sling, which supports and covers the inferior aspects of a tissue expander or implant. The inferior aspect of the acellular dermis is sutured to the chest wall to reestablish the IMF. The superior aspect is sutured to the pectoralis muscle, creating a subpectoral/sub-ADM implant pocket (Fig. 9.9). Over time, the acellular dermis is incorporated into the soft tissues, by

**Table 9.3** Meta-analysis-derived pooled complication rate for prosthetic breast reconstruction [43]

| Outcome [43] | Incidence (%) |
|---|---|
| Hematoma | 1.5 |
| Seroma | 3.5 |
| Infection | 4.7 |
| Mastectomy flap necrosis | 4.9 |
| Reconstructive failure | 3.8 |

vascular and fibroblast in-growth, theoretically reducing the risk for infection [34]. By enabling full release of the pectoralis major muscle from the IMF, use of ADM facilitates a larger, more defined pocket for tissue expander or implant placement. This allows for greater intraoperative expander fill volumes and more control over implant position. In the inferior pole this translates to greater lower pole fill and greater ptosis.

While there are many benefits to utilizing ADM, these must be weighed against the increased potential complications. While ADM is biologically inert and incorporates into the soft tissues over time, it is an additional foreign body that is implanted into the breast. Meta-analysis has demonstrated a twofold increase in complications when utilizing ADM in breast reconstruction [43]. Therefore, the risks and benefits of this procedure should be discussed with patients prior to surgery.

## Outcomes

Overall, prosthetic reconstruction is a reliable and generally simple option. According to a recent meta-analysis, the overall pooled complications rate is 14.0% [11.7–16.3%, 95% Confidence Interval] [43]. The most frequently reported complications include hematomas (1.5%), seromas (3.5%), infections (4.7%), and mastectomy flap necrosis (4.9%) (Table 9.3). Most complications are reasonably minor in nature and can be treated conservatively [44]; however, there is a 3.8% chance of reconstructive failure and explantation. For ADM-based reconstruction, complication rates average 15.4% [9.3–21.4%, 95% Confidence Interval] and there is an increased relative risk of overall complications of 2.05 compared to non-ADM prosthetic reconstruction [43].

## Abdomen-Based Flaps

For patients desiring autologous breast reconstruction, an abdominal flap is usually the first-line option, provided there is adequate lower abdominal soft tissue. Abdominal flaps are based upon the superior and inferior epigastric vessels that supply the rectus abdominus muscles and overlying abdominal tissue. These vessels are connected via a system of choke vessels [45], which allows the flap to be elevated as a pedicled flap based upon the superior epigastric pedicle or as a free flap based upon the inferior epigastric system. The pedicled flap is passed from the abdomen into the breast defect across the IMF while the free flap is completely separated and requires microvascular anastomosis of the inferior epigastric vessels to either the thoracodorsal or internal mammary systems.

In general, autologous reconstruction allows for reconstruction of a natural appearing and textured breast (Figs. 9.10a–c and 9.11a, b). Benefits of abdominal flap reconstruction include size, consistent vascular anatomy, and relatively low donor site morbidity. Additionally, as part of the procedure, patients receive an abdominoplasty with a favorably placed "tummy tuck" scar, which can often be hidden at or beneath the underwear line (Fig. 9.12). However, patients must be made aware of the potential for abdominal wall weakness or hernia after abdominal harvest.

Specific advantages of the pedicled transverse rectus abdominis myocutaneous (TRAM) flap include: predictable vascular supply, ease of harvest, avoidance of microvascular surgery, and shorter surgical time. Disadvantages involve the necessary sacrifice of rectus abdominis muscle, higher rates of fat necrosis (vs. free TRAM), limited arc of rotation, disruption of the IMF, smaller vascular territory of the superior epigastric system, and possible need for flap delay. Although there is a relatively higher rate of partial flap loss when compared to free tissue transfer, it should

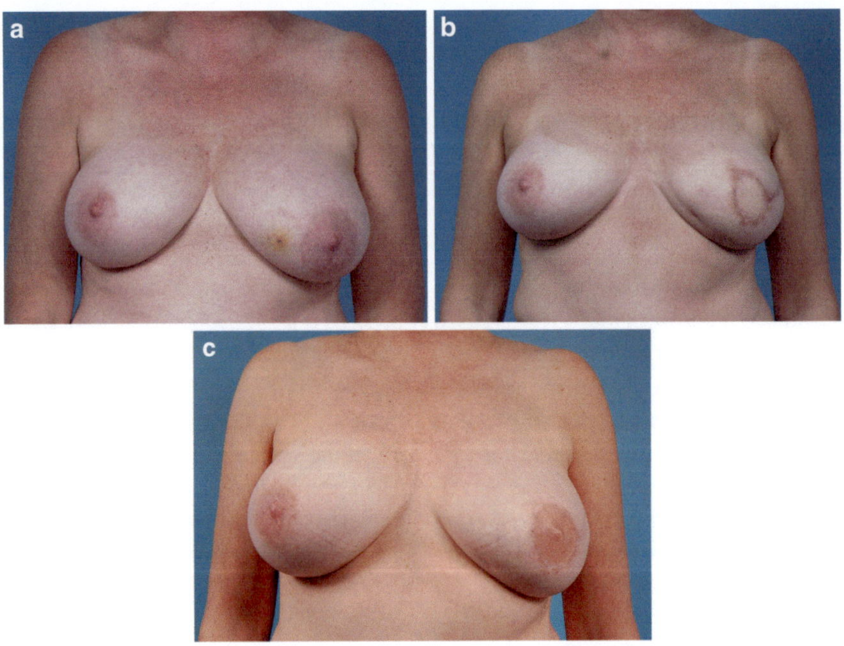

**Fig. 9.10** Unilateral free transverse rectus abdominus myocutaneous (TRAM) reconstruction following SSM. (**a**) Preoperative photograph. (**b**) Postoperative result demonstrating the aesthetic outcome of TRAM flap breast reconstruction after an optimally planned SSM incision. Note that the SSM performed with a periareolar incision with lateral extension allowed the flap skin paddle to be placed at the location of the nipple areolar complex (NAC). (**c**) Results following NAC reconstruction

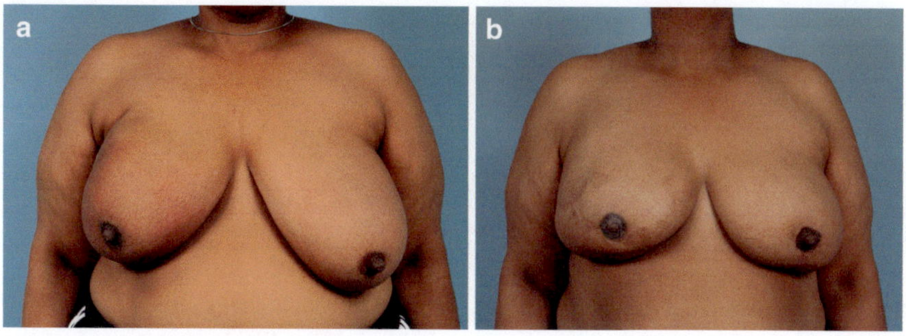


**Fig. 9.11** Unilateral deep inferior epigastric perforator flap reconstruction following SSM. (**a**) Preoperative photograph. (**b**) Postoperative result demonstrating the aesthetic outcome of DIEP flap breast reconstruction and nipple areolar complex reconstruction with contralateral breast reduction

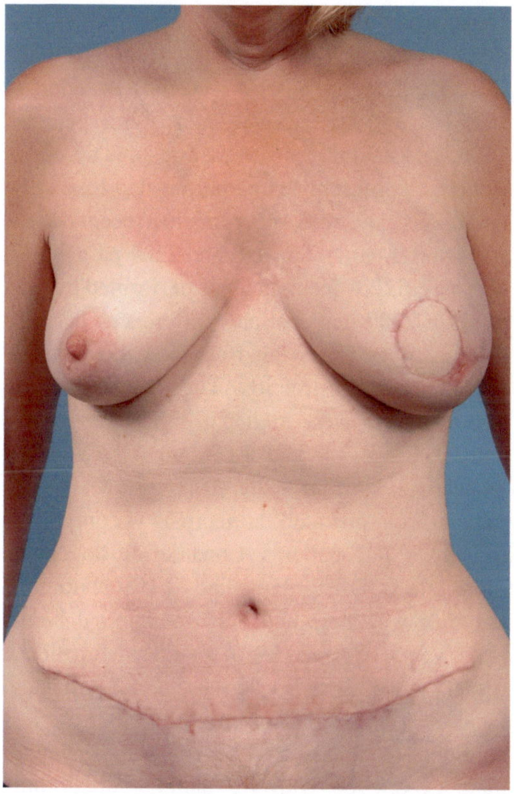

**Fig. 9.12** Abdominal scar following abdomen flap-based reconstruction. The abdominal incision is usually designed as an abdominoplasty or "tummy tuck" incision that is often well hidden in the underwear line. This is an example of an early scar with characteristic redness, which attenuates over time

be noted that total flap loss is extremely rare with a pedicled TRAM flap [46]. Delay of the flap, via ligation of the deep and superficial inferior epigastric systems 1 week prior to flap harvest, has been proven to significantly increase perfusion of the pedicled TRAM flap and to reduce complication rates [47]. Smokers and obese patients have significantly higher rates of complications with this procedure including fat necrosis, partial flap loss, and abdominal donor site morbidity [48].

A free TRAM flap is based upon the most robust blood supply of the abdomen: the deep inferior epigastric system. The blood vessels are large in caliber and the pedicle is long enough to allow for anastomosis to either the internal mammary or thoracodorsal systems. This flap can be elevated with the entire muscle or with a muscle sparing technique in which only the necessary portion of the muscle encompassing the vascular pedicle is taken. Advantages of the free TRAM include limited abdominal dissection, ability to preserve muscle, maximal flap perfusion allowing for a larger skin paddle, lower skin island placement and more easily concealed scars, maintenance of the IMF, and versatility at inset. In comparison to the pedicled TRAM, obese patients and smokers do not demonstrate increased flap complications when undergoing a free TRAM reconstruction. However, they are still at risk for complications such as abdominal or mastectomy skin flap loss, umbilicus loss, seromas, and infections. Also, when compared to normal weight patients, obese patients (BMI > 30) demonstrate significantly higher rates of overall complications [33]. Challenges specific to free tissue transfer include a higher total flap loss

**Table 9.4** Complications of abdomen-based autologous breast reconstruction [50, 53, 54]

| Outcome | TRAM [53] (%) | DIEP [53] (%) | SIEA [50, 54] (%) |
|---|---|---|---|
| Total flap loss | 1.0 | 2.0 | 5–7 |
| Partial flap loss | 1.8 | 2.5 | 0–5 |
| Fat necrosis | 4.9 | 10.1 | 1–14 |
| Abdominal bulge or weakness | 5.9 | 3.1 | 0 |
| Abdominal hernia | 3.9 | 0.8 | 0 |

when compared to pedicled TRAM or latissimus dorsi flap reconstruction, longer operative times, and the need for microvascular surgery.

While the free TRAM incorporates a segment of rectus abdominus muscle and fascia that carries perforating vessels to the skin, the deep inferior epigastric perforator (DIEP) flap isolates perforators and spares the anterior rectus sheath and muscle. Proponents of this technique report that saving the entire rectus muscle and fascia decreases donor site morbidity, such as loss of abdominal strength and development of hernias. However, other surgeons argue that dissection of perforators through the rectus abdominus dennervates the muscle, limiting the potential benefit of sparing the muscle.

DIEP flaps have a higher incidence of partial flap necrosis and require more revisions than TRAM flaps. This is likely due to the fact that small perforators are sacrificed in a DIEP flap during dissection of the main vascular supply, while they are preserved in a free TRAM. Therefore, patients should be advised that appropriate selection between a free TRAM and a DIEP flap depends on preoperative assessment and intraoperative findings.

The superficial inferior epigastric artery (SIEA) enters the abdomen above the rectus fascia [49]. Elevation of the SIEA flap does not violate abdominal fascia or the rectus abdominus muscle. Therefore, it truly limits donor site complications such as decreased abdominal wall strength and development of hernias. The major drawback to this flap is the highly variable size and presence of the SIEA as well as its smaller cutaneous vascular territory. The SIEA is present and of sufficient size in only 30–40% of patients [50, 51]. When performing autologous breast reconstruction from the abdomen, the SIEA flap can be attempted in all patients with the understanding that an intraoperative decision will be made as to whether there are vessels of sufficient caliber. If the SIEA cannot support the flap, then the surgeon can proceed to DIEP or TRAM flap reconstruction [54].

## Outcomes

Overall, abdominal flaps—whether pedicled or free—have good survival rates. With pedicled TRAMs, total flap loss is rare but some degree of ischemic compromise and partial flap loss or fat necrosis is expected. According to a recent review, 8.9% suffer partial flap loss and 2.5% palpable fat necrosis [52]. A meta-analysis performed by Man et al. in 2009 demonstrates differences between the outcomes following free TRAM and DIEP flap breast reconstruction. The total and partial flap loss rates were higher in DIEP flaps at 2.0 and 2.5% vs. 1.0 and 1.8% for TRAM flaps, respectively. Additionally, 10.1% of DIEP flap patients demonstrated fat necrosis vs. only 4.9% in TRAM flap patients. Considering donor site morbidities, DIEP flaps had 3.1% abdominal bulge or weakness and 0.8% abdominal hernia rates vs. 5.9% and 3.9% for TRAM patients, respectively [53]. SIEA flaps are performed under ideal anatomic conditions and therefore are less common. In Spiegel and Khan's 2007 review of their experience with 82 patients undergoing SIEA flap reconstruction, there were no abdominal hernias or bulges noted. The total and partial flap loss rates were 5.1% each. Fat necrosis was noted in 1% of the flaps and 3% went on to develop breast infections [54] (Table 9.4).

### Latissimus Dorsi Flap

The latissimus dorsi flap is a reliable, well-vascularized muscle, or myocutaneous flap that does not require microvascular surgery for ipsilateral breast reconstruction. The vascular pedicle is based upon the thoracodorsal system, which allows for easy rotation of the latissimus dorsi into the chest via a subcutaneous tunnel in the axilla. The volume of the latissimus dorsi flap can be increased by incorporating subcutaneous tissue with the flap or supplementation with an implant [56–59].

After careful planning of the incision, the latissimus dorsi is dissected free from its inferior and medial origins with or without a skin paddle. The thoracodorsal neurovascular pedicle is identified in the axilla near the insertion of the muscle and protected. Many surgeons will either disinsert the muscle at the humerus and/or divide the thoracodorsal nerve to limit movement in the breast from muscle contraction. A subcutaneous tunnel in the axilla is created to allow transposition of the muscle anteriorly into the chest. The flap is carefully inset into the mastectomy defect. When volume is desired, an implant or expander is placed beneath the muscle (in conjunction with pectoralis elevation as needed). The latissimus dorsi can then be secured to the chest wall and breast skin flaps circumscribing the prosthesis.

There are certain drawbacks to using the latissimus dorsi muscle. There is a significant risk for seroma formation at the donor site requiring prolonged drain maintenance. The donor site may leave unsightly scars. While the majority of patients do not experience functional limitations due to loss of the latissimus muscle, athletic individuals may complain of weakness in shoulder abduction and extension. Since the latissimus dorsi flap is relatively small, it is often used in conjunction with a tissue expander or implant, which increases the risk for potential complications.

### Outcomes

Latissimus dorsi flap breast reconstruction is considered a reliable flap with high survival rates (97.5–100%) [55, 56]. The durable nature of the thoracodorsal blood supply and the absence of microvascular technique minimize flap ischemic risk and complications. Traditionally, complication rates focus on donor site morbidity, which is beset by a 23–34% seroma rate [55, 57]. A recent comprehensive review by Losken et al. demonstrates a 34% overall *breast* complication rate (both with and without expander/implant) broken down into 7% major infection, 9.6% minor infection, 9.6% skin necrosis, 3.6% seroma, and 1% implant extrusion [55].

## Superior and Inferior Gluteal Artery Perforator Flaps

The superior and inferior gluteal arteries are branches of the internal iliac artery that supply the gluteal muscle and overlying tissues. Superior gluteal artery perforator (SGAP) and inferior gluteal artery perforator (IGAP) flaps can be designed based upon the perforators that arise through the muscle and supply the skin and subcutaneous tissue. The SGAP and IGAP flaps are indicated in breast reconstruction for patients who prefer a gluteal scar over an abdominal scar, those with insufficient abdominal tissue, those with abdominal scars precluding reliable flap transfer, or as a salvage procedure. An advantage of the gluteal flaps lies in the natural shape of the buttock, which more closely approximates a breast and therefore requires less shaping on the breast. It is important to note that these flaps are perforator-based flaps and therefore spare the muscle and cause no functional limitations. Smoking and prior liposuction of the donor site are absolute contraindications to the use of these flaps [58].

Compared to abdomen-based reconstruction, the gluteal perforator flaps have a smaller available skin paddle and a shorter pedicle length in most cases. The SGAP flap offers certain benefits over the IGAP flap as the sciatic and posterior femoral cutaneous nerves are protected during the harvest and the donor scar does not lie along a pressure-bearing region when the patient is seated. The inferior gluteal crease (IGAP), on the other hand, has a longer pedicle, which may allow for anastomosis within the axilla. Both flaps allow for a well-hidden scar either in the IGAP or just below the underwear line (SGAP).

### Outcomes

SGAP and IGAP flaps are known for their anatomic variability and difficult anastomoses. It is not surprising therefore that overall survival rates tend to be lower compared to standard TRAM flaps [59]. Total flap failure rates in the hands of experienced surgeons can be as low as 2%. Additionally, 15% will experience donor site seromas while 8% will have fat necrosis of the reconstructed breast [60].

## Nipple Reconstruction

Nipple areolar complex (NAC) reconstruction is a very important and final stage of breast reconstruction (Fig. 9.13). The NAC is the natural focal point of the breasts and its reconstruction leads to an increase in patient satisfaction with overall aesthetic outcome [17]. NAC reconstruction is typically performed 3–6 months after completion of the breast mound in order to allow the breast tissue to settle into its final shape. The aim of nipple reconstruction is to create a nipple-like mound of tissue at a symmetric and appropriate position on the breast. There are many local skin flap designs that effectively create a nipple mound. Regardless of the technique, all nipple mounds will shrink 50–75% over time. Therefore, some amount of overcorrection is necessary at the outset. Customized tattooing is performed 2–3 months later to create the appropriate color, size, and shape of the complete nipple areolar complex.

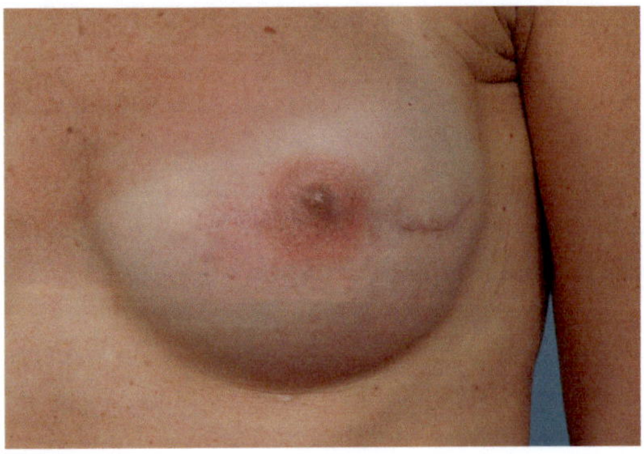

**Fig. 9.13** Nipple areolar complex (NAC) reconstruction. NAC reconstruction is the final stage of breast reconstruction. Numerous techniques have been described to reconstruct the NAC. In general the nipple mound is reconstructed via a local rearrangement flap and the areolar complex is tattooed at a later stage. NAC reconstruction positively affects aesthetic outcomes and patient psychological well-being

## Breast Conservation Therapy

Some high-risk patients are candidates for breast conservation therapy. The options for reconstruction for partial breast defects are dramatically different from those utilized in mastectomy reconstruction. In these cases, a combination of oncologic and reconstructive (i.e., oncoplastic) techniques may be combined to perform the lumpectomy and reconstruction simultaneously, such that the two procedures compliment each other [61, 62]. For example, following a lumpectomy, local tissue rearrangement can be completed in the form of a mastopexy or reduction mammaplasty in patients who desire a lift or reduction (Fig. 9.14a, b). The incisions and tissue removed during the reconstructive procedure are planned to incorporate the lumpectomy tissue. In these cases, location of the lumpectomy defect is critical in planning the reconstruction, as both the breast and reconstructive surgeons must predetermine the incisions and location of the parenchymal vascular pedicle.

In some scenarios, the tissue defect created by the lumpectomy is too large for standard oncoplastic parenchymal rearrangement. In these cases, one may consider bringing additional soft tissue to the breast in the form of a flap. In most cases, lumpectomy defects can be filled with a latissimus muscle flap. This muscle tends to reach the outer or upper quadrants of the breast. If a large lumpectomy defect is anticipated, then an "immediate-delayed" reconstruction can be planned wherein the latissimus muscle reconstruction is performed after final margins are pathologically confirmed (Fig. 9.15a, b). The latissimus can be delivered through a small axillary incision using endoscopic instruments for dissection [63]. Alternatively, there are cases of lumpectomy defects after radiation therapy with significant contracture and contour deformity. In these cases, a latissimus muscle with a cutaneous paddle may be required to correct both the volume and skin defect (Fig. 9.16a, b).

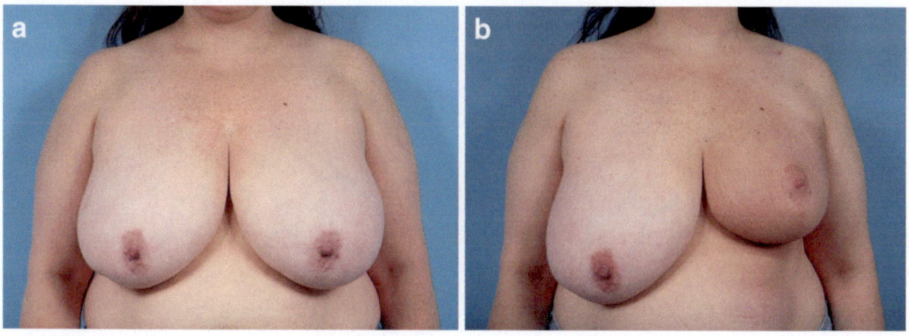

**Fig. 9.14** Left breast lumpectomy performed in conjunction with a breast reduction. (**a**) Preoperative photograph patient with ductal carcinoma in situ of the left breast who was scheduled to undergo breast conservation and adjuvant radiation, but desired a breast reduction. (**b**) Postoperative results after undergoing oncoplastic lumpectomy and breast reduction followed by radiation. The contralateral reduction procedure was delayed in this case due to the unpredictable effects of radiation on soft tissue contracture and increased risk for asymmetry

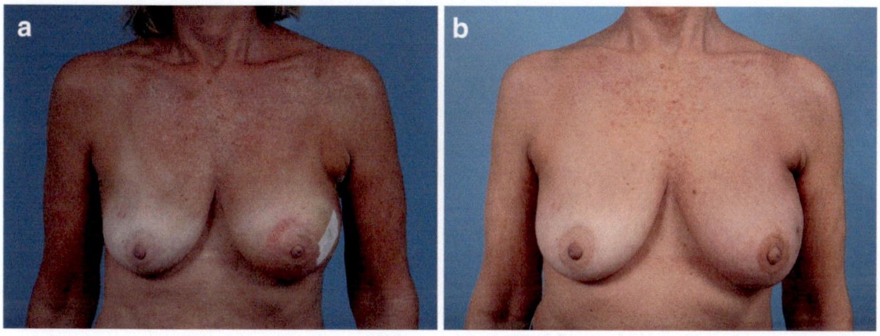

**Fig. 9.15** Muscle-only latissimus flap reconstruction following left breast lumpectomy. (**a**) Preoperative photograph. The patient decided to undergo breast conservation therapy. Due to the planned defect size, likelihood of deformity, and desire to maintain breast size, the patient elected to undergo an immediate muscle-only latissimus flap reconstruction. (**b**) Postoperative result demonstrating near normal contour of the breast after a muscle only latissimus flap reconstruction. In general, the latissimus flap provides adequate tissue for defects involving the upper or outer quadrants of the breast

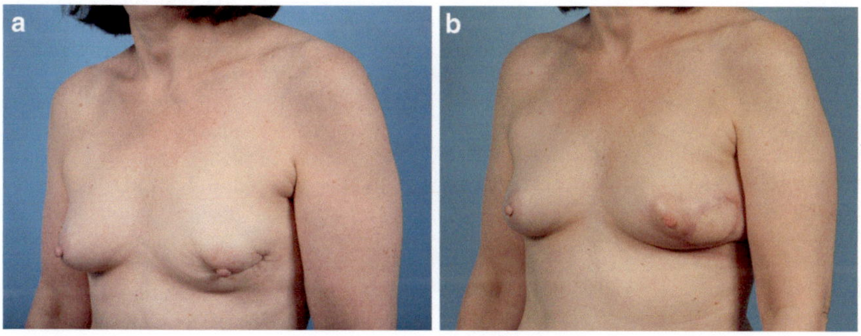

**Fig. 9.16** Myocutaneous latissimus flap reconstruction following left breast conservation therapy. (**a**) Preoperative photograph of a patient who underwent a lumpectomy. Postoperatively, the patient developed soft tissue and skin contracture of the lumpectomy defect. (**b**) Post-reconstruction result demonstrating near normal contour of the breast after a myocutaneous latissimus flap reconstruction. Note: the skin contracture necessitated incorporation of a skin paddle with the flap

## Conclusion

High-risk breast cancer patients pose a unique set of reconstructive challenges. While these patients tend to have bilateral mastectomies with a nipple sparing approach, options will vary according to the precise oncologic strategy outlined by the breast surgeon and the patient. With the thoughtful modification of standard prosthetic and autologous technique, high-risk patients can achieve reasonable reconstructive and aesthetic outcomes concomitant with definitive risk reduction surgery.

## References


1. Altekruse SF, Kosary C, Krapcho M, et al. SEER Cancer Statistics Review, 1975–2007. Bethesda, MD: National Cancer Institute; 2010.
2. Colditz GA, et al. Family history, age, and risk of breast cancer. Prospective data from the Nurses' Health Study. JAMA. 1993;270(3):338–43.
3. Sprague BL, Trentham-Dietz A. Prevalence of breast carcinoma in situ in the United States. JAMA. 2009;302(8):846–8.
4. Geiger AM, et al. A population-based study of bilateral prophylactic mastectomy efficacy in women at elevated risk for breast cancer in community practices. Arch Intern Med. 2005;165(5):516–20.
5. Kurian AW, Sigal BM, Plevritis SK. Survival analysis of cancer risk reduction strategies for BRCA1/2 mutation carriers. J Clin Oncol. 2010;28(2):222–31.
6. Metcalfe KA, et al. Prophylactic bilateral mastectomy: patterns of practice. Cancer. 2002;95(2):236–42.
7. Contant CM, et al. Clinical experience of prophylactic mastectomy followed by immediate breast reconstruction in women at hereditary risk of breast cancer (HB(O)C) or a proven BRCA1 and BRCA2 germ-line mutation. Eur J Surg Oncol. 2002;28(6):627–32.
8. Metcalfe KA, Semple JL, Narod SA. Satisfaction with breast reconstruction in women with bilateral prophylactic mastectomy: a descriptive study. Plast Reconstr Surg. 2004;114(2):360–6.
9. Spear SL, et al. Prophylactic mastectomy and reconstruction: clinical outcomes and patient satisfaction. Plast Reconstr Surg. 2008;122(1):1–9.
10. Rolnick SJP, Altschuler A, Nekhlyudov L, Elmore JG, Greene SM, Harris EL, et al. What women wish they knew before prophylactic mastectomy. Cancer Nurs. 2007;30(4):285–91.
11. Snell L, et al. Clarifying the expectations of patients undergoing implant breast reconstruction: a qualitative study. Plast Reconstr Surg. 2010;126(6): 1825–30.
12. Alderman AK, et al. Determinants of patient satisfaction in postmastectomy breast reconstruction. Plast Reconstr Surg. 2000;106(4):769–76.
13. Hu ES, et al. Patient-reported aesthetic satisfaction with breast reconstruction during the long-term survivorship Period. Plast Reconstr Surg. 2009;124(1): 1–8.
14. Bresser PJ, et al. Satisfaction with prophylactic mastectomy and breast reconstruction in genetically predisposed women. Plast Reconstr Surg. 2006;117(6):1675–82; discussion 1683–4.
15. Frost MH, et al. Long-term satisfaction and psychological and social function following bilateral prophylactic mastectomy. JAMA. 2000;284(3):319–24.
16. Gahm J, et al. Patient satisfaction with aesthetic outcome after bilateral prophylactic mastectomy and immediate reconstruction with implants. J Plast Reconstr Aesthet Surg. 2010;63(2):332–8.
17. Buck 2nd DW, et al. Patient-subjective cosmetic outcomes following the varying stages of tissue expander breast reconstruction: the importance of completion. Breast. 2010;19(6):521–6.
18. Simmons RM, et al. Analysis of nipple/areolar involvement with mastectomy: can the areola be preserved? Ann Surg Oncol. 2002;9(2):165–8.
19. Voltura AM, et al. Nipple-sparing mastectomy: critical assessment of 51 procedures and implications for selection criteria. Ann Surg Oncol. 2008;15(12):3396–401.
20. Cheung KL, et al. Subcutaneous mastectomy for primary breast cancer and ductal carcinoma in situ. Eur J Surg Oncol. 1997;23(4):343–7.
21. Hartmann LC, et al. Efficacy of bilateral prophylactic mastectomy in women with a family history of breast cancer. N Engl J Med. 1999;340(2):77–84.
22. Pennisi VR, Capozzi A. Subcutaneous mastectomy: an interim report on 1,244 patients. Ann Plast Surg. 1984;12(4):340–7.
23. Hartmann LC, et al. Efficacy of bilateral prophylactic mastectomy in BRCA1 and BRCA2 gene mutation carriers. J Natl Cancer Inst. 2001;93(21):1633–7.
24. Garcia-Etienne CA, et al. Nipple-sparing mastectomy: initial experience at the Memorial Sloan-Kettering Cancer Center and a comprehensive review of literature. Breast J. 2009;15(4):440–9.
25. Crowe Jr JP, et al. Nipple-sparing mastectomy: technique and results of 54 procedures. Arch Surg. 2004;139(2):148–50.
26. Stolier AJ, Sullivan SK, Dellacroce FJ. Technical considerations in nipple-sparing mastectomy: 82 consecutive cases without necrosis. Ann Surg Oncol. 2008;15(5):1341–7.
27. Rawlani V, Fiuk J, Johnson SA, et al. The effect of incision choice on outcomes of nipple-sparing mastectomy reconstruction. Can J Plast Surg. 2011;19: 129–33.
28. Psaila A, et al. Nipple sparing mastectomy with immediate breast reconstruction: a short term analysis of our experience. J Exp Clin Cancer Res. 2006;25(3): 309–12.

29. Komorowski AL, et al. Necrotic complications after nipple- and areola-sparing mastectomy. World J Surg. 2006;30(8):1410–3.
30. Bistoni G, et al. Nipple-sparing mastectomy. Preliminary results. J Exp Clin Cancer Res. 2006;25(4):495–7.
31. Verheyden CN. Nipple-sparing total mastectomy of large breasts: the role of tissue expansion. Plast Reconstr Surg. 1998;101(6):1494–500; discussion 1501–2.
32. Chang DW, et al. Effect of smoking on complications in patients undergoing free TRAM flap breast reconstruction. Plast Reconstr Surg. 2000;105(7):2374–80.
33. Chang DW, et al. Effect of obesity on flap and donor-site complications in free transverse rectus abdominis myocutaneous flap breast reconstruction. Plast Reconstr Surg. 2000;105(5):1640–8.
34. Rawlani V, et al. Tissue expander breast reconstruction using prehydrated human acellular dermis. Ann Plast Surg. 2011;66(6):593–7.
35. Spear SL, et al. Nipple-sparing mastectomy. Plast Reconstr Surg. 2009;123(6):1665–73.
36. Chopp D, Rawlani V, Ellis M, Johnson SA, Buck DW, Khan S, et al. A geometric analysis of mastectomy incisions: optimizing intra-operative breast volume. Can J Plast Surg. 2011;19(2):45–50.
37. Eldor L, Spiegel A. Breast reconstruction after bilateral prophylactic mastectomy in women at high risk for breast cancer. Breast J. 2009;15 Suppl 1:S81–9.
38. Meijers-Heijboer H, et al. Breast cancer after prophylactic bilateral mastectomy in women with a BRCA1 or BRCA2 mutation. N Engl J Med. 2001;345(3): 159–64.
39. D'Souza N, Darmanin G, Fedorowicz Z. Immediate versus delayed reconstruction following surgery for breast cancer. Cochrane Database Syst Rev. 2011;(7):CD008674.
40. Black D, et al. Detecting occult malignancy in prophylactic mastectomy: preoperative MRI versus sentinel lymph node biopsy. Ann Surg Oncol. 2007;14(9):2477–84.
41. Surgeons, A.S.o.P. Reconstructive breast surgery statistics 2010. 2010 Feburary 21. 2012. Available from: http://www.plasticsurgery.org/Documents/news-resources/statistics/2010-statisticss/Member-Surgeon-Data/2010-reconstructive-trends-statistics2.pdf.
42. Gurunluoglu R, et al. Current trends in breast reconstruction: survey of American Society of Plastic Surgeons 2010. Ann Plast Surg. 2011. DOI-10.1097/ SAP. 0b013e31822ed5ce.
43. Kim JY, et al. A meta-analysis of human acellular dermis and submuscular tissue expander breast reconstruction. Plast Reconstr Surg. 2012;129(1):28–41.
44. Spear SL, et al. The infected or exposed breast implant: management and treatment strategies. Plast Reconstr Surg. 2004;113(6):1634–44.
45. Moon HK, Taylor GI. The vascular anatomy of rectus abdominis musculocutaneous flaps based on the deep superior epigastric system. Plast Reconstr Surg. 1988;82(5):815–32.
46. Namnoum JD. An analysis of 920 pedicled and 286 free TRAM flap breast reconstructions, in Annual Meeting of the American Society of Plastic Surgeons. Orlando, FL; 2001.
47. Restifo RJ, et al. Surgical delay in TRAM flap breast reconstruction: a comparison of 7- and 14-day delay periods. Ann Plast Surg. 1997;38(4):330–3; discussion 333–4.
48. Nahabedian MY, et al. Breast reconstruction with the free TRAM or DIEP flap: patient selection, choice of flap, and outcome. Plast Reconstr Surg. 2002;110(2): 466–75; discussion 476–7.
49. Taylor GI, Daniel RK. The anatomy of several free flap donor sites. Plast Reconstr Surg. 1975;56(3): 243–53.
50. Chevray PM. Breast reconstruction with superficial inferior epigastric artery flaps: a prospective comparison with TRAM and DIEP flaps. Plast Reconstr Surg. 2004;114(5):1077–83; discussion 1084–5.
51. Allen RJ, Heitland A. Superficial inferior epigastric artery flap for breast reconstruction. Semin Plast Surg. 2002;15:35.
52. Atisha D, et al. The efficacy of the surgical delay procedure in pedicle TRAM breast reconstruction. Ann Plast Surg. 2009;63(4):383–8.
53. Man LX, Selber JC, Serletti JM. Abdominal wall following free TRAM or DIEP flap reconstruction: a meta-analysis and critical review. Plast Reconstr Surg. 2009;124(3):752–64.
54. Spiegel AJ, Khan FN. An Intraoperative algorithm for use of the SIEA flap for breast reconstruction. Plast Reconstr Surg. 2007;120(6):1450–9.
55. Losken A, et al. Outcomes evaluation following bilateral breast reconstruction using latissimus dorsi myocutaneous flaps. Ann Plast Surg. 2010;65(1):17–22.
56. Chang DW, et al. Autologous breast reconstruction with the extended latissimus dorsi flap. Plast Reconstr Surg. 2002;110(3):751–9; discussion 760–1.
57. Sternberg EG, et al. Latissimus dorsi flap remains an excellent choice for breast reconstruction. Ann Plast Surg. 2006;56(1):31–5.
58. Beckenstein MS, Grotting JC. Breast reconstruction with free-tissue transfer. Plast Reconstr Surg. 2001;108(5):1345–53; quiz 1354.
59. Werdin F, et al. Superior gluteal artery perforator flap in bilateral breast reconstruction. Ann Plast Surg. 2010;64(1):17–21.
60. LoTempio MM, Allen RJ. Breast reconstruction with SGAP and IGAP flaps. Plast Reconstr Surg. 2010;126(2):393–401.
61. Silverstein MJ. How I do it: oncoplastic breast-conservation surgery. Ann Surg Oncol. 2010;17 Suppl 3:242–4.
62. Whitworth P. Practical Oncoplastic Breast Surgery, in Society of Surgical Oncology Annual Cancer Symposium. San Antonio, TX; 2011.
63. Fine NA, Orgill DP, Pribaz JJ. Early clinical experience in endoscopic-assisted muscle flap harvest. Ann Plast Surg. 1994;33(5):465–9; discussion 469–72.

# 10 Management of Concomitant Risk

Megan E. Miller, Sarah M. Nielsen, and Swati A. Kulkarni

## Introduction

Breast cancer risk has been well-characterized for a number of genetic syndromes including carriers of *BRCA1/BRCA2*, *p53*, and *PTEN* mutations. This chapter will focus primarily on the risk of developing other malignancies in those individuals or family members with a genetic predisposition to breast cancer (Table 10.1). Screening protocols and risk reduction strategies will also be reviewed for individual malignancies where appropriate.

## *BRCA1/BRCA2* Mutation Carriers

Hereditary breast and ovarian cancer (HOBC) syndrome, characterized by a markedly increased risk of breast and ovarian cancer with an early age of onset, is caused by mutations in the breast cancer susceptibility genes *(BRCA) 1 and 2*. *BRCA 1 and 2* are tumor suppressor genes which function in the repair of DNA strand breaks; mutations are inherited in an autosomal-dominant fashion with high penetrance [1]. *BRCA1/2* mutations have also been associated with an increased risk of ovarian, prostate, pancreatic, colorectal, and gastric cancer, and melanoma. The following sections review the evidence for cancer risk at each site and provide recommendations regarding clinical patient management (Table 10.2).

M.E. Miller, M.D. (✉) • S.A. Kulkarni, M.D.
Department of Surgery, University of Chicago Medical Center, 5841 S. Maryland Avenue, MC 6040, Chicago, IL 60637, USA
e-mail: megan.miller2@uchospitals.edu; skulkarni@surgery.bsd.uchicago.edu

S.M. Nielsen, M.S, C.G.C.
Department of Hematology/Oncology, University of Chicago Medical Center, 5841 S. Maryland Avenue, MC 2115, Chicago, IL 60637, USA
e-mail: snielsen@medicine.bsd.uchicago.edu

### Ovarian Cancer

In contrast to the general population (1–2% lifetime risk), estimates of ovarian cancer range from 37 to 62% in *BRCA1* mutation carriers, and from 11 to 23% in *BRCA2* mutation carriers [2–5]. Meta-analysis of ovarian cancer screening in women at high genetic risk, including *BRCA1/2* carriers, shows an increased incidence of high-grade serous cancers for which there is no recognizable precursor [6].

*Screening Recommendations* Current options for the early detection of ovarian cancer include transvaginal ultrasound (TVU) and measurement of serum CA-125 levels. In premenopausal women, TVU is recommended during day 1–10 of the menstrual cycle and CA-125 levels after day 5 of the menstrual cycle [1]. This screening regimen should begin at age 35, or 5–10 years earlier than the earliest age of first diagnosis of ovarian cancer in the family, and should be performed every 6 months. Recent studies find ovarian cancer screening for *BRCA* mutation carriers

N.M. Hansen (ed.), *Management of the Patient at High Risk for Breast Cancer*, DOI 10.1007/978-1-4614-5891-3_10, © Springer Science+Business Media New York 2013

**Table 10.1** Hereditary cancer syndromes associated with an increased risk of breast cancer [1–5, 12, 21–23, 27, 31, 35, 37, 49, 56, 65, 74, 80, 84]

| Syndrome | Gene(s) | Inheritance | Related cancer risks (lifetime) |
|---|---|---|---|
| Hereditary breast and ovarian cancer | *BRCA1*<br>*BRCA2* | Autosomal dominant | Ovarian: 27–54%<br>Melanoma: 5–7%<br>Prostate: 20–80%<br>Gastric: <5%<br>Pancreatic: 3–5% |
| Cowden | *PTEN* | Autosomal dominant | Thyroid: 35%<br>Colorectal: 10%<br>Endometrial: 28%<br>Melanoma: 6%<br>Kidney: 34% |
| Li–Fraumeni | *p53* | Autosomal dominant | Absolute lifetime risks for LFS-associated cancers are unknown<br>Sarcoma brain<br>Leukemia adrenocortical<br>Colorectal pancreas<br>Any childhood cancer |
| Peutz-Jeghers | *STK11* | Autosomal dominant | Colorectal: 39%<br>Lung: 15–17%<br>Small bowel: 29%<br>Uterine: 9%<br>Gastric: 13%<br>Ovarian: 18–21%<br>Pancreatic: 11–36%<br>Cervical: 10% |
| Fanconi anemia | At least 15 *FANC* genes | Autosomal recessive | Absolute lifetime risks for FA-associated cancers are unknown<br>AML<br>Skin<br>Brain<br>Kidney<br>Esophageal<br>Liver |
| Hereditary diffuse gastric cancer | *CDH1* | Autosomal dominant | Diffuse gastric: 80% |
| Ataxia telangiectasia | *ATM* | Autosomal recessive | Absolute lifetime risks for AT-associated cancers are unknown<br>Acute leukemia<br>Pancreatic<br>Lymphoma<br>Gastric<br>Ovarian<br>Liver<br>Salivary glands<br>Oral cavity |

may be of limited value, based on low sensitivity and low positive predictive value in asymptomatic women at high risk [7, 8].

*Risk Reduction Strategies* Prophylactic bilateral salpingo-oophorectomy (PBSO) is recommended for *BRCA1/2* carriers after the completion of childbearing and ideally by age 35–40 years [1]. This recommendation is based on studies of surveillance compared with PBSO in which the mean age of diagnosis of ovarian cancer was 50.8 years [9]. Results of a recent meta-analysis of ten

**Table 10.2** Lifetime risk of concomitant cancers in *BRCA1/2* mutation carriers [1–5, 12, 21–23, 27, 31, 35, 37]

| Cancer site | General population (%) | *BRCA1* (%) | *BRCA2* (%) | Screening recommendations | Risk reduction strategies |
|---|---|---|---|---|---|
| Ovarian | 1–2 | 37–62 | 11–23 | Transvaginal ultrasound and serum CA-125 levels at age 35 | Bilateral salpingo-oophorectomy at age 35–40 |
| Prostate | 10–17 | 18–57 | 28–80 | PSA and DRE annually at age 40 | |
| Pancreatic | 1.3 | 2.9–4.7 | 4.6–5.0 | EUS or other imaging annually starting at age 40 | Limit smoking and alcohol; weight loss |
| Melanoma | 1.8–2.7 | Not increased from general population | 4.6–6.9 | Full-body skin examination by dermatologist or experienced practitioner annually at age 10 | Limit UV and radiation exposure |

studies involving *BRCA1/2* mutation carriers demonstrated an 80% reduction in the risk of ovarian or fallopian cancer following PBSO [10]. Other studies focusing on the risk reduction of ovarian cancer alone after PBSO estimate a 95% decreased risk; ovarian cancer-specific mortality is also reduced after PBSO in *BRCA1/2* mutation carriers [9, 11].

Historic studies on incidence of cancer in *BRCA* mutation carriers identify risks of other gynecological cancers, including those of the fallopian tubes, uterus, endometrium, and cervix [12, 13]. "Primary" peritoneal cancer is a common late sequelae of locally advanced or metastatic ovarian cancer [13]. Even after PSBO, 4.3% of women developed peritoneal cancer within 20 years [3].

*Surgical Options* Laparoscopic PBSO is the surgical procedure of choice. A complete survey of the abdomen and pelvis should be done, including all visceral and peritoneal surfaces. Any suspicious areas by inspection or palpation should be biopsied with frozen section as appropriate [14]. All ovarian tissue should be removed, if necessary en bloc with surrounding adhesive tissue to ensure complete resection. As much of the fallopian tube should be removed as possible, but small amounts of the intramural (interstitial) portion may be left in situ without increasing the risk of malignancy [15]. If there are additional gynecological indications, hysterectomy can be performed simultaneously for reduction of cancer risk, but it should not be considered routine [16]. *BRCA1/2* carriers considering risk reduction surgery should be counseled regarding surgically-induced menopause. Symptoms can be mediated with the use of hormone replacement therapy (HRT); despite concern about the use of HRT in *BRCA* mutation carriers, current data suggest that HRT does not negate the reduction in breast cancer risk derived from PBSO [1, 17].

*Chemoprevention* Case–control studies demonstrate that oral contraceptives (OCPs) reduce the risk of ovarian cancer by 45–50% in *BRCA1* mutation carriers and by 60% in *BRCA2* carriers, with risks decreasing with longer duration of use [18, 19]. A recent meta-analysis of *BRCA* mutation carriers with ($N$=1,503) and without ($N$=6,315) ovarian cancer, the use of OCPs reduced the risk of ovarian cancer by 50% in *BRCA1/2* mutation carriers [20]. For each additional 10 years of OCP use, there was a significantly reduced ovarian cancer risk (RR 0.64). When used for 5 or more years, OCPs may be used for ovarian cancer risk-reduction [18–20]. However, PBSO is still recommended for optimal risk reduction [1].

## Prostate Cancer

Male carriers of *BRCA1/2* mutations are at an increased risk of prostate cancer. The risk is mediated by ethnicity, age, and mutation type.

The Breast Cancer Linkage Consortium (BCLC) studies report a relative risk of 1.82–3.33 for prostate cancer in *BRCA1* carriers [13, 21]. For *BRCA2* carriers, the relative risk is between four and sevenfold [22, 23]. *BRCA2* mutations have been associated with a lower mean age at diagnosis, more advanced tumor stage, higher tumor grade, and shorter median survival time [24, 25].

*Screening Recommendations and Risk Reduction Strategies* The American Cancer Society recommends offering standard screening with prostate-specific antigen test (PSA) and digital rectal examination to men with a known or likely *BRCA1* or 2 mutation starting at age 40 or 45 years [26]. A multicenter, international study entitled IMPACT (Identification of Men with a Genetic Predisposition to Prostate Cancer: Targeted screening in *BRCA1/2* carriers and controls) was recently undertaken to determine the efficacy of prostate cancer screening in men with *BRCA* mutations [27]. Prostate cancer was diagnosed as a result of screening in 3.3% of patients, compared with the annual incidence of 0.1–1% in the general population [28]; 9 of the 11 cancers were found in *BRCA* mutation carriers. These data provide convincing evidence that screening PSA has a high positive predictive value in *BRCA* patients. Based on the available data, there are no clear recommendations for risk-reduction strategies beyond beginning screening at age 40 in high-risk individuals, including those with *BRCA1/2* mutations.

## Melanoma

Several studies have suggested a link between mutations in *BRCA2* and melanoma. The BCLC study on 3,728 individuals from 173 breast-ovarian cancer families reported a relative risk of cutaneous malignant melanoma of 2.58 [22]. An odds ratio of 4 for *BRCA2* mutations was reported in Ashkenazi patients with ocular melanoma, and other studies of breast cancer families have found an increased incidence of ocular or cutaneous melanoma [29, 30]

*Screening Recommendations and Risk Reduction Strategies* The Melanoma Genetics Consortium recommends that high-risk individuals have a baseline skin examination by a trained health care provider beginning at age 10, with follow up every 6 months until the nevus pattern is stable and the patient is competent for self-surveillance, and then annual follow up [31].

*BRCA2* is down-regulated in a dose-dependent manner by UV radiation in human cells and is involved in a DNA-damaging signaling pathway induced by UV exposure [32]. Further, expression of wild-type *BRCA2* can protect cells from UV-induced cell death. The standard recommendation to those at increased melanoma risk, due to personal and/or family history, or to genetic factors, is to reduce or eliminate sun exposure and UV radiation.

## Pancreatic Cancer

Several studies have demonstrated that *BRCA* mutations increase the risk of pancreatic adenocarcinoma [33, 34]. Compared to the general population risk of 1.3%, the cumulative age-adjusted lifetime risk of pancreatic cancer is 3.6% in *BRCA1* carriers and 4.9% in *BRCA2* carriers [5, 12, 35]. Given the phenotypic aggressiveness of pancreatic cancer, lack of early symptoms, and frequent late-stage at diagnosis, *BRCA* mutation carriers may derive particular benefit from screening protocols and risk reduction strategies.

*Screening Recommendations and Risk Reduction Strategies* Currently, there is no consensus on the most suitable modality for pancreatic surveillance, and regimens are largely institution-specific [36]. Commonly ordered screening tests include CEA, CA 19–9, liver function tests, amylase, lipase, CT scans, and MRCP. More invasive tests include EUS and ERCP [37, 38]. *BRCA1/2* mutation carriers with a family history of pancreatic cancer should undergo screening starting at age 40, or 10 years prior to the diagnosis of pancreatic cancer in the affected family member, whichever is earlier [37]. The American

Gastroenterology Association recommends spiral CT as the initial screening investigation, with follow-up EUS and CA 19–9 measurements if CT is non-diagnostic [39]. If results are abnormal or there is interval development of suspicious characteristics, such as pancreatic or biliary ductal dilation, a mass, or a discrete lesion, subsequent screening should proceed every 3–6 months [36, 37]. In addition, practitioners should educate patients about modifiable risk factors such as smoking and assist in planning appropriate lifestyle modifications [40].

## Gastric Cancer

Some epidemiologic studies have reported an increased risk of gastric cancer associated with *BRCA1/2* mutations, with RR 2.0–6.9 depending on the particular study population [12, 22]. Other studies have not identified a risk greater than that in the general population [21, 23]. Given the conflicting data, gastric cancer screening with endoscopy can be considered in *BRCA1/2* mutation carriers with a family history of gastric cancer, and should start at age 40, or 5–10 years prior to the earliest age of diagnosis [41]. Risk reduction with dietary modification, avoidance of tobacco, and prompt treatment of premalignant conditions such as *H. pylori* and mucosal dysplasia should be implemented.

## Colorectal Cancer

A two to four fold increased risk of colorectal cancer associated with *BRCA1/2* mutations was found in several of the early BCLC and population-based series [12, 21]. However, follow-up studies examining over 2,500 patients with a diagnosis of colorectal cancer have not demonstrated an increased risk associated with *BRCA* mutations [42, 43]. Recommended screening in *BRCA1/2* mutation carriers is therefore the same as the general population, with earlier and more frequent testing based on personal and/or family history of the disease.

## Cowden Syndrome

Cowden Syndrome (CS) is an autosomal dominant cancer predisposition syndrome caused by germline mutations in the tumor suppressor gene phosphate and tensin homologue on chromosome ten (*PTEN*). CS is the prototype of the *PTEN* hamartoma tumor syndrome (PHTS), which includes four clinically distinct syndromes: CS, Bannayan-Riley-Ruvalcaba syndrome, Proteus syndrome, and Proteus-like syndrome [44]. CS is usually identified in adulthood by the characteristic multiple disorganized benign growths, or hamartomas, especially of the skin and mucous membranes. These pathognomonic lesions, present in over 90% of patients with CS, include trichilemmomas, papillomatous papules, and acral and plantar keratoses. Other common findings in CS are macrocephaly, Lhermitte-Duclos disease (dysplastic gangliogliocytoma of the cerebellum), megencephaly, and dolicoencephaly [44–46]. The criteria for CS have been updated several times since their inception in 1996. Germline *PTEN* mutations have been found in approximately 85% of patients who meet the clinical criteria for CS, and mutations in the *PTEN* promoter have been identified in approximately 7% of patients meeting clinical criteria without an identifiable mutation [47, 48] (Table 10.3).

*Cancer Risks* Results from the first prospective study of lifetime cancer risks in the *PTEN* mutation carriers were recently published and the new risk estimates are significantly elevated from those historically quoted [49] (Table 10.4). Following breast cancer, thyroid disease is the second most common manifestation of CS, affecting between two-thirds and three-quarters of patients [45, 50]. The benign thyroid conditions associated with CS include follicular adenomas, adenomatous nodules, and multinodular goiter [44]. It is now known that patients with CS have a 35% lifetime risk of developing epithelial thyroid cancer, typically with follicular pathology [49, 51]. The average age of onset (38 years) is earlier than that of the general population; even

**Table 10.3** Diagnostic criteria for Cowden syndrome (CS) [44, 45, 50]

| Pathognomonic criteria | Major criteria | Minor criteria |
|---|---|---|
| Mucocutaneous lesions:<br>Trichilemmomas, facial<br>Acral keratoses<br>Papillomatous lesions<br>Mucosal lesions<br>Lhermitte-Duclos Disease (LDD) | Breast carcinoma, invasive<br>Thyroid carcinoma, especially follicular<br>Macrocephaly (>97% percentile)<br>Endometrial carcinoma | Other thyroid lesions, i.e. adenoma, multinodular goiter, Hashimoto's thyroiditis<br>Developmental delay<br>GI hamartomas/polyposis<br>Fibrocystic disease of the breast<br>Lipomas<br>Fibromas<br>Genito-urinary tumors (renal cell carcinoma, uterine fibroids) or malformations (bicornuate uterus) |
| An operational diagnosis of Cowden syndrome can be made if an individual meets any of the following: | | |
| 1. Pathognomonic mucocutaneous lesions alone if there are: | Six or more facial papules, of which three or more must be trichilemmomas, or<br>Cutaneous facial papules and oral mucosal papillomatosis, or<br>Oral mucosal papillomatosis and acral keratoses, or<br>Six or more palmo-plantar keratoses | |
| 2. Two major criteria but one must be macrocephaly or Lhermitte-Duclos syndrome | | |
| 3. One major and two minor criteria | | |
| 4. Four minor criteria | | |
| In a family where one individual is diagnosed with CS by genetic status or clinical criteria, other members can be diagnosed if they meet any of the following: | | |
| 1. Pathognomonic criteria | | |
| 2. Any one major criteria with or without minor criteria | | |
| 3. Two minor criteria | | |

children with CS have developed thyroid cancer, though interestingly all these cases demonstrated papillary pathology [49, 51].

Abnormalities of the genitourinary tract are common in CS patients. Women have an approximately 28% lifetime risk of developing endometrial cancer and up to 50% of women develop multiple large uterine fibroids [49, 51, 52]. Additionally, Tan et al. recently reported renal cell carcinoma (papillary subtype) has a lifetime risk as high as 34% in CS [49].

Benign and malignant tumors of the skin, brain, and gastrointestinal tract are also seen with increased frequency in CS patients [44, 52]. The skin and brain findings associated with CS tend to be benign in nature, though of note, there is a 6% lifetime risk for melanoma in CS carriers [49]. Recent studies have systematically assessed polyp burden and colorectal cancer risk in patients with CS. Greater than 90% of CS patients who received colonoscopies were found to have polyps. The polyps were most often hyperplastic and located in the colon, but ganglioneuromatous and adenomatous polyps were also found in the esophagus, stomach, duodenum, jejunum, ileum and rectum. In one series, colorectal cancer was identified in 13% of patients, all of whom were diagnosed at less than 50 years old [53]. Overall, the lifetime risk of colorectal cancer in CS patients is estimated to be 10% [44, 45, 49].

*Screening Recommendations and Risk Reduction Strategies* Of the four *PTEN* hamartoma tumor syndromes, an increased risk of malignancy has been found only in Cowden syndrome. However, since they are all associated with germline mutations in *PTEN*, some experts advise all individuals with PHTS to follow the same cancer surveillance strategies as those for CS [44, 45]. Current screening guidelines specify cancer surveillance for known *PTEN* mutation carriers, those who meet clinical criteria, and close relatives of *PTEN* mutation carriers who have not undergone genetic testing. Surveillance should be individualized according to personal and/or family history [1].

**Table 10.4** Risk of cancer and associated conditions in Cowden syndrome [49, 51, 53]

| Cancer | Lifetime risk (%) | Mean age of onset (yrs.) | Pathology | Associated conditions |
|---|---|---|---|---|
| Thyroid | 35 | 37.5 | Follicular | Follicular adenomas, adenomatous nodules, multinodular goiter |
| Endometrial | 28 | 40–45 | Adenocarcinoma | Uterine fibroids, genitourinary malformations |
| Renal | 34 | 40 | Papillary, chromophobe | Unknown |
| Colorectal | 10 | 40 | Adenocarcinoma, signet ring | GI polyps of mixed histology, primarily hyperplastic |
| Melanoma | 6 | Unknown | Unknown | Unknown |

Comprehensive physical examinations should be performed annually beginning at age 18, or 5 years prior to the earliest age at diagnosis of malignancy in the family [1, 44]. Careful attention should be given to dermatological changes with a low threshold for referral to a dermatologist. Thyroid exam and baseline ultrasound should be initiated at diagnosis of CS or upon finding an associated mutation, as even children with CS are at risk for thyroid cancer [49, 51]. Based on recent prospective data revealing a higher risk for endometrial cancer than previously thought, a more aggressive regimen is being recommended, including endometrial biopsies for premenopausal women on an annual basis starting at age 30, or 5 years prior to the earliest age of diagnosis of endometrial cancer in the family. For postmenopausal women, annual TVU with biopsy of any suspicious areas is recommended [44, 49]. Due to updated reported risk estimates regarding renal cell carcinoma (RCC), biannual renal ultrasound/MRI in addition to annual urinalysis with cytology is now being recommended for individuals with CS [49, 50]. New guidelines for colorectal cancer surveillance have been developed. Colonoscopies should begin at age 35–40, or 5 years younger than the earliest age of colon cancer onset in the family. The recommended screening interval is biannually, though heavy polyp burden may necessitate more frequent screenings [49, 51].

The malignant tumors associated with CS are diverse and vary by age at onset and anatomic location, making risk-reduction recommendations largely ineffective. Decisions about risk reduction should be made on a case-by-case basis, taking personal and family history of both benign and malignant neoplasms into consideration.

## Li–Fraumeni Syndrome

Li–Fraumeni Syndrome (LFS) is a rare familial cancer syndrome caused by germline mutations in the *p53* tumor suppressor gene [54]. Transmission has been shown to be autosomal dominant. However, only 50–70% of families meeting the classical LFS criteria have a *p53* mutation, suggesting that there may be alternative mutations, either in the promoter or in different genes altogether, that are responsible for LFS [55] (Table 10.5).

*Cancer Risks* Soft tissue sarcomas, premenopausal breast cancer, adrenocortical carcinoma, and brain tumors account for the majority of cancers in patients with germline *p53* mutations, and at least one of these cancers has been found in one or more members of all families with a mutation in *p53* [56, 57]. Other cancers commonly associated with LFS are osteosarcomas, colon cancer, leukemia, and early onset of any childhood cancer, particularly adrenocortical carcinoma (ACC), rhabdomyosarcoma, and brain tumors (i.e., choroid plexus tumors) [55, 58, 59]. Some studies have demonstrated an increased incidence of melanoma, germ cell tumors, Wilms' tumor, lymphoma, lung cancer, and gastrointestinal and endocrine tumors [60, 61].

For patients with a known germline *p53* mutation, the estimated cancer risk is 30% by age 20 and 95% by age 70 [61, 62]. Chompret et al. estimate the lifetime risk of developing cancer in *p53* mutation carriers is 73% for males and nearly 100% for females, with the high incidence of breast cancer in female carriers accounting for

**Table 10.5** Clinical criteria for the diagnosis of Li–Fraumeni syndrome (LFS) [55–60]

| Clinical criteria | Description |
|---|---|
| Classic LFS 1988 | Individual diagnosed with sarcoma prior to age 45, and<br>A first-degree relative with cancer prior to age 45, and<br>Another first- or second-degree relative with cancer diagnosed prior to age 45 OR with sarcoma at any age |
| Chompret et al. [55] | Individual with sarcoma, brain tumor, breast cancer, or ACC prior to age 36, and at least one first- or second-degree relative with cancer (other than breast cancer if the individual has breast cancer) prior to age 46, or a relative with multiple primary cancers at any age; OR<br>Individual with multiple primary tumors, two of which are sarcoma, brain tumor, breast cancer, and/or ACC, with the initial cancer prior to age 36, regardless of family history, OR<br>Individual with ACC at any age, regardless of family history |
| Eeles [59] | In families that do not meet classic LFS criteria:<br>Two different tumors from the extended LFS spectrum (sarcoma, brain tumor, breast cancer, ACC, leukemia, melanoma, pancreatic cancer, prostate cancer) in two first- or second-degree relatives at any age |
| Birch [58] | In families that do not meet classic LFS criteria:<br>Individual with any childhood cancer, sarcoma, brain tumor, or ACC diagnosed prior to age 45, AND<br>A first- or second-degree relative with a LFS-type tumor (sarcoma, brain tumor, breast cancer, ACC, or leukemia) diagnosed at any age, AND<br>A first- or second-degree relative with any cancer diagnosed prior to age 60 |

the accounting for the gender-related discrepancy [55]. Patients with LFS who survive their first cancer have a markedly increased risk of developing multiple primary neoplasms as they age. After the primary diagnosis of cancer, approximately 15% of LFS patients develop a second cancer, 4% a third cancer, and 2% eventually develop a fourth cancer [63]. Younger age at diagnosis of the first cancer is associated with greater subsequent cancer risk, with a relative risk of 83 for those initially diagnosed prior to age 19 [63]. The exceedingly high lifetime risk of cancer for *p53* mutation carriers includes all malignancies, almost a quarter of which are outside the spectrum of LFS tumor types [61]. It is difficult to estimate the risk of each specific cancer associated with LFS due to phenotypic variability and controversy surrounding the clinical criteria [56].

*Screening Recommendations and Risk Reduction Strategies* The diverse range of tumors and ages of onset argue against the implementation of potentially invasive, repetitive, and costly screening tests for germline *p53* mutation carriers [63]. In fact, clinical surveillance strategies have previously been discouraged for patients with LFS secondary to a lack of evidence of benefit from the early detection of malignancies [64]. Screening guidelines for *p53* mutation carriers recommend a comprehensive annual physical exam starting at age 20–25 years with a high index of suspicion for rare cancers and subsequent primary neoplasms in cancer survivors [1]. Screening for colorectal cancer with colonoscopy should be considered every 2–5 years starting at age 25 [1]. Initiating screening at these early ages is based on the characteristically young age of cancer diagnosis, at an average of 21.9 years (range 4 months to 49 years) for *p53* mutation carriers and 31.6 years in those meeting LFS criteria without a mutation [56]. In a recent review of inherited cancer syndromes, D'Orazio adds the recommendation of annual urinalysis and complete blood count (CBC) [65]. These tests, which screen for ACC and leukemia, are more frequently utilized in the pediatric population, but may be considered in adult *p53* mutation carriers with a family history of these malignancies.

Some groups advocate more formalized and aggressive screening regimens based on recent data. Masciari et al. implemented an imaging surveillance program utilizing

F18-fluorodeoxyglucose–positron emission tomography/computed tomography (FDG-PET/CT) in which a diagnosis of cancer was made in 20% of patients [66]. Villani et al. suggest surveillance with annual brain MRI, annual whole-body MRI, biannual ultrasound of the abdomen and pelvis, and CBC, LDH, and ESR every 4 months. Survival at follow-up was 20% in the non-surveillance group and 100% in the surveillance group ($p=0.0417$) [64]. While whole-body PET-CT or MRI may be considered in some high-risk LFS patients, larger trials are necessary prior to making evidenced-based recommendations.

Several studies have shown that radiation treatment significantly increases the risk of secondary malignancies in *p53* mutation carriers, specifically for tumors that develop within the radiation field [57, 63]. While it is not always possible to avoid radiation in the treatment of a primary malignancy, knowledge of *p53* mutation status could inform decisions about dose, duration, and extent of radiation field to limit exposure. Similarly, limiting UV exposure is prudent given the increased risk of melanoma found in some studies of *p53* mutation carriers [61].

Individualized screening in *p53* mutation carriers should be based on personal and/or family tumor history. Additional imaging and biochemical studies should be supplemented when warranted clinically or upon presentation of signs or symptoms of particular cancers. The diversity of tumor types in LFS and the inability to predict an individual's risk of a particular cancer limit the utility of risk reduction strategies.

## Peutz-Jeghers Syndrome/*STK11* Mutation

Peutz-Jeghers syndrome (PJS) is caused by mutations in the *STK11* gene and transmitted in an autosomal dominant fashion. A recent systematic review of 1,644 PJS patients from 20 cohort studies complied and analyzed the wide ranges of cancer risks reported in the literature [67]. In addition to breast cancer, which has a lifetime risk of 32–54%, the most frequently reported cancers overall are colorectal cancer, followed by small bowel, stomach, and pancreatic cancer [67]. Of note, PJS patients more frequently develop sex cord ovarian tumors with annular tubules, rather than epithelial subtype [68]. Male children with PJS have an increased risk of Sertoli cell tumors [69] (Table 10.6).

*Screening Recommendations and Risk Reduction Strategies* Regular surveillance is recommended for patients with PJS based on the high risk of benign intestinal complications (intussusception, obstruction, infarction, and bleeding) and malignant disease [67, 70]. Several series have demonstrated a low incidence of neoplasms in

**Table 10.6** Peutz-Jeghers syndrome: cancer risk and surveillance guidelines, NCCN 2011 [1]

| Site (% risk) | Screening procedure and interval | Initiation age |
|---|---|---|
| Breast (45–50) | Mammogram and breast MRI annually; clinical breast exam every 6 months | 25 years |
| Colon (39) | Colonoscopy every 2–3 years | Late teens |
| Stomach (2) | Upper endoscopy every 2–3 years | Late teens |
| Pancreas (11–36) | Magnetic resonance cholangiopancreatography (MRCP) and/or endoscopic ultrasound (EUS) every 1–2 years<br>CA 19–9 every 1–2 years | 25–30 years |
| Small intestine (13) | Small bowel visualization (CT enterography, small bowel enteroclysis) baseline at 8–10 years; follow-up interval based on findings but at least by age 18, then every 2–3 years; individualize based on symptoms | 8–10 years |
| Ovary (18–21),<br>Cervix (10), Uterus (9) | Pelvic examination and PAP smear annually<br>Consider transvaginal ultrasound | 18–20 years |
| Testes | Annual testicular exam and observation for feminizing changes | 10 years |
| Lung (15–17) | Provide education about symptoms and smoking cessation<br>No other specific recommendations have been made | |

polypectomy specimens [71, 72]. Nonetheless, endoscopic polypectomy for polyps greater than 10–15 mm is recommended for patients with PJS [73]. Intraoperative enteroscopy has been recommended in patients undergoing laparotomy, as it increases the rate of polypectomy and has greater sensitivity to detect all polyps, resulting in a "clean sweep" to decrease the rate of repeat laparotomy [73, 74]. Several pharmacologic therapies that target the mTOR pathway are being evaluated in clinical trials to determine if there is a decrease in polyp burden and a concomitant reduction in malignancies [70].

## Hereditary Diffuse Gastric Cancer/ *CDH1* Mutation

Autosomal dominant germline mutations of the tumor suppressor gene *CDH1*, which encodes the protein e-cadherin, have been implicated as the genetic basis of hereditary diffuse gastric cancer (HDGC) and invasive lobular breast carcinoma [75]. The lifetime risk of gastric cancer in HDCG kindreds is estimated at 80% with an average age of onset of 40 years [76, 77]. The hallmark of HDGC is a pattern of isolated, mucin-filled signet ring cells scattered throughout the gastric mucosa [77].

*Screening Recommendations* The screening recommendation for patients with a *CDH1* germline mutation, untested family members, and those at increased risk due to clinical criteria is endoscopic surveillance every 6–12 months [76, 77]. Using a white light high definition endoscope, the mucosa should be carefully inspected on inflation and deflation, and minimum of 30 biopsies obtained [76, 77]. Increased risk for colon cancer has been suggested in HDGC families but not confirmed. In families with *CDH1* mutations and a positive history of colon cancer, colonoscopy should begin 10 years prior to the youngest age at colon cancer diagnosis, or age 40, whichever comes first, and repeated every 3–5 years depending on findings [76].

*Risk Reduction Strategies* Prophylactic gastrectomy is recommended for known *CDH1* germline mutation carriers [76]. This is based on the inability to reliably detect the characteristically diffuse and isolated gastric cancer cells and their submucosal pattern of spread at endoscopy [77]. Gastrectomy is not recommended until age 20 due to the significant morbidity related to postoperative changes in digestion and nutrition [77, 78]. The procedure of choice is a total gastrectomy and D1 lymphadenectomy with Roux-en-Y reconstruction [76, 78].

## Low Penetrance Mutations

The following syndromes are associated with a relatively low risk of breast cancer and other malignancies. There are no specific screening recommendations or risk reduction strategies for these syndromes outside of a clinical trial. Management of these patients should be dictated by family and personal history of cancer. Nibrin (*NBN*) and Ataxia telangiectasia-mutated (*ATM*) mutations are known to increase sensitivity to radiation and chemotherapy, which may produce toxicity or induce further DNA damage, potentially increasing subsequent malignancy risks [79]. This should be taken into consideration when treating these patients for breast cancer or other malignancies, potentially by decreasing doses or utilizing alternative therapies when possible.

## Ataxia Telangiectasia/*ATM*

Ataxia telangiectasia (AT) is an autosomal recessive disorder with an incidence of 1 in 100,000. AT is characterized by ataxia, progressive dysphagia, immune deficiency, and pulmonary disease [80]. The incidence of malignancy in homozygotes is 1% per year after age 10, 85% of which are lymphomas and acute leukemias [81]. The heterozygous mutation carrier rate is much higher, estimated at 2% in the general population, and has been linked to an increased risk of breast cancer with a relative risk of 2.4–6.3 [80, 82, 83]. A meta-analysis by Easton et al. reported a pooled relative risk of 1.9 for risk for malignancies other than breast cancer in *ATM* carriers [84].

Thompson et al. demonstrated a potential excess risk of colorectal and stomach cancer, although overall numbers were small [82].

## Fanconi's Anemia/*PALB2* Mutations

Fanconi's anemia (FA) is a rare autosomal recessive disorder. The hallmark feature is an increased sensitivity to chromosomal breakage upon cellular exposure to DNA interstrand cross-linking agents, such as alkylating chemotherapeutic drugs [85, 86]. A common link between breast cancer susceptibility and FA was demonstrated in 2002, when one of the FA proteins, FANCD1, was found to be the same protein encoded by the *BRCA2* gene [87]. An additional FA protein, FACNC/*PALB2*, is critical for BRCA2's chromatin localization and recruitment to DNA damage sites, making it an important mediator of *BRCA2*-mediated tumor suppression [88] (Fig. 10.1).

Fanconi's anemia is typically diagnosed in childhood, secondary to phenotypes including abnormalities of the skin, arms, head, eyes, kidneys, and ears; short stature; and developmental disability [86]. Aplastic anemia generally develops during the first decade of life, with a cumulative risk of 90% by the age of 40 [89]. There is an increased risk of pancreatic cancer in individuals with *PALB2* mutations, particularly in families with a history of breast cancer [90]. It has been suggested that families with both breast and pancreatic cancer undergo genetic testing for *PALB2*, as the mutation is more likely to be found in this particular context [88].

## Nijmegen Breakage Syndrome/*NBN* Mutation

The Nijmegen Breakage syndrome (NBS) is an autosomal recessive disorder caused by mutation in the *NBN* gene, which encodes for the protein nibrin [91]. Nibrin has been identified at the crossroads of several pathways associated with breast cancer susceptibility [92]. Patients with NBS are at an increased risk of growth retardation, immunodeficiency, microcephaly, sensitivity to radiation and malignancy, with 40% developing cancer before the age of 20 [91, 93].

Individuals who are heterozygous for *NBN* mutations are phenotypically normal but carry an increased risk of developing cancer. Several studies in Eastern European families with a history of breast cancer have demonstrated an increased risk of breast cancer in heterozygous *NBN* mutation carriers [92, 94]. *NBN* mutations have been associated with hematologic malignancies, as well as head and neck, colorectal, gastric, renal, brain, and prostate cancers [94, 95]. However, overall numbers are small and risk estimates for malignancies by anatomic site cannot be made.

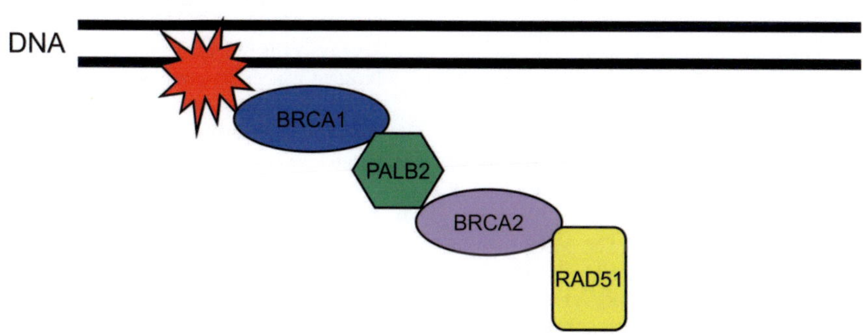


**Fig. 10.1** The role of *PALB2* in the *BRCA1/2* complex. *PALB2* (also known as FANCN) physically links *BRCA1* and *BRCA2* (also known as FANCD1) and aids in the recruitment of the complex to sites of DNA damage. The interaction of this complex with the enzyme RAD51 initiates homologous recombination, an important function in tumor suppressor activity

In conclusion, breast cancer risk has been well characterized for a number of genetic syndromes, but these syndromes are also associated with an increased risk of concomitant malignancies. Physicians and patients need to be familiar with these risks so that timely and appropriate screening can be completed to ensure that these other potential malignancies are not overlooked.

## References


1. National Comprehensive Cancer Network. Genetic/familial high-risk assessment: breast and ovarian cancer. NCCN Clinical Practice Guidelines in Oncology. NCCN.org, 2011.
2. Antoniou A, Pharoah PD, Narod S, et al. Average risks of breast and ovarian cancer associated with *BRCA1* or *BRCA2* mutations detected in case series unselected for family history: a combined analysis of 22 studies. Am J Hum Genet. 2003;72:1117–30.
3. Finch A, Beiner M, Lubinski J, et al. Salpingo-oophorectomy and the risk of ovarian, fallopian tube, and peritoneal cancers in women with a BRCA1 or BRCA2 mutation. JAMA. 2006;296:185–92.
4. King MC, Marks JH, Mandell JB. Breast and ovarian cancer risks due to inherited mutations in BRCA1 and BRCA2. Science. 2003;302:643–6.
5. Reis LAGKC, Hankey BF, Miller BK, editors. SEER cancer statistics review, 1973–1995. Bethesda, MD: National Cancer Institute; 1998.
6. Hogg R, Friedlander M. Biology of epithelial ovarian cancer: implications for screening women at high genetic risk. J Clin Oncol. 2004;22:1315–27.
7. Stirling D, Evans DG, Pichert G, et al. Screening for familial ovarian cancer: failure of current protocols to detect ovarian cancer at an early stage according to the international Federation of gynecology and obstetrics system. J Clin Oncol. 2005;23:5588–96.
8. Woodward ER, Sleightholme HV, Considine AM, et al. Annual surveillance by CA125 and transvaginal ultrasound for ovarian cancer in both high-risk and population risk women is ineffective. BJOG. 2007;114:1500–9.
9. Rebbeck TR, Lynch HT, Neuhausen SL, et al. Prophylactic oophorectomy in carriers of BRCA1 or BRCA2 mutations. N Engl J Med. 2002;346:1616–22.
10. Rebbeck TR, Kauff ND, Domchek SM. Meta-analysis of risk reduction estimates associated with risk-reducing salpingo-oophorectomy in BRCA1 or BRCA2 mutation carriers. J Natl Cancer Inst. 2009;101:80–7.
11. Domchek SM, Friebel TM, Neuhausen SL, et al. Mortality after bilateral salpingo-oophorectomy in BRCA1 and BRCA2 mutation carriers: a prospective cohort study. Lancet Oncol. 2006;7:223–9.
12. Brose MS, Rebbeck TR, Calzone KA, et al. Cancer risk estimates for BRCA1 mutation carriers identified in a risk evaluation program. J Natl Cancer Inst. 2002;94:1365–72.
13. Thompson D, Easton DF. Cancer incidence in BRCA1 mutation carriers. J Natl Cancer Inst. 2002;94:1358–65.
14. Rabban JT, Mackey A, Powell CB, et al. Correlation of macroscopic and microscopic pathology in risk reducing salpingo-oophorectomy: implications for intraoperative specimen evaluation. Gynecol Oncol. 2011;121:466–71.
15. Guillem JG, Wood WC, Moley JF, et al. ASCO/SSO review of current role of risk-reducing surgery in common hereditary cancer syndromes. J Clin Oncol. 2006;24:4642–60.
16. Gabriel CA, Tigges-Cardwell J, Stopfer J, et al. Use of total abdominal hysterectomy and hormone replacement therapy in BRCA1 and BRCA2 mutation carriers undergoing risk-reducing salpingo-oophorectomy. Fam Cancer. 2009;8:23–8.
17. Eisen A, Lubinski J, Klijn J, et al. Breast cancer risk following bilateral oophorectomy in BRCA1 and BRCA2 mutation carriers: an international case–control study. J Clin Oncol. 2005;23:7491–6.
18. McLaughlin JR, Risch HA, Lubinski J, et al. Reproductive risk factors for ovarian cancer in carriers of BRCA1 or BRCA2 mutations: a case–control study. Lancet Oncol. 2007;8:26–34.
19. Narod SA, Risch H, Moslehi R, et al. Oral contraceptives and the risk of hereditary ovarian cancer. Hereditary ovarian cancer clinical study group. N Engl J Med. 1998;339:424–8.
20. Iodice S, Barile M, Rotmensz N, et al. Oral contraceptive use and breast or ovarian cancer risk in BRCA1/2 carriers: a meta-analysis. Eur J Cancer. 2010;46:2275–84.
21. Ford D, Easton DF, Bishop DT, et al. Risks of cancer in BRCA1-mutation carriers. Breast Cancer Linkage Consortium. Lancet. 1994;343:692–5.
22. Cancer risks in BRCA2 mutation carriers. The Breast Cancer Linkage Consortium. J Natl Cancer Inst. 1999;91:1310–6.
23. van Asperen CJ, Brohet RM, Meijers-Heijboer EJ, et al. Cancer risks in BRCA2 families: estimates for sites other than breast and ovary. J Med Genet. 2005;42:711–9.
24. Tryggvadottir L, Vidarsdottir L, Thorgeirsson T, et al. Prostate cancer progression and survival in BRCA2 mutation carriers. J Natl Cancer Inst. 2007;99:929–35.
25. Narod SA, Neuhausen S, Vichodez G, et al. Rapid progression of prostate cancer in men with a BRCA2 mutation. Br J Cancer. 2008;99:371–4.
26. Wolf AM, Wender RC, Etzioni RB, et al. American Cancer Society guideline for the early detection of prostate cancer: update 2010. CA Cancer J Clin. 2010;60:70–98.
27. Mitra AV, Bancroft EK, Barbachano Y, et al. Targeted prostate cancer screening in men with mutations in BRCA1 and BRCA2 detects aggressive prostate cancer: preliminary analysis of the results of the IMPACT study. BJU Int. 2011;107:28–39.
28. Hankey BF, Ries LA, Edwards BK. The surveillance, epidemiology, and end results program: a national

resource. Cancer Epidemiol, Biomarkers Prev. 1999;8: 1117–21.
29. Goggins W, Gao W, Tsao H. Association between female breast cancer and cutaneous melanoma. Int J Canc. 2004;111:792–4.
30. Iscovich J, Abdulrazik M, Cour C, et al. Prevalence of the BRCA2 6174 del T mutation in Israeli uveal melanoma patients. Int J Canc. 2002;98:42–4.
31. Kefford RF, Newton Bishop JA, Bergman W, et al. Counseling and DNA testing for individuals perceived to be genetically predisposed to melanoma: a consensus statement of the Melanoma Genetics Consortium. J Clin Oncol. 1999;17:3245–51.
32. Wang SC, Makino K, Su LK, et al. Ultraviolet irradiation induces BRCA2 protein depletion through a p53-independent and protein synthesis-dependent pathway. Cancer Res. 2001;61:2838–42.
33. Hahn SA, Greenhalf B, Ellis I, et al. BRCA2 germline mutations in familial pancreatic carcinoma. J Natl Cancer Inst. 2003;95:214–21.
34. Murphy KM, Brune KA, Griffin C, et al. Evaluation of candidate genes MAP2K4, MADH4, ACVR1B, and BRCA2 in familial pancreatic cancer: deleterious BRCA2 mutations in 17%. Cancer Res. 2002;62: 3789–93.
35. Ferrone CR, Levine DA, Tang LH, et al. BRCA germline mutations in Jewish patients with pancreatic adenocarcinoma. J Clin Oncol. 2009;27:433–8.
36. Langer P, Kann PH, Fendrich V, et al. Five years of prospective screening of high-risk individuals from families with familial pancreatic cancer. Gut. 2009;58:1410–8.
37. Canto MI, Goggins M, Hruban RH, et al. Screening for early pancreatic neoplasia in high-risk individuals: a prospective controlled study. Clin Gastroenterol Hepatol. 2006;4:766–81; quiz 665.
38. Poley JW, Kluijt I, Gouma DJ, et al. The yield of first-time endoscopic ultrasonography in screening individuals at a high risk of developing pancreatic cancer. Am J Gastroenterol. 2009;104:2175–81.
39. American Gastroenterological Association medical position statement: epidemiology, diagnosis, and treatment of pancreatic ductal adenocarcinoma. Gastroenterology. 1999;117:1463–84.
40. Thiebaut AC, Jiao L, Silverman DT, et al. Dietary fatty acids and pancreatic cancer in the NIH-AARP diet and health study. J Natl Cancer Inst. 2009;101:1001–11.
41. Mohamad HB, Apffelstaedt JP. Counseling for male BRCA mutation carriers: a review. Breast. 2008;17: 441–50.
42. Niell BL, Rennert G, Bonner JD, et al. BRCA1 and BRCA2 founder mutations and the risk of colorectal cancer. J Natl Cancer Inst. 2004;96:15–21.
43. Struewing JP, Hartge P, Wacholder S, et al. The risk of cancer associated with specific mutations of BRCA1 and BRCA2 among Ashkenazi Jews. N Engl J Med. 1997;336:1401–8.
44. Hobert JA, Eng C. PTEN hamartoma tumor syndrome: an overview. Genet Med. 2009;11:687–94.
45. Eng C. Will the real Cowden syndrome please stand up: revised diagnostic criteria. J Med Genet. 2000;37: 828–30.
46. Zbuk KM, Eng C. Hamartomatous polyposis syndromes. Nat Clin Pract Gastroenterol Hepatol. 2007;4:492–502.
47. Marsh DJ, Coulon V, Lunetta KL, et al. Mutation spectrum and genotype-phenotype analyses in Cowden disease and Bannayan-Zonana syndrome, two hamartoma syndromes with germline PTEN mutation. Hum Mol Genet. 1998;7:507–15.
48. Zhou XP, Waite KA, Pilarski R, et al. Germline PTEN promoter mutations and deletions in Cowden/Bannayan-Riley-Ruvalcaba syndrome result in aberrant PTEN protein and dysregulation of the phosphoinositol-3-kinase/Akt pathway. Am J Hum Genet. 2003;73:404–11.
49. Tan MH, Mester JL, Ngeow J, et al. Lifetime cancer risks in individuals with germline PTEN mutations. Clin Cancer Res. 2012;18:400–7.
50. Pilarski R, Eng C. Will the real Cowden syndrome please stand up (again)? Expanding mutational and clinical spectra of the PTEN hamartoma tumour syndrome. J Med Genet. 2004;41:323–6.
51. Ngeow J, Mester J, Rybicki LA, et al. Incidence and clinical characteristics of thyroid cancer in prospective series of individuals with Cowden and Cowden-like syndrome characterized by germline PTEN, SDH, or KLLN alterations. J Clin Endocrinol Metab. 2011;96:E2063–71.
52. Pilarski R, Stephens JA, Noss R, et al. Predicting PTEN mutations: an evaluation of Cowden syndrome and Bannayan-Riley-Ruvalcaba syndrome clinical features. J Med Genet. 2011;48:505–12.
53. Heald B, Mester J, Rybicki L, et al. Frequent gastrointestinal polyps and colorectal adenocarcinomas in a prospective series of PTEN mutation carriers. Gastroenterology. 2010;139:1927–33.
54. Malkin D, Li FP, Strong LC, et al. Germ line p53 mutations in a familial syndrome of breast cancer, sarcomas, and other neoplasms. Science. 1990;250: 1233–8.
55. Chompret A, Brugieres L, Ronsin M, et al. P53 germline mutations in childhood cancers and cancer risk for carrier individuals. Br J Cancer. 2000;82:1932–7.
56. Gonzalez KD, Noltner KA, Buzin CH, et al. Beyond Li Fraumeni syndrome: clinical characteristics of families with p53 germline mutations. J Clin Oncol. 2009;27:1250–6.
57. Li FP, Fraumeni Jr JF, Mulvihill JJ, et al. A cancer family syndrome in twenty-four kindreds. Cancer Res. 1988;48:5358–62.
58. Birch JM, Hartley AL, Tricker KJ, et al. Prevalence and diversity of constitutional mutations in the p53 gene among 21 Li-Fraumeni families. Cancer Res. 1994;54:1298–304.
59. Eeles RA. Germline mutations in the TP53 gene. Cancer Surv. 1995;25:101–24.
60. Chompret A, Abel A, Stoppa-Lyonnet D, et al. Sensitivity and predictive value of criteria for p53 germline mutation screening. J Med Genet. 2001;38:43–7.
61. Nichols KE, Malkin D, Garber JE, et al. Germ-line p53 mutations predispose to a wide spectrum of early-onset cancers. Cancer Epidemiol Biomarkers Prev. 2001;10: 83–7.

62. Lustbader ED, Williams WR, Bondy ML, et al. Segregation analysis of cancer in families of childhood soft-tissue-sarcoma patients. Am J Hum Genet. 1992;51:344–56.
63. Hisada M, Garber JE, Fung CY, et al. Multiple primary cancers in families with Li-Fraumeni syndrome. J Natl Cancer Inst. 1998;90:606–11.
64. Villani A, Tabori U, Schiffman J, et al. Biochemical and imaging surveillance in germline TP53 mutation carriers with Li-Fraumeni syndrome: a prospective observational study. Lancet Oncol. 2011;12:559–67.
65. D'Orazio JA. Inherited cancer syndromes in children and young adults. J Pediatr Hematol Oncol. 2010;32: 195–228.
66. Masciari S, Van den Abbeele AD, Diller LR, et al. F18-fluorodeoxyglucose-positron emission tomography/computed tomography screening in Li-Fraumeni syndrome. JAMA. 2008;299:1315–9.
67. van Lier MG, Wagner A, Mathus-Vliegen EM, et al. High cancer risk in Peutz-Jeghers syndrome: a systematic review and surveillance recommendations. Am J Gastroenterol. 2010;105:1258–64; author reply 65.
68. Young RH, Welch WR, Dickersin GR, et al. Ovarian sex cord tumor with annular tubules: review of 74 cases including 27 with Peutz-Jeghers syndrome and four with adenoma malignum of the cervix. Cancer. 1982;50:1384–402.
69. Giardiello FM, Trimbath JD. Peutz-Jeghers syndrome and management recommendations. Clin Gastroenterol Hepatol. 2006;4:408–15.
70. Beggs AD, Latchford AR, Vasen HF, et al. Peutz-Jeghers syndrome: a systematic review and recommendations for management. Gut. 2010;59: 975–86.
71. Giardiello FM, Welsh SB, Hamilton SR, et al. Increased risk of cancer in the Peutz-Jeghers syndrome. N Engl J Med. 1987;316:1511–4.
72. Latchford AR, Neale KF, Spigelman AD, et al. Features of duodenal cancer in patients with familial adenomatous polyposis. Clin Gastroenterol Hepatol. 2009;7:659–63.
73. van Lier MG, Mathus-Vliegen EM, Wagner A, et al. High cumulative risk of intussusception in patients with Peutz-Jeghers syndrome: time to update surveillance guidelines? Am J Gastroenterol. 2011;106: 940–5.
74. Edwards DP, Khosraviani K, Stafferton R, et al. Long-term results of polyp clearance by intraoperative enteroscopy in the Peutz-Jeghers syndrome. Dis Colon Rectum. 2003;46:48–50.
75. Guilford P, Hopkins J, Harraway J, et al. E-cadherin germline mutations in familial gastric cancer. Nature. 1998;392:402–5.
76. Fitzgerald RC, Hardwick R, Huntsman D, et al. Hereditary diffuse gastric cancer: updated consensus guidelines for clinical management and directions for future research. J Med Genet. 2010;47:436–44.
77. Guilford P, Humar B, Blair V. Hereditary diffuse gastric cancer: translation of CDH1 germline mutations into clinical practice. Gastric Cancer. 2010;13:1–10.
78. Blair V, Martin I, Shaw D, et al. Hereditary diffuse gastric cancer: diagnosis and management. Clin Gastroenterol Hepatol. 2006;4:262–75.
79. Pollard JM, Gatti RA. Clinical radiation sensitivity with DNA repair disorders: an overview. Int J Radiat Oncol Biol Phys. 2009;74:1323–31.
80. Swift M, Morrell D, Cromartie E, et al. The incidence and gene frequency of ataxia-telangiectasia in the United States. Am J Hum Genet. 1986;39:573–83.
81. Morrell D, Cromartie E, Swift M. Mortality and cancer incidence in 263 patients with ataxia-telangiectasia. J Natl Cancer Inst. 1986;77:89–92.
82. Thompson D, Duedal S, Kirner J, et al. Cancer risks and mortality in heterozygous ATM mutation carriers. J Natl Cancer Inst. 2005;97:813–22.
83. Swift M, Reitnauer PJ, Morrell D, et al. Breast and other cancers in families with ataxia-telangiectasia. N Engl J Med. 1987;316:1289–94.
84. Easton DF. Cancer risks in A-T heterozygotes. Int J Radiat Biol. 1994;66:S177–82.
85. Bagby GC, Alter BP. Fanconi anemia. Semin Hematol. 2006;43:147–56.
86. D'Andrea AD. Susceptibility pathways in Fanconi's anemia and breast cancer. N Engl J Med. 2010;362: 1909–19.
87. Howlett NG, Taniguchi T, Olson S, et al. Biallelic inactivation of BRCA2 in Fanconi anemia. Science. 2002;297:606–9.
88. Tischkowitz M, Xia B. PALB2/FANCN: recombining cancer and Fanconi anemia. Cancer Res. 2010;70: 7353–9.
89. Alter BP, Greene MH, Velazquez I, et al. Cancer in Fanconi anemia. Blood. 2003;101:2072.
90. Jones S, Hruban RH, Kamiyama M, et al. Exomic sequencing identifies PALB2 as a pancreatic cancer susceptibility gene. Science. 2009;324:217.
91. Howlett NG, Scuric Z, D'Andrea AD, et al. Impaired DNA double strand break repair in cells from Nijmegen breakage syndrome patients. DNA Repair (Amst). 2006;5:251–7.
92. Desjardins S, Beauparlant JC, Labrie Y, et al. Variations in the NBN/NBS1 gene and the risk of breast cancer in non-BRCA1/2 French Canadian families with high risk of breast cancer. BMC Cancer. 2009;9:181.
93. Seemanova E. An increased risk for malignant neoplasms in heterozygotes for a syndrome of microcephaly, normal intelligence, growth retardation, remarkable facies, immunodeficiency and chromosomal instability. Mutat Res. 1990;238:321–4.
94. Nowak J, Mosor M, Ziolkowska I, et al. Heterozygous carriers of the I171V mutation of the NBS1 gene have a significantly increased risk of solid malignant tumours. Eur J Cancer. 2008;44:627–30.
95. Seemanova E, Jarolim P, Seeman P, et al. Cancer risk of heterozygotes with the NBN founder mutation. J Natl Cancer Inst. 2007;99:1875–80.

# Psychological Implications of Testing Positive for the BRCA Gene

# 11

Timothy Pearman

## Introduction

Breast cancer is the most common cancer in American women with approximately 230,000 cases diagnosed annually [1]. Women in the United States have a 1 in 8 chance of developing the disease. While most cases of breast cancer do not have a strong familial component, it is estimated that approximately 5–10% of cases of breast cancer are due to a known genetic factor [2]. In women with a known BRCA 1 or 2 mutation, 40–66% will eventually develop breast cancer (compared to 10–12% in the general population) [3]. In response, The American College of Medical Genetics published guidelines for genetic testing for breast and ovarian cancer in 1999.

Since that time, research has investigated the emotional impact of both testing and being identified as high risk, coping with testing results generated, and coping among women choosing not to have this testing. This chapter will briefly review the recommendations of the American College of Medical Genetics and review literature on distress and psychological functioning in women at high risk for breast cancer. In addition, we will review coping strategies, the role of family support, self-esteem and communication, and finally touch upon research investigating the impact of support groups and enhanced counseling approaches on psychological functioning in this population.

The process of risk assessment begins with an interview eliciting a detailed three-generation family cancer history. In doing so, counselors are able to determine whether increased risk for breast cancer is apparent. Initial discussions should educate patients, and also address questions, concerns, and expectations regarding the implications of genetic testing and outcomes. In sum, increased risk for a mutation in BRCA1/2 genes is suspected if there are three or more affected first or second degree relatives on the same side of the family, regardless of age at diagnosis, or less than three relatives if one patient was diagnosed at age 45 or less. In addition, if a family member has been identified with a mutation, there are one or more cases of ovarian cancer and one or more cases of breast cancer on the same side of the family, or multiple primary or bilateral breast cancers in the patient or one family member, the patient is considered at risk. Finally, if there is any breast cancer in a male patient or relative, or the patient is of

Timothy Pearman, Ph.D. (✉)
Supportive Oncology, Robert H. Lurie Comprehensive Cancer Center of Northwestern University, 250 E. Superior Street, Suite 520, Chicago, IL 60611, USA

Department of Medical Social Sciences, Department of Psychiatry & Behavioral Sciences, Northwestern University Feinberg School of Medicine, 250 E. Superior Street, Suite 520, Chicago, IL 60611, USA
e-mail: t-pearman@northwestern.edu

N.M. Hansen (ed.), *Management of the Patient at High Risk for Breast Cancer*,
DOI 10.1007/978-1-4614-5891-3_11, 

certain ethnic backgrounds (e.g., Ashkenazi Jewish descent), the patient is considered at risk.

The second stage of the process is discussion and education so that the patient can make an informed choice about pursuing genetic testing. The potential risks and benefits should be addressed, as well as possible outcomes of testing (positive, negative, or uncertain test results). Part of this discussion should include discussion of psychological risks, and also the difficulty of assuring the confidentiality of results and the possibility of discrimination by insurers and employers.

Finally, once adequate time has been given for the patient to evaluate the next steps, informed consent is obtained and testing initiated with a blood draw. Following the testing, all individuals tested must receive their results in person, regardless of the results. Individuals found to have a mutation are provided with a full explanation and interpretation of the test result, psychological support, and information concerning testing of relatives. They are also given information regarding prevention and early detection. For individuals receiving information about a mutation of uncertain significance, testing of additional family members is indicated to assess the significance of the variation.

A final note: women already diagnosed with breast cancer may receive genetic testing as well. The information in this chapter does not address genetic testing concerns of this group of women and is beyond the scope of this chapter. Interested readers are referred to a recent literature review of this population for further information [4].

## Psychological Impact of High-Risk Status

Interestingly, the literature on the emotional impact of high-risk status has been conflicting [5]. Some studies have found no distress in women at high risk [6] and other studies have found significant distress in this population, with some studies finding up to 43% of women displaying significant levels of distress [7]. In addition, some studies have found that individuals' preexisting functioning is related to distress levels related to genetic testing [8]. Other factors such as personality style, stage of life with respect to child bearing, and previous experience of family members with genetic testing and cancer can also impact distress levels [9].

Another key aspect to distress may be inconclusive test results. Inconclusive results comprise approximately 80% of all genetic test findings [10]. As a result, many women who have sought genetic testing are left with ambivalence and dissatisfaction with their test results. There are two types of inconclusive results that are possible: uncertain negative results and uncertain positive results. Uncertain negative results occur when an individual at high risk for a familial mutation receives a negative genetic test result. This can occur due to an undetected mutation (false negative) or a mutation in an as yet unknown gene. Uncertain positive results (variants of unknown significance) occur when a mutation is discovered but it is unknown as to the impact of this mutation on future cancer risk [11].

The potential impact of genetic testing may also affect an entire family system at large. Patients who test positive must decide whether to inform their siblings, children, and parents. This can be a very distressing process, especially in families with strained interpersonal relationships [12]. Individuals with children are faced with many complicated decisions: What is the best way to tell a child? At what age should a child be told? Which family members should be included in the discussion? These decisions can seem overwhelming and there are no solid developmental standards to guide these decisions at present.

Also interesting is that most studies have found that levels of distress do not seem to differ between women affected and unaffected by a known genetic mutation, but instead seem related to simply being at familial high risk. Power et al. [5] found that high levels of distress were present in approximately 20% of women undergoing genetic testing, regardless of mutation status. As a point of comparison, significant levels of distress are thought to be present in approximately 40% of cancer patients, so while these numbers do not approach that level, they are indicative of a high level of need for psychological screening and intervention in this population. One difference between affected and unaffected groups may be somatization symptoms. Women with inconclusive mutations in this study seemed to express their distress by manifesting somatic symptoms (as opposed to depression or anxiety) more frequently than women with no known hereditary risk or those of high-risk status.

## Time Course and Coping

A recent study evaluated a group of 155 women tested for BRCA1/2 mutations, and found that mutation carriers endorsed more depressive symptoms, negative mood, and cancer-specific distress relative to non-mutation carriers at 1 and 6 months after test receipt [13]. However, this study noted significant change over time, such that women positive for BRCA1/2 mutations showed significantly decreasing levels of distress and mood disturbance by 12 months following test receipt, consistent with the literature noted above. Also of interest, neither having a previous cancer diagnosis, nor receiving a true negative vs. uninformative negative result predicted reactions to genetic testing.

The fact that distress was elevated among mutation carriers in the immediate (6-month) period following testing but returned to near baseline by 12 months suggests two things in particular. First, it appears that activities such as making decisions regarding prophylactic treatment, telling family members about test results, etc., are very stressful to women with known mutations and that these decisions are made fairly rapidly. Second, it appears that women with known mutation adapt fairly well over time, such that their distress levels approach baseline (and also the levels of non-mutation carriers) by 1 year post-testing.

Notably, only one study to date has measured psychological impact and distress related to testing over a longer time period [14]. This study found that anxiety and depressive symptoms increased significantly in both BRCA1/2 positive and negative women from 1 year to approximately 5 years post-testing. These symptoms were predicted by cancer-specific distress, having lost a relative to breast or ovarian cancer, and less open communication about the test results, suggesting that a woman's environment, as well as ways in which a woman copes with positive or negative test results, may have significant impact on distress.

## Family Support, Self-Esteem, Communication and Distress

A recent study of 222 high-risk women found that several variables predicted psychological distress [15]. It was observed that both personal and social resources played a role in adjustment to a diagnosis of high-risk status. Specifically, self-esteem was associated with less general distress, whereas feeling stigmatized was associated with more cancer-specific and general distress. Self-esteem also mediated the relationships between social support and general distress. Support from family and friends was positively associated with self-esteem, which in turn was inversely related to general distress. This is consistent with other studies of cancer coping. Further, it was found that women who communicated openly regarding hereditary breast cancer risk had the lowest levels of self-reported vulnerability. Not surprisingly, support from a significant other was directly associated with less general distress. Finally, a woman's response to high-risk status (prophylactic mastectomy, prophylactic salpingo-oopherectomy or surveillance alone) did not appear related to cancer-specific or overall distress, with groups having similar mean scores in all domains.

Another study found similar results in 237 women carrying a BRCA1/2 mutation [16]. This study measured the impact of self-esteem, mastery, and perceived stigma on adjustment. Women were between 4 months and 8 years post-notification of carrier status. In this study, time since receiving test results, affected status, having undergone prophylactic mastectomy or prophylactic oophorectomy was not associated with demographic or psychological variables. Self-esteem and feelings of mastery were associated with fewer intrusive thoughts, whereas stigma was associated with more. The authors conclude that cancer-specific distress may be explained by past and ongoing experiences of cancer in the family and personality variables rather than by the time since testing.

The findings above were replicated and elaborated on in a study that found women who felt supported by their families were more likely to engage in open communication regarding risk [17]. This open communication in turn was associated with lower levels of both cancer-specific and general distress. The study concluded that if communication about hereditary risk is hampered, women tend to feel isolated and alone in their worries and emotions, and experience increased distress. The authors posit that such "protective buffering" by family members, while well intended, is not likely to be helpful.

The impact of preexisting anxiety and feelings of stigma related to testing results was also seen in a study of 111 women carrying a BRCA1 mutation [18]. This study showed that women who experienced high levels of anxiety pre-testing continued to experience high levels of anxiety up to 1 year post-testing. Pre-test anxiety appeared more predictive of post-test anxiety than did actual mutation status. The authors suggest that healthcare providers screen for high levels of anxiety pre-testing and develop interventions to address these risk factors for post-testing distress.

Another contributor to distress over time is coping style. A study of 126 women at increased familial risk of breast cancer looked at this variable and found that use of avoidant coping and initial levels of distress were unique predictors of distress over a 6 month period post-testing [19]. Avoidant coping is described as the use of denial, self-distraction, detachment, and substance use in coping with a stressor. Also, over the study period, coping styles appeared stable, and results of genetic testing did not seem to impact coping style. It is worth mentioning that this study was performed on all Caucasian women, so it is difficult to ascertain if there are racial or other demographic differences in coping.

Another study of 91 Italian women found that coping strategies in general appeared similar to those of the general population, suggesting that coping strategies may be fairly stable and not dependent upon disease status, genetic risk or other medical variables [20]. This finding begs the question of whether interventions geared toward decreasing the use of negative coping strategies (i.e., avoidance) and increasing the use of active coping strategies could assist in decreasing distress in women at risk for significant psychological distress as a result of genetic testing.

## Education and Supportive Interventions

Very few studies to date have addressed the potentially beneficial impact of psycho-educational groups and other interventions on well-being and coping of high-risk women. In one study [21] female BRCA mutation carriers were approached by a social worker after learning about their test results and offered participation in an educational support group. Data was collected regarding emotional well-being, breast cancer risk knowledge and perception, risk management behavior and family communication before and after group participation. The results were generally nonsignificant; women perceived their breast cancer risk as high and experienced a very high frequency of cancer thoughts at both pre- and post-testing.

Interestingly, communication with the family of origin was significantly reduced at the time of post-testing compared to pre-intervention. Women reported being very highly satisfied with the group in terms of their decision-making processes regarding cancer surveillance or prophylactic surgery. One obvious limitation of this study is the lack of a control group of high risk women who did not receive the intervention, so it is unknown if this data represents the natural course of coping with high risk status, or indicates a negative impact of group intervention in terms of emotional distress.

Another trial evaluated an individual intervention that the researchers described as "enhanced counseling" [22]. In this trial, women were randomly assigned to either the enhanced counseling group or control condition (standard counseling plus general health information to control for time and attention.) The enhanced group intervention was designed to promote cognitive and affective processing of cancer risk information. Women in the enhanced counseling group exhibited greater knowledge than women in the control group 1 week after the intervention. In addition, the intervention was found to be emotionally beneficial for women testing positive for a genetic mutation. Specifically, these women experienced lower levels of distress than women in the control group who tested positive.

Interestingly, the impact of an enhanced "decision support" intervention has not been found to decrease psychological distress [23]. In this study, 214 women undergoing BRCA1/2 testing were randomly assigned to the usual care condition or to the enhanced decision aid condition. Women receiving the enhanced decision support aid were significantly more distressed in the short-term. However, both usual care and decision aid conditions were similar in anxiety by 1 year follow up.

## Conclusions and Future Directions

Overall, women at high risk for hereditary breast cancer display levels of distress and psychological/emotional functioning that are similar to those in the general population. Nonetheless, a significant minority (approximately 20%) experience significantly elevated distress, regardless of actual genetic mutation status. A number of moderators appear to influence the risk that a woman will experience significant distress. These risks include self-esteem and mastery, with high self-esteem and mastery leading to decreased cancer-specific distress. Also, coping style appears to be important, with women utilizing an avoidant coping style experiencing more distress. Finally, social support and family communication appear important, with women experiencing high social support, and increased communication within the family having lower levels of psychological distress over time.

The impact of time since high risk assessment has been somewhat controversial. Most studies have found that women being evaluated for high risk status experience an initial increase in distress followed by a period of adaptation, which lasts up to 1 year. After 1 year, the impact of high risk status on distress and coping is unclear. At least one study has found that cancer-specific distress is increased from year 1 to year 5 post-testing. And at least one study has found that cancer-specific distress remains fairly constant up to 8 years post-testing. More research is clearly needed to determine the impact of time since assessment on distress, as little research has investigated this in women further than 1 year after assessment of risk status.

Given the fact that a number of family, interpersonal and medical variables can influence the risk that a woman will be significantly distressed following genetic testing, it is important to begin to develop screening measures to assess distress in this population. One recent study (24) has attempted to do so. This study developed a measure called the Genetic Risk Assessment Coping Evaluation (GRACE). More effort will be needed to replicate this measure. Any screening measure will need to focus highly on pre-test levels of anxiety, since pre-test levels of anxiety have been the most significant predictor of post-test anxiety. Interestingly, most studies have found that pre-test anxiety is an even more powerful predictor of post-test distress than is actual genetic risk status.

After screening measures are developed, the next issue will be to develop tailored interventions for women at high risk for distress. Thus far interventions to reduce distress have focused on providing more information to women in the hopes that "more will be better." Unfortunately, this does not appear to have been the case, and in some cases, women receiving more information appear to be at increased risk for distress, at least in the short term (up to 1 year). Therefore, it will be important that future research attempt to focus not only on the role of information in moderating distress, but also address the impact of coping style, self-esteem and feelings of stigmatization and mastery in any future interventions.

A final note is that almost all of the research in this area has been performed on women who were relatively affluent and Caucasian.

This is due to a number of factors, including perhaps most importantly restrictions in insurance coverage for genetic testing. As genetic testing becomes more prevalent and more widely covered by all public and private insurance plans, research will need to focus more on different ethnic and socioeconomic groups, as it should not be assumed that all groups will display similar patterns of distress, coping and psychological health in relation to high risk status.

## References


1. ACS Cancer Facts and Figures. Available at: http://www.cancer.org/Research/CancerFactsFigures/CancerFactsFigures/cancer-facts-figures-2011 (2011). Accessed 2 Dec 2011.
2. Genetic susceptibility to breast and ovarian cancer: assessment, counseling and testing guidelines. American College of Medical Genetics; 1999. http://www.ncbi.nlm.nih.gov/pubmed?term=Genetic%20susceptibility%20to%20breast%20and%20ovarian%20cancer%3A%20assessment%2C%20counseling%20and%20testing%20guidelines.%20American%20College%20of%20Medical%20Genetics%3B%201999.
3. Chen S, Parmigiani G. Meta-analysis of BRCA1 and BRCA2 penetrance. J Clin Oncol. 2007;25:1329–33.
4. Schlich-Bakker KJ, ten Kroode HFJ, Ausems MGEM. A literature review of the psychological impact of genetic testing on breast cancer patients. Patient Educ Couns. 2008;62:13–20.
5. Power TE, Robinson JW, Bridge P, Bernier FP, Gilchrist DM. Distress and psychosocial needs of a heterogeneous high risk familial cancer population. J Genet Couns. 2011;20:249–69.
6. Dagan E, Shochat T. Quality of life in asymptomatic BRCA1/2 mutation carriers. Prev Med. 2009;48:193–6.
7. Watson M, Lloyd SM, Eeles R, et al. Psycho social impact of testing (by linkage) for the BRCA1 breast cancer gene: an investigation of two families in the research setting. Psychooncology. 1996;5:233–9.
8. Vadaparampil ST, Miree CA, Wilson C, Jacobsen PB. Psychosocial and behavioral impact of genetic counseling and testing. Breast Dis. 2006;27:98–108.
9. Meiser B. Psychological impact of genetic testing for cancer susceptibility: an update of the literature. Psychooncology. 2005;14:1060–74.
10. Armes JE, Venter DJ. The pathology of inherited breast cancer. Pathology. 2002;34:309–14.
11. Vink GR, van Asperen CJ, Devilee P, Breuning MH, Bakker E. Unclassified variants in disease-causing genes: nonuniformity of genetic testing and counseling, a proposal for guidelines. Eur J Hum Genet. 2004;13:525–7.
12. Di Propspero LS, Seminsky M, Honeyford J, Doan B, Franssen E, Meschino W, et al. Psychosocial issues following a positive result of genetic testing for BRCA1 and BRCA2 mutations: findings from a focus group and a needs-assessment survey. Can Med Assoc J. 2001;164:1005–9.
13. Beran TM, Stanton AL, Kwan L, Seldon J, Bower JE, Vodermaier A, Ganz PA. The trajectory of psychological impact in BRCA1/2 genetic testing: does time heal? Ann Behav Med. 2008;36:107–16.
14. van Oostrom I, Meijers-Heijboer H, Lodder LN. Long-term psychological impact of carrying a BRCA1/2 mutation and prophylactic surgery: a 5-year follow up study. J Clin Oncol. 2003;21:3867–74.
15. den Heijer M, Vos J, Seynaeve C, Vanheusden K, Duivenvoorden HJ, Tilanus-Linthorst M, Menke-Pluymers MBE, Tibben A. The impact of social and personal resources on psychological distress in women at risk for hereditary breast cancer. Psycho-Oncology. 2010; doi:10.1879.
16. den Heijer M, Seynaeve C, Vanheusden K, Duivenvoorden HJ, Bartels CCM, Menke-Pluymers MBE, Tibben A. Psychological distress in women at risk for hereditary breast cancer: the role of family communication and perceived social support. Psycho-Oncology. 2010; doi:10.1850.
17. Ertmanski S, Metcalfe K, Trempala J, Glowacka MD, Lubinski J, Narod SA, Gronwald J. Identification of patients at high risk of psychological distress after BRCA1 genetic testing. Genet Test Mol Biomarkers. 2009;13(3):325–30.
18. Dougall AL, Smith AW, Somers TJ, Posluszny DM, Rubinstein WS, Baum A. Coping with genetic testing for breast cancer susceptibility. Psychosom Med. 2009;71:98–105.
19. Annunziata MA, Muzzatti B, Narciso D, Mella S, Viel A, Bidoli E, Dolcetti R. Mood state profile and coping strategies after BRCA-1/2 genetic test disclosure: a retrospective study in Italy. Support Care Cancer. 2011;19:733–5.
20. Landsbergen KM, Brunner HG, Manders P, Hoogerbrugge N, Prins JB. Educational support groups for BRCA mutation carriers satisfy need for information but do not affect emotional distress. Genet Couns. 2010;21(4):423–37.
21. Roussi P, Sherman KA, Miller S, Buzagio J, Daly M, Taylor A, Ross E, Godwin A. Enhanced counseling for women undergoing BRCA ½ testing: impact on knowledge and psychological distress-results from a randomised clinical trial. Psychol Health. 2010;25(4):401–15.
22. Hooker GW, Leventhal KG, DeMarco T, Peshkin BN, Finch C, Wahl E, Joines JR, Brown K, Valdimarsdottir H, Schwartz MD. Longitudinal changes in patient distress following interactive decision aid use among BRCA1/2 carriers: a randomized clinical trial. Med Decis Making. 2011;31(3):412–21.
23. Phelps C, Bennett P, Jones H, Hood K, Brain K, Murray A. The development of a cancer genetic-specific measure of coping: the GRACE. Psychooncology. 2010;19(8):847–54.

# The High-Tech High Risk Clinic

# 12

Brian Drohan, Constance Roche, and Kevin S. Hughes

## Introduction

The high risk clinic is an important component of any comprehensive medical system. An effective high risk clinic employs knowledgeable staff, with the ability to assess risk, appropriately counsel, provide, and interpret cancer predisposition genetic testing, and make recommendations and assist individuals to adopt risk reduction strategies. After almost two decades after the cloning of the BRCA genes, and commercial availability and insurance coverage for testing, only a fraction of BRCA mutation carriers have been identified. We address the task of employing twenty first century technology to match the recent advances in genetics and to anticipate implementation of systems to accommodate the large numbers of individuals who will be identified as high risk. Specifically, this chapter will discuss HughesRiskApps (HRA), an integrated, open access software package originated at the Massachusetts General Hospital (MGH) and the Newton Wellesley Hospital (NWH), and that is undergoing continued enhancements through grants, philanthropy and an active user group.

B. Drohan, Ph.D. (✉) • C. Roche, M.S.N.
• K.S. Hughes, M.D., F.A.C.S. (✉)
Avon Comprehensive Breast Evaluation Center, Massachusetts General Hospital, 55 Fruit Street, Yawkey 7, Boston, MA 02114, USA
e-mail: bdrohan@partners.org; kshughes@partners.org

There is no doubt that a high risk clinic is an important component of a breast center, a cancer center, or indeed any comprehensive medical system. The purpose of the service is to identify individuals at elevated risk for cancer and to encourage management strategies to decrease the morbidity and mortality of the disease. The need for breast cancer risk assessment has long been recognized and much has been written about how to develop and implement a program [1]. There is clear evidence that measures to identify, screen, and provide prevention strategies can decrease the occurrence of breast and ovarian cancer and, in the case of breast cancer, to detect disease at an earlier, more treatable stage.

An effective high risk clinic employs knowledgeable staff, with the ability to assess risk, appropriately counsel, provide, and interpret cancer predisposition genetic testing, and make recommendations and assist individuals to adopt risk reduction strategies.

Sadly, almost two decades after the cloning of the BRCA genes, and commercial availability and insurance coverage for testing, only a fraction of BRCA mutation carriers have been identified. The prevailing approach that relies on referral of individuals for assessment, testing, and counseling has failed to identify most high risk individuals [2].

In this chapter, we assume that the reader acknowledges the need for a risk assessment clinic and has available educated staff and ancillary resources to provide the service. We address the task of employing twenty first century technology

N.M. Hansen (ed.), *Management of the Patient at High Risk for Breast Cancer*,
DOI 10.1007/978-1-4614-5891-3_12, © Springer Science+Business Media New York 2013

to match the recent advances in genetics and to anticipate implementation of systems to accommodate the large numbers of individuals who will be identified as high risk. It is time to take advantage of available technology and the vast scientific knowledge base and to make an impact on cancer prevention.

Clinicians who manage high risk patients have adopted modern software technologies to collect data, draw pedigrees, and run risk models [3], yet they confront the limitations of technology, specifically, the lack of interoperability and the unmet need for specialization in the Electronic Health Record (EHR). EHR's remain mired in nineteenth century approaches to data collection, often acting as little more than computerized file cabinets holding electronic versions of free text notes.

Interoperability refers to the ability of one software package to share information with other software packages. Most software products currently used in risk clinics are not interoperable, forcing duplicate data entry. Risk clinicians enter the same data into a pedigree drawing program, and then into programs to run models such as BRCAPRO. In addition, most high risk clinics also maintain a database to manage demographics, potentially tripling data entry. Patient data entry has barely been leveraged. In fact, patients who take 15–30 min to enter their family history at home into "My Family Health Portrait" [4] are asked to print out the resulting pedigree on paper and bring it in to the risk assessment appointment where it can be transcribed into the risk clinic software programs. Thus, the same data is entered four times, once by the patient and three times by the high risk professional or staff. On the other hand, high risk clinicians are already taking advantage of Clinical Decision Support (CDS) in the form of the pedigree, and risk models. CDS is the use of computer software to analyze clinical data and to present suggested actions to the clinician in a way that makes the clinician want to undertake that action, often using a visualization.

It is unfortunate that at a time when risk clinics are poised to leap ahead into the twenty first century, they are being asked instead to embrace the EHR, losing their capability to draw pedigrees, run risk models, or manage their data in a way that allows quality control and participation in what ASCO (American Society of Clinical Oncology) has called the Rapid Learning Health Care System. In this chapter we will discuss the next generation of high risk software.

The role of technology can be realized in all phases of the high risk clinic activities: identification of high risk patients, preparation prior to the clinic visit at home and later in the waiting area, the visit itself, genetic testing, and follow-up, in addition to the administrative actions prior to, during, and following each visit. In an attempt to interweave these artificial divisions, we will discuss software packages that bridge the divide between one function and the next, and discuss opportunities to improve the process further in the future.

Specifically, this chapter will discuss HRA, an integrated, open access software package originated at the MGH and the NWH, and that is undergoing continued enhancements through grants, philanthropy, and an active user group.

## Identification of High Risk Patients

Currently the identification of high risk patients requires the clinician to remember and act upon long and convoluted guidelines, typically in the midst of a busy clinic. As a result, the majority of patients with BRCA mutations have yet to be identified, despite the availability of genetic testing since 1996. Efforts to deal with this problem have included education of professionals and the lay public, paper tools, and software approaches. Education has been extensively implemented, yet to date we have estimated that approximately 5%of carriers have been identified [5]. Paper tools such as FHAT [6] or printouts of the NCCN guidelines [7] have the advantage of ease of implementation, but require several minutes of clinician time to calculate the level of risk for hereditary breast-ovarian cancer. While these represent clever approaches, these paper forms have not been adopted due to the increased work required of the clinician and due to their narrow scope (i.e., a separate tool would be required for every hereditary disease that a practice wished to identify, overwhelming the primary clinician).

A much more promising approach is the use of patient entered data followed by CDS to identify patients at risk for any hereditary condition. One such approach is available via the internet using "My Generations," which allows patient entered data, and produces pedigree drawing and risk assessment calculations. Another program is the surgeon generals' tool "My Family Health Portrait," which allows individuals to enter their family history and to draw a pedigree. This software does not produce risk calculations, but the output follows a standardized format known as an HL7 message. An HL7 message can be imported into any HL7 compliant software [8], representing the best opportunity currently available for the sharing of family history data between EHRs in sufficient resolution to perform risk assessment and CDS. Such interoperability has already been demonstrated using tools such as My Family Health Portrait, HRA, CancerGene, and Progeny [9], yet a much greater potential exists with use of the Microsoft HealthVault personal health record platform.

HRA uses the approach of patient entered data prior to a mammogram screening or provider visit using Tablets. This primary care level Tablet captures general risk information and family history limited to which relatives have had cancer and at what age, and a family structure (number of various relative types). Once family history has been entered, the major cancer risk models are run automatically, including BRCAPRO, Claus, Gail, Myriad, MMRPRO, CCRAT, and PREMM [10–12]. Prior to entering the patient exam room, the clinician receives a printout that shows a pedigree, the risk model calculations and suggestions as to whether genetic consultation or testing is indicated. In addition, the system can be set to generate letters to patients suggesting they make a risk clinic appointment, with a copy sent to their referring clinician. This system is in use at the breast imaging centers at NWH and Barnabas Health Hospitals. At NWH, 115,445 unique patient family histories have been collected since 2007. There is a fairly consistent average of a little more than 25 individuals a week identified as being at risk and sent letters regarding making an appointment at the high risk center. At St. Barnabas, the system has been in use since 2009, with similar results. Despite the autonomy of the system and the limited work on the part of the staff, there remains the challenge of following up and assuring that identified patients attend an appointment, receive recommendations and have the opportunity to engage in risk reduction measures.

## Preparation Prior to the Clinic Visit at and in the Waiting Area

Most high risk clinics send patients a letter prior to the visit, providing information about what to expect at the visit, directions to the clinic, and paper forms to complete prior to the visit. These letters are typically premade forms with the patient's information and address added ad hoc, or templates requiring clerical staff to type in the patient-specific information. The ideal software would identify patients whose appointments are pending in the near future, and automatically generate letters, directions, and forms to be sent to the patient. These could be emailed, or sent by standard overland mail.

In the waiting area, typically patients fill out paper forms in addition to, or instead of, those sent to their homes in advance. In some clinics, support staff will interview the patient and keypunch their data into both pedigree drawing software (Progeny [13], Cyrillic [14], etc.) and redundantly into risk model software (CancerGene [15], Boadicea [16], Tyrer-Cuzick [17]). There are relatively few clinics that have been able to manage the IT hurdles necessary to integrate these types of tools into an efficient workflow. With HRA, the patients enter their data into a tablet pc computer survey (Fig. 12.1). The risk clinic tablet survey collects a more robust family history than the mammography and primary care surveys, as it collect names, ages, and vital status of each relative, as well as the types of cancers and ages of diagnoses of each. The patient entered data is then used to run risk models, draw a pedigree, and the clinical workflow surrounding genetic testing and other risk management decisions.

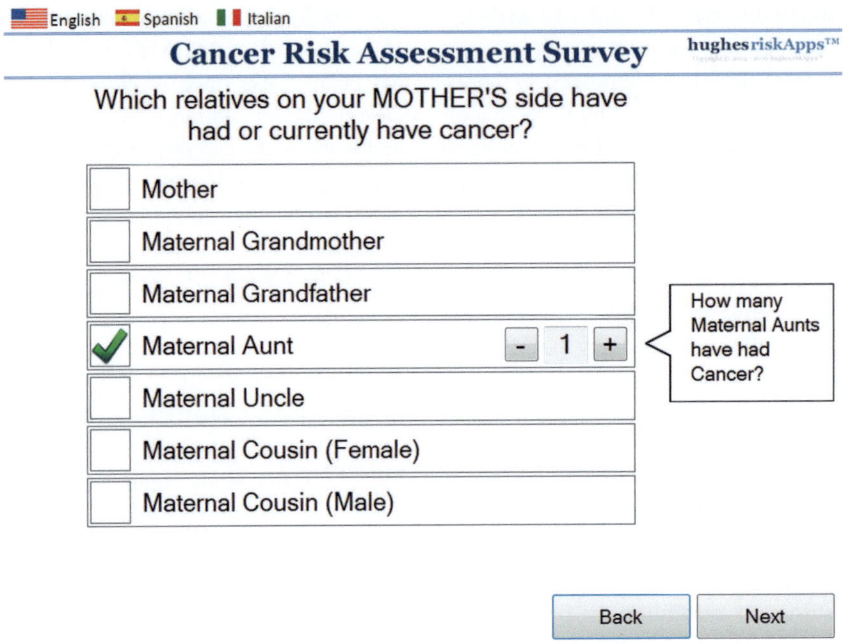


**Fig. 12.1** A sample tablet survey screen showing the step in collecting family history of cancer in which we identify the maternal relatives who have had cancer. Subsequent screens go on to collect which cancers each relative had, and the estimated age of onset

## The Visit

If the family history has not been entered into a pedigree drawing package and into the risk model software by the patient or support staff, the counselor may do this during the visit, or see the patient without a pedigree or risk calculations, planning to make up that deficiency after the visit. If the data has been entered by the patient or staff, the risk counselor can view the results and discuss with the patient. As errors or additions are identified, the counselor must make corrections and/or enhancements in both software packages. Alternatively, using HRA, the counselor can review and edit the patient-entered data once and immediately rerun the risk models and review the corrected pedigree, all during the visit. In addition, HRA uses CDS to suggest management options to the counselor (Fig. 12.2). The tool can take the standards of care for genetic testing and calculate risk model results for each relative in the family, ultimately displaying a recommendation in the context of several comparative health voutcomes. The breast and ovarian cancer risk is shown using four different possible scenarios, based on (1) BRCAPRO estimation before testing, (2) with positive BRCA testing, (3) with negative testing, and (4) for a woman of that age in the general population. This view helps the counselor see the potential effect of testing and helps him or her better explain to the patient the value of testing. By providing a sorted list with those at the highest risk level on top, it highlights the cases in which it is best to test the closest living affected family member, and all those in the family that could benefit from testing (Fig. 12.3).

## Genetic Testing

At the conclusion of the visit, the counselor and patient develop clear plans for the next steps, including genetic testing when indicated. If a relative is the logical family member to have testing

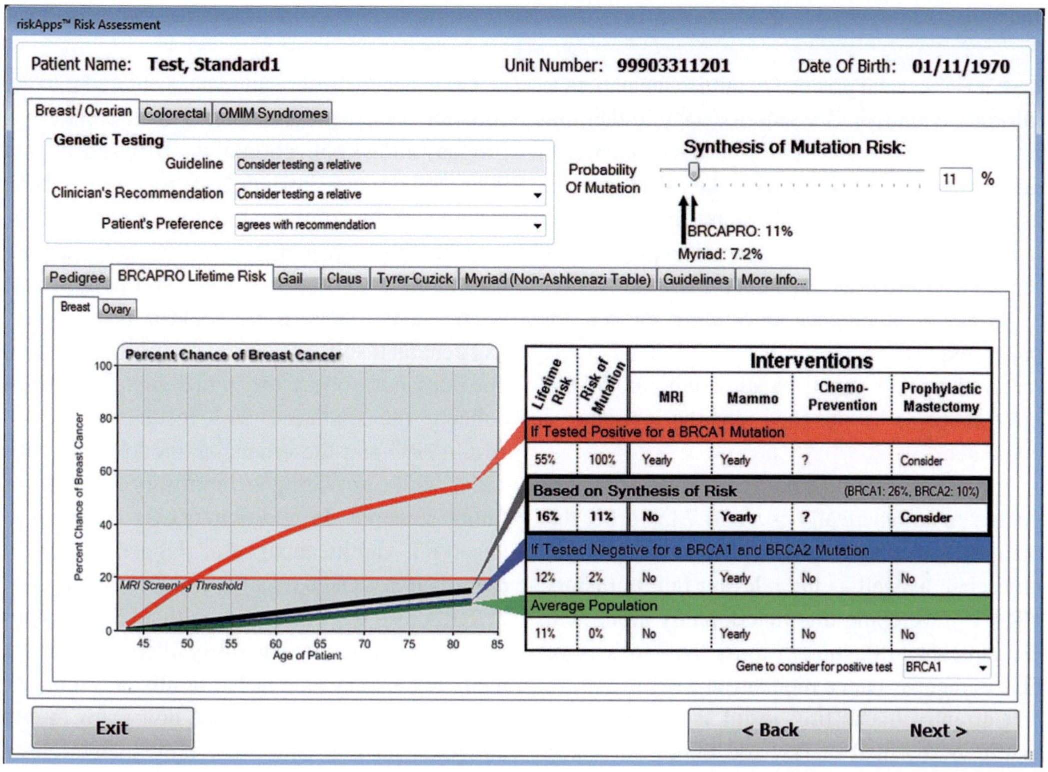


**Fig. 12.2** A view of the future risk of breast cancer based on the various outcomes of the decision regarding genetic testing, with the corresponding recommendations for the standard breast interventions

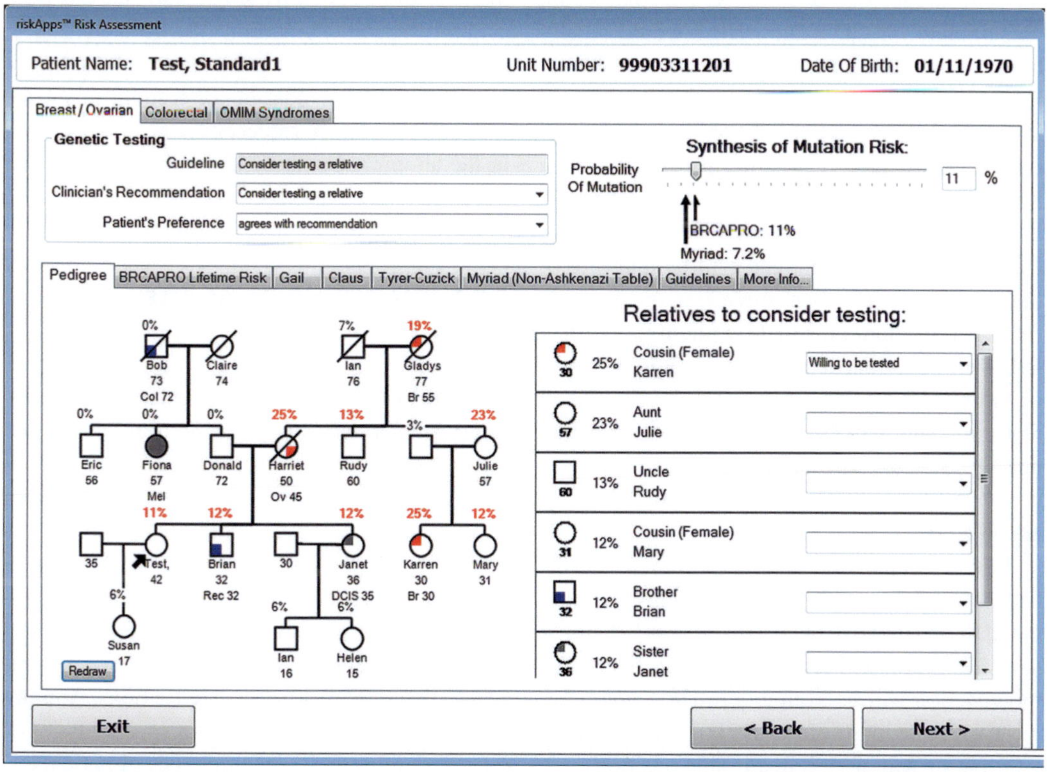


**Fig. 12.3** A typical pedigree for an at risk patient showing the risk of mutation for every individual in the family, the genetic testing recommendation from the CDS algorithm, and a sorted list of who in the family is eligible for testing

first, it is the usual practice to advise the patient to inform the relative. A counselor local to the relative may be suggested. HRA produces a letter to the relative that explains why she or he is being asked to test and lists local counselors. This letter is handed to the patient, who can then pass it on to the relative, avoiding any HIPAA issues.

Typically, when genetic testing is elected, the paper requisition is completed by hand. Once received by the genetic testing laboratory, that information is keypunched into the laboratory's computer.

In the ideal world, that requisition would be generated automatically as an HL7 lab order that includes the demographic information, ordering physician, as well as the relevant family history. HRA is developing this functionality along with GeneInsight [18], though most labs are not yet able to receive such a requisition.

Currently the testing result is received as a hard copy by mail or fax, and the result is keypunched into the risk clinic software (e.g., HRA) or is scanned into the EHR. In 2008, the American health Information Community (AHIC) identified the core data set for family history [19] that would be sufficient for CDS The EHR's would ideally have robust family history sections, capable of holding this data (which includes the genetic testing result for any relative). To our knowledge, no current EHR has been able to achieve this. Scanning into the EHR is a dangerous approach, as rudimentary CDS included in many EHRs lacks the ability to read, and will be unaware of the mutation status when suggesting the patient's risk level. In addition, with or without CDS, most EHRs may bury the genetic test result in the notes or the results section, increasing the likelihood that clinicians will be unaware of the patient's genetic status. No EHR currently manages genetic test result as structured data, though pilots are underway.

Ideally, genetic testing labs should send results back in HL7 messages that can be imported into the EHR and into risk clinic software as structured data. Pilots are in process. It is highly likely that this function will be available in HRA and other niche software long before an EHR can digest this information and place it in a usable position.

Once genetic test result data is entered into the software package, it is managed in different ways. Progeny allows collection of the BRCA result but does not rerun risk models. (Progeny has been customized by some centers to run risk models, but as each instance of Progeny is highly customized to the local needs of the user, this approach is not easily generalized). CancerGene can collect general results (deleterious or polymorphism) but does not collect the actual mutation. HRA collects the mutation and result and reruns BRCAPRO and the other risk models automatically, while providing a repository of data for future research. In addition, VUSs (variants of uncertain significance) are flagged to allow reevaluation as new data becomes available.

HRA also tracks families with a known mutation in order to help identify high risk family members, listing each tested family and showing which mutation type is present, how many family members have been tested, how many family members are candidates for testing (risk of mutation 10%or greater, over age 18, and alive). It is currently not uncommon for only one family member to be tested by single site analysis once a family specific mutation has been identified. Considering the high probability of finding a mutation, and low cost of the testing, this often missed opportunity represents low hanging fruit in the attempt at making a significant impact on public health.

## Administrative Actions After the Visit

Typically, the counselor sends letters to the referring providers and/or the patients following the visit. The generation of these letters is time consuming, often done by cutting and pasting from templates. HRA can be configured several ways depending on the clinical workflow. One option is to use the recommendations stored in the computer by the clinician with the help of CDS to drive the generation of letters built from paragraphs that reflect individualized actions. Another is to create a set of templates for specific types of outcomes relevant to specific types of patients.

## Summary

As in most areas of medicine, software and CDS can make the high risk clinic more efficient and easier to monitor for quality control and improvement. Every risk clinic should be using a pedigree program and a risk models program. Some examples of software have been provided, with an obvious slant toward our solution, which tries to knit the various functions together into a coherent whole.

## References

1. Vogel VG, editor. Management of patient at high risk for breast cancer. Malden, MA: Blackwood Scientific, Inc.; 2001.
2. Ozanne EM, Loberg A, Hughes S, Lawrence C, Drohan B, Semine A, et al. Identification and management of women at high risk for hereditary breast/ovarian cancer syndrome. Breast J. 2009;15(2):155–62.
3. Crane RM, Raymond B. Fulfilling the potential of clinical information systems. Perm J. 2003;7:62–7.
4. https://familyhistory.hhs.gov/fhh-web/home.action. Accessed April 2012.
5. Drohan B, Roche CA, Cusack Jr JC, Hughes KS. Hereditary breast and ovarian cancer and other hereditary syndromes: using technology to identify carriers. Ann Surg Oncol. 2012;19(6):1732–7.
6. Gilpin CA, Carson N, Hunter AG. A preliminary validation of a family history assessment form to select women at risk for breast or ovarian cancer for referral to a genetics center. Clin Genet. 2000;58(4):299–308.
7. http://www.nccn.org/professionals/physician_gls/f_guidelines.asp#detection. Last Accessed 8th Mar 2012.
8. Shabo A, Hughes KS. Family history information exchange services using HL7 clinical genomics standard specifications. Int J Semant Web Inf Syst. 2005;1(4):44–67.
9. http://www.hughesriskapps.com/. Last Accessed 8th Mar 2012.
10. Euhus DM. Understanding mathematical models for breast cancer risk assessment and counseling. Breast J. 2001;7(4):224–32. Review.
11. http://www.cancer.gov/colorectalcancerrisk/. Accessed 8th Mar 2012.
12. Kastrinos F, Steyerberg EW, Mercado R, Balmaña J, Holter S, Gallinger S, et al. The PREMM(1,2,6) model predicts risk of MLH1, MSH2, and MSH6 germline mutations based on cancer history. Gastroenterology. 2011;140(1):73–81. Epub 2010 Aug 19.
13. http://www.progenygenetics.com/. Accessed 8th Mar 2012.
14. http://www.cyrillicsoftware.com/. Accessed 8th Mar 2012.
15. http://www4.utsouthwestern.edu/breasthealth/cagene/. Accessed 8th Mar 2012.
16. http://www.srl.cam.ac.uk/genepi/boadicea/boadicea_intro.html. Accessed 8th Mar 2012.
17. http://www.ems-trials.org/riskevaluator/. Accessed 8th Mar 2012.
18. http://pcpgm.partners.org/it-solutions/geneinsight. Accessed 8th Mar 2012.
19. Feero WG, Bigley MB, Brinner KM, et al. New standards and enhanced utility for family health history information in the electronic health record: an update from the American Health Information Community's Family Health History Multi-Stakeholder Workgroup. J Am Med Inform Assoc. 2008;15(6):723–8.

# 13 Current and Future Direction in Basic and Translational Research

Susan M. Love

As this book clearly outlines, the use of modern mammographic screening combined with the ability to easily test for the BRCA breast cancer susceptibility genes have increased the focus on identification of the high risk patient and her options for prevention. Nonetheless mammographic screening is best at identifying high risk lesions that have developed microcalcifications. Non-calcifying precancerous disease remains for the most part, undetected. By the same token genetic testing only identifies the women with the genes we know about and misses all of those for whom we as of yet have no genetic marker. Clearly the fact that most women who develop breast cancer have neither of these findings indicates that we have far to go in the identification of women at risk for breast cancer.

Similarly our approaches to prevention are crude at best. While removing ovaries and breasts will indeed reduce the risk of subsequent cancer they are gross whole organ approaches not without significant clinical and psychological morbidity. Systemic hormonal chemoprevention has been demonstrated to reduce risk as well at least for estrogen positive cancers, but uptake has been disappointing. The ideal for prevention would be to identify a causal agent that can be avoided or vaccinated against, as has been done in cancer of the cervix. However, many years following the identification of mouse mammary tumor virus, there has yet to be compelling data for an infectious cause. Some investigators have moved to attempts to harness the immune system to prevent disease which will be reviewed. Finally the major barriers to developing new approaches to prevention will be discussed.

It is clear that there is an enormous need to both better identify women at risk and to prevent their developing subsequent cancer. The major barrier to developing new approaches to prevention involves the limitations of imaging. In this chapter I will focus primarily on the breast and how exploiting its unique anatomy and physiology may hold the key to these goals.

## Where Does Breast Cancer Start?

Wellings et al. [1] studies in human breasts in 1975 have been widely accepted as demonstrating that all breast cancer begins at the junction of the duct and lobule or the terminal duct lobular unit (TDLU).

This has been interpreted to mean that cancer is multicentric in origin and could not begin in a ductal tree despite reports to the contrary dating back as far as James Ewing [2] in 1940. Although the reported incidence of multicentricity ranges from 0 to 78% depending on the criteria used, researchers who have used techniques of whole breast sectioning such as Holland et al. [3] and more recently Mai et al. [4] have concluded that

S.M. Love, M.D. M.B.A. (✉)
Dr. Susan Love Research Foundation, 2811 Wilshire Blvd, Suite 500, Santa Monica, CA 90403, USA
e-mail: slove@dslrf.org

N.M. Hansen (ed.), *Management of the Patient at High Risk for Breast Cancer*,
DOI 10.1007/978-1-4614-5891-3_13, 

the in situ component is most often located in a single ductal tree or lobe. Teboul, using large-field ultrasound, also recognized breast carcinoma as a malignant diffuse disease involving the whole epithelium of the affected lobe [5]. Recent work by Tibor Tot on whole mount specimens has confirmed the limitation of cancer to one ductal system. He recently hypothesized that DCIS [6] and consequently breast cancer in general is a lobar disease with simultaneous or asynchronous, and often multiple in situ tumor foci localized within a single lobe thus suggesting the anatomy behind multifocality.

Researchers who have explored the clonality of mammary epithelium and early proliferative lesions without regard to the underlying anatomy have demonstrated loss of heterozygosity (LOH) with contiguous patches of normal appearing mammary epithelium [7–12]. Kurose et al. [13] using modern techniques of laser capture microdissection were able to take it a step further as they analyzed both the epithelial cells and stroma of 41 sporadic invasive adenocarcinomas of the breast. They demonstrated LOH in ranging from 25 to 69% in epithelial cells and 17–61% in the stroma cells respectively. They propose a genetic model of multi-step carcinogenesis for the breast involving first the epithelial and then the stromal cells.

Tsai et al. [14] point out that “finding that a tumor has a single inactivated X chromosome indicates only that the initial events leading to the tumor occurred at some time in development after X chromosome inactivation. These events could have occurred before maturity of the breast so that many epithelial cells, all containing the same inactive X chromosome and initiating genetic abnormalities representing their independent evolution into a tumor after the initiating events.” The potential of predifferentiation initiation of breast cancer is raised by the extensive epidemiological data showing increased breast cancer incidence among women who received radiation before mammary gland differentiation. Children treated with low doses of radiation for benign conditions such as enlarged thymus [15], skin hemangiomas [16], tinea capitis [17], and tuberculosis [18] have been demonstrated to have an increased in subsequent breast cancer sometimes as much as threefold. The highest increase in breast cancer risk was seen in individuals younger than age 14 when treated with multiple fluoroscopies for the management of pulmonary tuberculosis [19] and in women who were younger than age 10 at the time of exposure to atomic bomb irradiation [20]. These predifferentiation stem cells may be uniquely sensitive to other agents in addition to radiation as suggested by the increased risk of breast cancer in women over 40 who received diethylstilbestrol (DES) while in utero. This leads to the hypothesis espoused by Tibor Tot that the initial lesion may occur to a stem cell destined to develop into a whole duct. This could be in utero or at least prior to puberty resulting in the whole duct being clonal and abnormal, a sick lobe.

Further evidence that clonality predates proliferation comes from Diallo et al. [21]. To their surprise X chromosome inactivation analysis revealed a monoclonal origin of all the informative cases of DCIS, ADH and papilloma analyzed. There were no differences between neoplastic lesions such as DCIS and hyperplastic lesions such as ADH of usual type and papillomas. They noted that all the TDLUs analyzed in this study were also monoclonal in origin supporting the earlier reports of Tsai who demonstrated that entire lobules and larger ducts are monoclonal with opposite alleles inactivated within the same breast. They concluded that the breast is organized into distinct regions or patches in which all the epithelial cells show the same X chromosome inactivation pattern. More recently Vicini and Goldstein [22] have described monomorphic epithelial proliferations extending adjacent to cancers, further suggesting that the “sick lobe” may have large patches of transformed but not yet premalignant disease. One could easily make the leap that these clonal patches represent one lobe or ductal system, though direct proof is still missing due in part to the difficulty of tracking an arborizing three dimensional lobe on a two dimensional slide.

Despite all the studies implying that the individual lobes or ductal systems are the units of interest in preventing and treating breast cancer there is still controversy in the literature as to their number and distribution in a breast. Most surgical textbooks state without attribution that

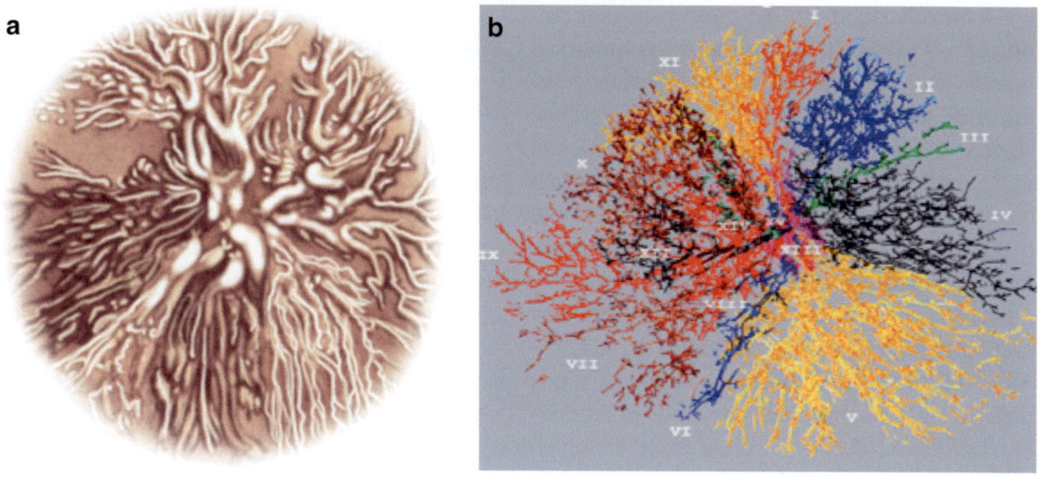


**Fig. 13.1** (**a**) Duct anatomy and distribution a. Astley Cooper. (**b**) Duct anatomy and distribution Going's computerized mode

there are 15–20 ductal openings on the nipple, but no scientific source for this pronouncement has been identified. The study of breast duct anatomy dates back to 1845, with Cooper's studies injecting colored wax into the ducts of over 200 breasts of women who died during lactation [23] (Fig. 13.1). He described human breast tissue as organized into separate lobes consisting of one central duct, its peripheral branches, and associated glandular tissue.

A continuing source of controversy in subsequent studies has been the number of lobes per breast. Reports of breast and nipple duct anatomy vary depending on whether the study focused on openings on the nipple that can be cannulated in vivo [5, 24–26] or in vitro and followed into functional ducts in the breast or the number of duct profiles seen on cross-sections of the nipple [27–30] the former acknowledging 5–9 openings on the nipple and the latter identifying 15–20 "duct appearing" structures. Some of the debate may in fact be semantic as when Teboul and Halliwell described 15–20 ducts converging on 5–8 milk pores in a series of more than 6,000 breasts studied via ultrasound and ductoscopy [5]. Moffat and Going's [27] three-dimensional (3D) computer model of a single autopsy breast traced ten complete nonanastamosing ductal systems (Fig. 13.1). Using six separate approaches, Love and Barsky [24] found that more than 90% of the nipples examined in their studies contained

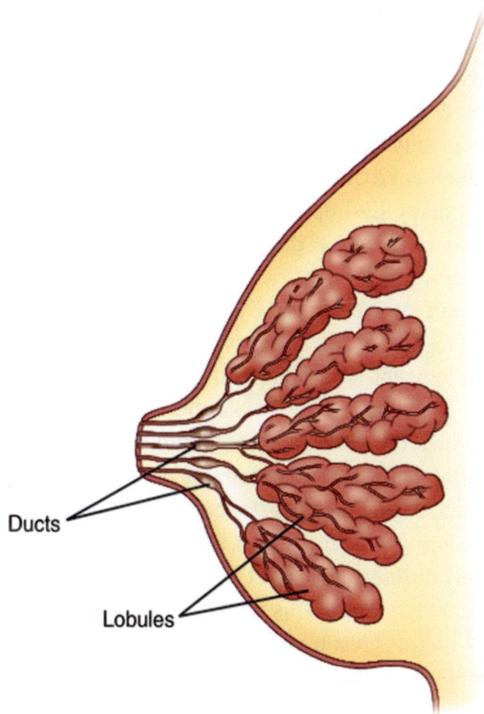


**Fig. 13.2** Distribution of the ducts

5–9 ductal orifices. They were able to document as well that the location of the ductal orifice predicts the location of the ductal system it serves. That is, the central ducts lead to lobes in the center of the breast and the peripheral ones to the appropriate peripheral lobes (Fig. 13.2).

One explanation for the discrepant observation of 5–9 vs. 15–20 ducts may be the additional tubular structures that mimic the appearance of ducts behind the nipple, but do not contribute significantly to the ductal lobular infrastructure of the breast. The nature of these additional structures and their role in breast physiology and pathology has yet to be described and it could be that they represent ductal branching close to the nipple surface, rudimentary undeveloped ducts or even ducts with associated sebaceous glands [31–33]. Collectively however, these data suggest that there are 5–12 significant, independent, arborizing lactiferous ductal systems, each of which cover a finite portion of the breast geography, and can be accessed from the nipple.

The distribution of the ducts is usually depicted radially with each duct occupying the same sized segment of the breast. Primary data supporting this model is rarely quoted and Astley Cooper himself presented evidence against it. His dissections demonstrated that different ductal systems vary greatly in size and may lie over or under one another, intertwining like the roots of a tree. Love and Barsky [24] described a central group and a peripheral group of ducts and Going and Moffat [27] described a breast where three lobes occupied one half of the breast. Other unanswered questions regarding the anatomy of the ducts include what happens after a woman finishes breastfeeding. The process of involution has been well described but there is no description of the reconstitution of the ductal system for the next child. Is the pattern the same developed from residual stem cells lining a path through the stroma? Or completely different generated from rudimentary ducts behind the nipple? This remains to be explored.

With this presumptive evidence that the unit of risk is not the breast as a whole but a single sick lobe or ductal system, are there ways we can use this information to screen for risk and then treat the lobe in question?

## Access to the Ductal Systems

While the anatomy of the ductal systems may still be in question, it is clear that they are readily accessible at least to infants.

## Nipple Aspirate Fluid

Nipple aspirate fluid (NAF) refers to the drops of fluid that can often be obtained through breast massage and a simple suction device (Fig. 13.3). Although this is successful in 80% of non-lactating Caucasian women, it can usually be elicited from only one or two ducts (Fig. 13.3). This fluid, considered a way of interrogating the duct, has been widely studied for potential cellular and non-cellular markers of breast cancer risk. It has not been established as of yet whether this fluid

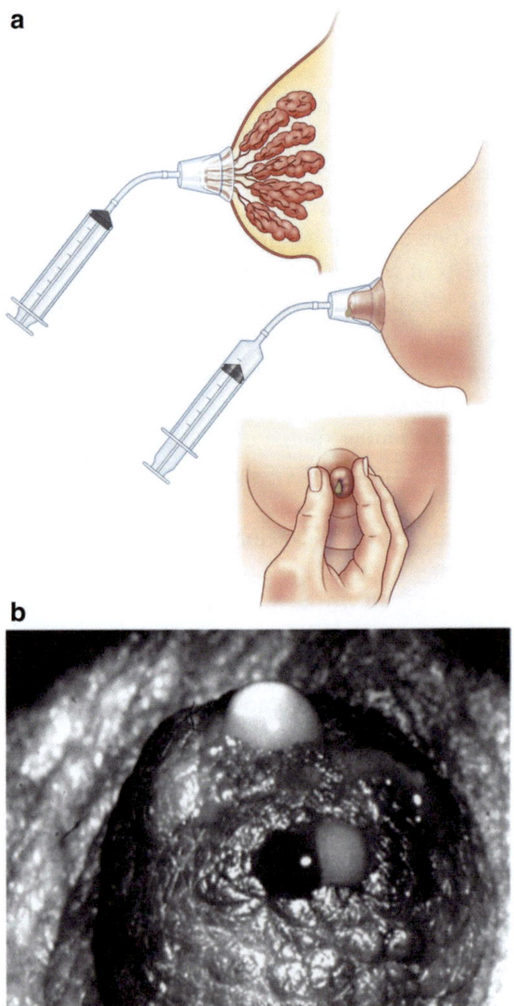


**Fig. 13.3** (**a**) Nipple aspiration. (**b**) Nipple showing drops of NAF

represents the whole breast or only the duct from which it was obtained. Its etiology is also not clear, as it could be overflow of normal ductal fluid obtained from a particularly accessible or extensive duct or represent a pathological process such as a low grade inflammation. It is clearly different from galactorrhea and spontaneous nipple discharge with or without blood, which is pathological representing a papilloma, papillomatosis and occasionally cancer. While the different color seen from different ducts (Fig. 13.3) would suggest that it represents a local etiology, the epidemiology of NAF production would suggest a systemic process [33]. It is more commonly elicited from women aged 35–50 years, of non-Asian ethnic origin, who experienced early age of menarche, and who have lactated. Moreover, reductions in NAF yield are associated with selective estrogen receptor modulators and oophorectomy [34, 35]. This would suggest that systemic hormonal stimulation of the breast leads to NAF production, but does not explain why only a few ducts produce it. It is certainly possible that as with pathological discharge, some NAF is systemic in origin while other types represent local pathology. Sanchez et al. [36] used polyacrylamide gel electrophoresis to analyze NAF protein banding patterns and delineated two types. One was more similar to milk, and was found in women who had given birth in the last 4 years or were on oral contraceptives. This type was also more common in women with breast cancer. The other type closely resembled cyst fluid with regard to color and components, and was more common in women with benign disease. Other studies have demonstrated intraductal papillary processes as the source of atypical cells in NAF, suggesting that local as well as systemic factors influence NAF production, both of which need to be taken into account in our thinking.

## Ductal Lavage

In an attempt to better access the whole breast, technologies for duct cannulation, including catheters and ductoscopes, have been developed. The first reported lavage, referred to as a "rinse," was performed by LeBorgne [37] in Uruguay in 1953. He dilated the ducts, instilled saline, and then massaged fluid out manually. Sartorius et al. [38] combined lavage with contrast ductography to collect the fluid as NAF after imaging. Love developed an intraductal catheter, which used a double lumen to maintain the patency of the duct while lavaging it [39] (Fig. 13.4). These first-generation devices have allowed proof of principle.

Several studies involving the intraductal delivery of dyes to demarcate the path of lavage fluids have demonstrated permeation of the lobular-alveolar portion of the ductal systems [40–42]. Moreover, the procedure has collected lavage cells exhibiting cytological features of lobular

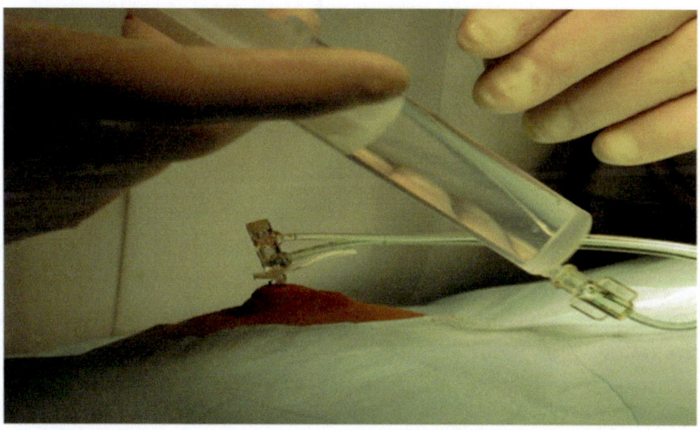

**Fig. 13.4** Ductal lavage

carcinoma in situ (LCIS) from a patient with pathology-confirmed LCIS [40]. In addition, lavage study participants have reported feeling the cooler (room) temperature of the lavage saline circulating within chest wall and axial regions (unpublished observations). Collectively, these data suggest that epithelial cells can be collected from the terminal reaches of the mammary tree, and that these samples can be used to detect malignant cells in a subset of women with breast cancer, albeit with low sensitivity.

Initially, the presumption was made that the duct that secreted most actively and, therefore, was most readily accessible, would be the "sentinel" duct, representing the status of the breast [39]. In fact, if NAF represents a field defect within the whole breast, one would expect that sampling any duct with NAF in a breast with cancer would demonstrate atypical cells. Studies by Khan et al. [41] and Brogi et al. [40] have demonstrated that this is not the case. Another assumption was that the fluid yielding ducts would be the ones most likely to harbor atypical and malignant cells. On the contrary, several investigations [42–44] have demonstrated atypical cells in non-discharging ducts at a rate similar to their incidence in discharging ducts. These findings are not surprising since spontaneous serosanguinous or watery discharge represents in situ or invasive cancer only about 5% of the time. Much of the data generated from the analysis of NAF fluid and cancer risk may be a result of pooling fluid from several different pathological mechanisms, potentially in the same breast. A recent study by Wood et al. [45] found that nipple aspiration fluid was more commonly expressed in cancerous compared with unaffected breasts, and overall sensitivity for detecting marked atypia or malignant cells in affected breasts was similar to previous studies, at approximately 17%.

The hope that ductal lavage would be the answer to screening ducts for cancer may have been overly optimistic. Sartorius et al. [38] postulated in 1977 that with increasingly large invasive cancers, the ducts might become obstructed and epithelial cells with higher-grade atypia may extravasate into surrounding tissues rather than shed into the ductal system. If this were the case, early noninvasive lesions such as DCIS would be more likely to yield atypical epithelial cells in lavage specimen. In a follow-up study, Khan et al. [46] included only women with calcifications on mammogram, thus increasing the probability of DCIS lesions. Of the ten women diagnosed histologically with DCIS, only one woman produced nipple fluid from a DCIS-bearing duct, and the cytology was benign. These findings corroborate results of the earlier studies and suggest low overall utility for cytologic evaluation of ductal lavage, even in the setting of known DCIS.

The technology has additional limitations, however. One technical challenge is that it is not always possible to tell whether a duct has been perforated in the process of cannulation. Thus, some lavages may actually represent a sampling of stroma rather than ductal fluid. For this reason we have tried lavaging under direct vision with a ductoscope [47] which can help with these distinctions but is time consuming, and appropriate scopes are not readily available. Most recently we have used ultrasound to monitor the procedure documenting a 7% perforation rate in healthy women [47].

In fact, the microenvironment of each duct may be distinct with regard to many properties. Bhandare et al. [43] have shown different estrogen and estrogen precursor levels in different ducts. Figure 13.2 shows NAF from several ducts in one nipple and the different colors of secretion suggest that indeed the fluid from separate ducts has distinct properties. Our unpublished observations have suggested independence and variability between ducts, but as with Khan and colleagues' data, these findings were obtained with lavage. A critical goal is to define interductal variation at the genetic, biochemical and cellular levels within the normal and diseased breast. We are currently analyzing a lavage study using ductoscopy to confirm the anatomy and comparing hormone, protein, cell and biomarker levels in at least three ducts per woman in an attempt to answer this question. It does appear that cytology is not the same in all the ducts, and it is certainly possible that some ductal contents are local, whereas others relate to the whole breast.

## Ductoscopy

Clearly, another way to exploit the access provided by the ductal system is through direct endoscopic visualization of the ductal tree, which may afford a novel approach to intraductal lesions such as DCIS. Although mammary ductoscopy has not yet garnered widespread use, tremendous improvements in endoscope technology in the past decade have allowed for unprecedented visualization and access to the intraluminal duct (Fig. 13.5a). Both in the United States and Asia, ductoscopy has had the greatest utility in the setting of pathologic nipple discharge. Currently available endoscopes measure 0.55–0.9 cm in external diameter, often with a working side port that allows for snaring and extraction of ductal lesions [48]. Investigators have shown that ductoscopic-guided extraction is effective for benign intraductal papillomas, but less effective in removing malignant lesions, including DCIS.

In evaluation of abnormal nipple discharge, ductoscopy has been shown to be of benefit by avoiding the need for preoperative ductogram. One series reported that 61% of ducts with discharge had abnormal endoscopic findings that were surgically excised with ductoscopic guidance [49]. Of the six cancers diagnosed, four had had negative preoperative radiographic work-up. In patients with known DCIS or breast cancer, ductoscopic guidance has been shown to improve reexcision rates. Dooley [50] have had extensive experience with this technique, and in their hands, lumpectomy for early-stage cancers guided by ductoscopy had a markedly reduced likelihood of local failure compared with standard lumpectomy techniques.

Ductoscopy can be monitored in real time with ultrasound allowing the anatomy to be appreciated as well (Fig. 13.5b). While it may have potential in identifying pre-cancerous lesions, the need to scope every duct precludes it being used for screening.

## Ductal Fluid for Screening

Seminal studies by Page and Dupont demonstrated that a diagnosis of histological atypia via surgical biopsy is associated with a fivefold increase in relative risk for future invasive breast cancer development [51, 52]. Cytological atypia diagnosed in fluids obtained by nipple aspiration and random periareolar fine needle aspiration is associated with a similar two to fivefold increase [53–55]. Because a diagnosis of atypia through a variety of modalities has consistently been associated with elevated risk for breast cancer development, it was assumed that it would also be a reliable marker in ductal lavage. However, there are a number of challenges associated with the cytological evaluation of ductal lavage samples. To date, long-term follow-up has not been completed for lavage studies, and the prognostic significance of atypia detected by this technique remains undefined. It has been argued that

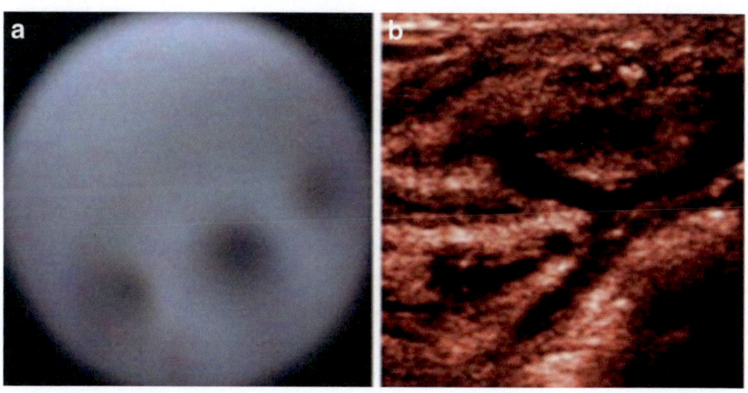

**Fig. 13.5** (**a**) Ductoscopy showing a trifurcation. (**b**) Ultrasound confirmation of the trifurcation

extrapolation from NAF studies may be inappropriate given that it is unknown what proportion of the cells collected by lavage represent naturally exfoliated cells vs. intact cells that are dislodged as the result of the procedure. However, sampling via the random periareolar fine needle aspiration technique is independent of naturally occurring exfoliation and yet reveals a striking association between cytological atypia and short-term risk [55] although not specifically in the area sampled. It is also true that cytological atypia on ductal lavage may not represent pathological atypical hyperplasia [56] but still could be a marker of risk. A more critical issue, associated with the diagnosis of atypia by any modality, is that despite the elevation of relative risk, the majority of women diagnosed with histological or cytological atypical hyperplasia do not develop breast cancer [53, 57]. In addition, most of the women who developed breast cancer in NAF studies with long-term follow-up had not been diagnosed with atypia [54]. A long term study, Serial Evaluation of Ductal Epithelium (SEDE), designed to answer this question was halted prematurely but an attempt is being made to complete the follow up. Additional challenges associated with exfoliative breast cytology stem from the fact that it is a subjective procedure often plagued by low reproducibility and poor inter-observer agreement, particularly with regard to the classification of atypical hyperplasia [58].

## Molecular Biomarkers in Lavage Fluid

Due to the relatively low yield of cytologic evaluation for breast cancer diagnosis, many groups have now focused on molecular biomarkers in ductal lavage fluid to identify characteristics specific to precancerous and cancerous lesions of the breast. Current studies analyzing genetic, epigenetic, and proteomic attributes of cells in ductal lavage fluid have suggested that biomarker analysis may be a more sensitive tool than cytology alone, because molecular biomarker changes often precede morphologic alterations and their detection might lead to earlier identification of breasts at risk for malignant change.

Some investigators have used fluorescence in situ hybridization (FISH) to detect genomic abnormalities by identifying aneusomy of chromosomes within ductal lavage cells, as changes in copy numbers of chromosomes 1, 8, 11, and 17 have been shown to be associated with both preinvasive and invasive breast lesions. King et al. [34] described aneusomy for these chromosomes in 71% of the specimens from malignant cases and in 11% from benign cases, for a sensitivity of 71% and specificity of 89%. Krishnamurthy et al. [59] evaluated the utility of using FISH as an adjunct to cytologic evaluation. They confirmed chromosomal aneuploidy in all of the malignant and markedly atypical cases, but found aneusomy in only one case described by cytology as mildly atypical. The authors concluded that FISH-based detection of chromosomal aneuploidy could potentially be used as an adjunct to cytologic evaluation in confirming both benign and malignant diagnoses. Adduci et al. [60] utilized array-based comparative genomic hybridization (CGH) in primary surgical specimens then tested matched ductal lavage specimens with region-specific FISH probes to determine whether similar chromosomal alterations were present in both specimens. Although only 11% of cytology samples were characterized as malignant, 55% of samples showed biomarker changes that were identical to those found in the primary surgical specimen. This study clearly demonstrated the increased sensitivity of molecular probes over cytology for detection of malignancy in ductal lavage samples.

Genomic and epigenomic markers have also been examined. Using quantitative fluorescence image analysis, Zhang et al. [61] evaluated lavage specimens from women with both benign and malignant findings and demonstrated 100% sensitivity in detecting cancer using DNA5cER and G-actin expression. Others have shown that evaluation of methylation may also have more sensitivity for cancer detection than cytology: Krassenstein et al. [62] used a panel of six loci to detect hypermethylation of CpG islands in matched tissue and nipple aspiration fluid samples. They detected hypermethylation in all of the malignant tissue and 82% of the fluid samples. Fackler et al. [63] utilized quantitative multiplex methylation-specific polymerase chain reaction (QM-PCR) to evaluate promoter methylation events in a panel of genes believed to be associated with increased breast cancer risk. In their evaluation of QM-PCR vs. cytologic evaluation, QM-PCR had double the rate of detection of cancer cells.

While many proteins [64, 65], carbohydrates [64–67], and hormones [64, 68] have been described in ductal fluid none have been validated in a way which allows them to be clinically useful. For this reason proteomic analyses using the surface-enhanced laser desorption and ionization-time of light/mass spectrometry (SELDI-TOF-MS) technique have been conducted on lavage fluid with success. Sauter et al. [69] prospectively collected nipple aspiration fluid from women scheduled for diagnostic breast biopsy and identified three protein peaks associated with the pathologic categories of atypical ductal hyperplasia, DCIS, and invasive disease. Pavlou et al. [70] reported more recently on an analysis of the whole proteome of NAF in women scheduled for breast biopsy. While 336 proteins were shared by women with and without cancer, there were 441 that were restricted to the women with cancer suggesting that NAF may well be able to predict cancer risk.

At this time, the overall utility of nipple fluid as a tool for risk assessment and early detection of breast cancer remains controversial. While the ability to access the fluid bathing the site of cancer initiation is tantalizing we still lack enough understanding of the physiology of ductal fluid to fully exploit its utility.

## Intraductal Therapy

Because as we have described most breast cancers arise from ductal epithelial cells in one lobe, enormous opportunities exist in targeting therapy directly into the ductal system. Additionally, intraductal therapy is less likely to cause systemic toxicity and adverse effects. Investigation of the role that the intraductal route may play in the treatment and prevention of breast cancer is in its infancy.

It has been shown that paclitaxel prevents tumor growth in the MNU-induced rat breast cancer model [71]. The bulk of the preclinical data, however, comes from Murata [72]. They demonstrated that intraductal pegylated liposomal doxorubicin (PLD) is associated with a potent protective effect both in the MNU-induced rat model and in the spontaneous Her2/neu transgenic mouse model. Results from the study demonstrated that not only was the intraductal administration of chemopreventive or chemotherapeutic drugs significantly more effective in preventing tumor development and promoting tumor regression, but there were also lower circulating levels of the agents and, as a result, no evidence of systemic toxicity. 4-hydroxytamoxifen was found to be as effective as subcutaneous tamoxifen in the prevention of tumors, and intraductal administration of PLD caused complete regression in 24 of 25 tumors with a tumor-free 3-month follow-up period. PLD was also found to be protective against tumor formation. Toxicity studies showed no myelosuppression and peak levels of drug were significantly lower for intraductal vs. intravenous injection. The preclinical research was expanded to determine the effects of intraductal administration of other anticancer agents, including 5-fluorouracil (5-FU), carboplatin, nanoparticle albumin-bound paclitaxel (nab-paclitaxel), and methotrexate, on treatment of early and established tumors in a chemically induced rat carcinogenesis model. They did not observe major systemic side effects in rats that were treated with the equivalent (5-FU) or higher doses of a clinical human dose (PLD, carboplatin, methotrexate, or nab-paclitaxel). Treatment with 5-FU was associated with the greatest antitumor effects among the five agents, as evidenced by the lowest number of neoplastic events and a low Ki-67 labeling index. The observed transient hair thinning in rats in response to intraductal 5-FU indicates that a systemic concentration is achieved, which may be explained by the agent's small molecular weight and short half-life. Further, intraductal 5-FU administered to four ducts resulted in protection of the remaining eight uninjected mammary glands from tumor development (72% tumor-free mammary glands), and with greater efficacy than that seen in rats after intravenous administration of 5-FU (51% tumor-free

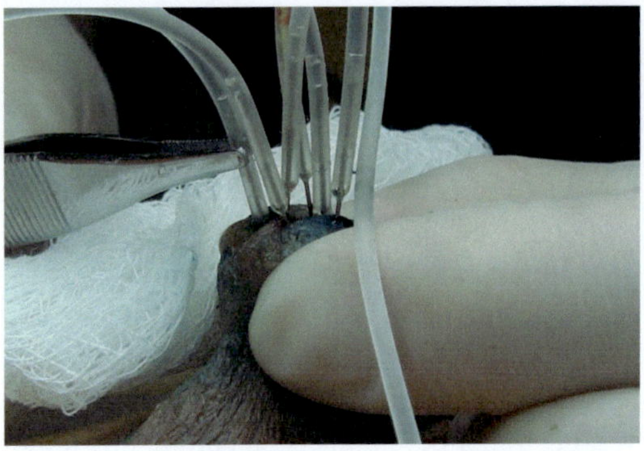

**Fig. 13.6** Cannulas in duct from multiple duct study

mammary glands). Thus, intraductal 5-FU was superior to intravenous 5-FU in preventing mammary tumorigenesis in the injected mammary glands and also showed efficacy in the uninjected glands in the same animal, implicating the participation of a systemic factor in tumor prevention with this particular agent.

These preclinical studies show that carboplatin, 5-FU, and PLD are suitable for further intraductal testing in clinical trials. At the same time, their clinical trial data with PLD support the feasibility of intraductal administration of agents. Stearns et al. demonstrated that administering PLD into one duct of women awaiting a mastectomy was safe and associated with minimal side effects. Nevertheless, the clinical trial is associated with several limitations and should be regarded as a proof-of-principle study. First, they evaluated only a few dose levels in a small number of women ($n = 17$). Second, they administered PLD once into one ductal system. Safety should be investigated with longer observation period in women who are awaiting mastectomy and lumpectomy or those at high risk who are considering prevention options.

Since the use of this approach for prevention would require instillation of the drug into the majority of ducts in a breast, Love et al. [73, 74] conducted a Phase I dose-escalation study in Beijing, China to determine safety and evaluate histopathologic response to either intraductal carboplatin or PLD instilled into 5–8 ducts in 31 women 2–7 days prior to mastectomy for breast cancer (Fig. 13.6). The procedure was done under local anesthesia with only mild breast discomfort during drug delivery. Three dose levels were used, with the highest level approaching the dose used intravenously. This total dose was divided among the cannulated ducts. Of note there was no attempt to determine whether a duct was intact or had been perforated during the procedure. Assuming our reported perforation rate of 7%, we assume that some of the drug may have extravasated. After planned mastectomy, the treated ducts were instilled with gelatin mixed with India ink for identification purposes (Fig. 13.7a). Nonetheless at the highest doses of PLD, patients experienced only tenderness, mild erythema and breast swelling, but no serious adverse events were noted. In the carboplatin group, both inflammatory responses and epithelial changes increased in a dose-dependent fashion. In the PLD group, no inflammatory changes were seen, but there was a marked increase of epithelial response to PLD treatment compared with the carboplatin-treated patients, including epithelial attenuation in the terminal ductal-lobular units (Fig. 13.8). A review of mastectomy specimens revealed that the drugs were distributed widely throughout the ductal systems and reached the TDLUs (Fig. 13.7b).

On the basis of this work Love and Mahoney [75] have tested intraductal PLD in the neo-adjuvant setting for DCIS. In patients with core biopsy-proven DCIS, the involved ductal orifice was cannulated and confirmed on ductogram prior to instilling 20 mg of PLD (10 $cm^3$) intraductally. The women were followed for 6-weeks before scheduled surgery. The study end points were regression of the lesion on surgical pathology, decreased markers in ductal fluid, and changes on MRI before and after treatment. The study was completed with 13 women receiving the full drug dose into the duct harboring DCIS, with two women reporting mild to moderate breast inflammatory reactions that responded to anti-inflammatory medications. Initial evaluation of histology of surgical specimens has confirmed a tissue response of inflammation, squamous metaplasia, and fat necrosis. Although women in this study underwent surgery, the long-term implications of the trial may be to facilitate future treat-

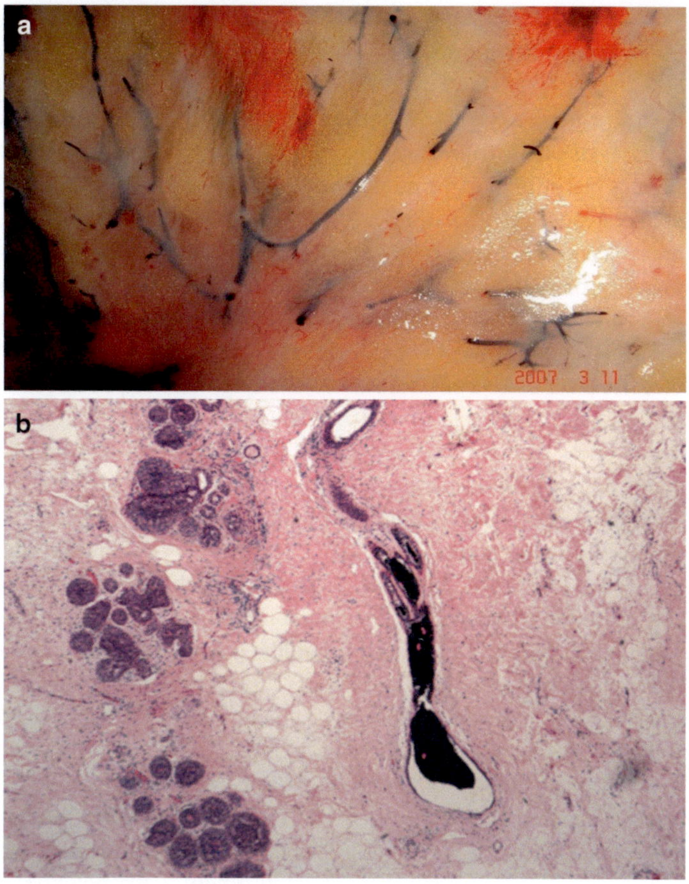


**Fig. 13.7** (**a**) Surgical specimen showing dye in treated ducts. (**b**) Dye in terminal ductal-lobular units of treated duct

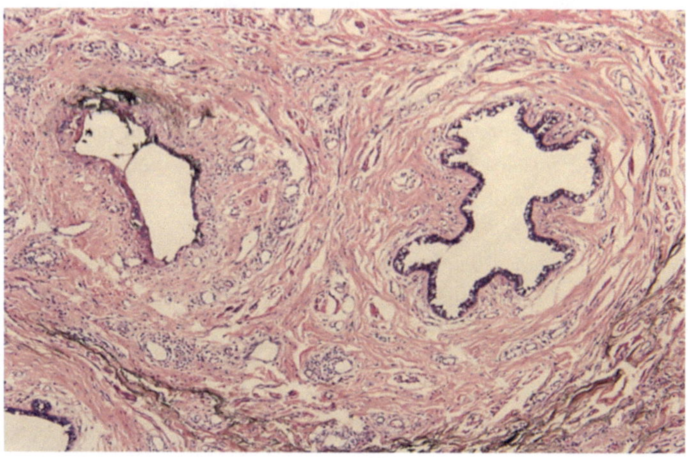

**Fig. 13.8** Treated duct

ment of DCIS with intraductal therapy alone. In addition, if this approach is effective in stripping cancer precursor cells from the ducts, intraductal injection of ablative agents in unaffected, high-risk women may allow for true loco-regional chemoprevention.

## Breast Cancer Etiology

If we are going to be able to prevent the majority of cases of breast cancer, it may well be time to refocus our efforts on the etiology of the disease. While genes and radiation are among known breast cancer causes, other etiologies for the majority of cases are still unknown. Infections and chronic inflammation have been linked to some cancers but studies of infectious causes of breast cancer have been limited to looking for specific viral signatures in invasive cancers. The breast ducts are intimately associated with cutaneous and oral microorganisms during lactation and sexual activity, and could well harbor infectious agents that contribute to carcinogenesis.

1936, Dr. John Joseph Bittner, a geneticist and cancer biologist working at the Jackson laboratory in Bar Harbor Maine, established the theory that a cancerous agent or "milk factor," could be transmitted by cancerous mothers to young mice from a virus in their mother's milk [76]. The majority of mammary tumors in mice are caused by mouse mammary tumor virus (MMTV); nonetheless evidence for viral etiologies of human breast cancer has been controversial. Interestingly, MMTV-like gene sequences have been identified in the human breast tumors, with 38% of breast cancer tissue from American women testing positive for MMTV-like genes [77–79]. In studies of Australian breast cancer patients, prevalence of MMTV-like genes correlated with severity of cancer, with invasive breast cancer tissues expressing higher levels of MMTV-like genes compared to noninvasive breast cancer tissues. Furthermore, MMTV-like genes were rarely found in normal breast tissue. Taken together, these data show that the presence of MMTV-like genes in breast tumors correlates with an invasive phenotype and provides evidence that a virus may be associated with human breast tumorigenesis [80].

DNA from human papillomavirus (HPV), most commonly associated with cervical cancer, has been detected by some groups in cancerous breast tissues [81–83]. However, others have failed to find a link between HPV infection and breast cancer [84, 85]. The ubiquitous human herpes virus Epstein-Barr virus (EBV) has varying presence in breast cancer cells. While some groups report identification of tumors with up to 50% EBV-positivity [86–88], other groups have failed to detect EBV in breast cancer tissues altogether [89, 90].

While none of this work is definitive it should not be dismissed since as the example of cancer of the cervix shows so well. The potential of a preventative vaccine based on an infectious cause remains a possibility and needs further exploration.

## Preventative Vaccines

With the increased knowledge regarding the immune system and the absence of a defined etiology of breast cancer there has been increased interest in developing a vaccine to either prevent breast cancer or treat the earliest stages. Most research has focused on therapeutic vaccines [91] aimed at eliciting an antigen-specific immune response against tumor antigens. Thus far the animal models have been more encouraging than the human studies. Two groups are focusing on the potential of various tumor antigens to elicit significant immunologic memory to prevent recurrence of cancer once it has been clinically removed. Disis [92] and Clive et al. [93] both tested a vaccine utilizing HER-2/neu peptides to explore the efficacy of the vaccine in killing tumor cells that express HER-2/neu. Disis and colleagues created a vaccine based on recombinant HER-2/neu intracellular domain protein in patients with HER-2/neu positive cancers [94]. Peoples et al. [95], used a HER-2/neu peptide derived from the protein's extracellular domain (E75-peptide vaccine) and tested the vaccine in node-positive and node-negative patients that were rendered disease-free after current therapies. This team [96] found that their HER-2/neu E75 peptide vaccine stimulates specific immunity in disease-free breast cancer patients, albeit the immunity wanes with time. A vaccine booster is safe and effective, with the greatest effect observed when given at 6 months after completion of the primary vaccination series.

While this work is interesting the ultimate goal is prevention all together. This has led to increasing interest, in moving to treatment of DCIS or prevention which could prove to be simpler and more effective. Proof of this concept has been demonstrated in animal models and work is ongoing to establish the validity in humans. A single vaccination with the antigen alpha-lactalbumin prevented breast cancer tumors from forming in mice [97]. Other researchers have focused on human mucin 1 (MUC1), a protein that is overexpressed in 90% of human breast cancers. Several studies have demonstrated the ability of MUC1-based vaccines to elicit an effective antitumor immune response in vivo and clinical trials are currently underway to determine if this response translates into prevention of tumor growth in humans [98].

Dr. Czerniecki and colleagues at the University of Pennsylvania are currently conducting a randomized phase I/II trial of HER-2/neu pulsed DC1 vaccine for patients with DCIS [87, 88, 99, 100]. This trial is studying the safety and efficacy of the vaccine in treating patients with DCIS who have not had any prior definitive treatment. Dr. Czerniecki's trial will shed light on the efficacy of a potential vaccine in patients whose immune systems have not been suppressed through prior conventional treatments.

These approaches while exciting, will require extensive testing in women to demonstrate both safety and efficacy.

## Major Challenge

In our focus on prevention of breast cancer and the work described in this chapter it is clear that a major challenge to progress is the limitation of our technology. The clinical community recognizes that most noninvasive disease will not progress and therefore does not need to be eradicated; however, the lack of an accurate method to monitor the extent and status of disease over time whether by imaging or a systemic marker has been a barrier to the adoption of less radical approaches. Mammography is limited to visualizing calcifications and MRI, while able to identify some DCIS, has not proved to be a good monitoring tool. As a result, watchful waiting has not been seriously tested nor have non-surgical approaches such as hormonal therapy, anti-HER2/neu approaches, vaccines or intraductal drug instillation been tried. The major barrier to less invasive approaches to preventing breast cancer or treating precancerous lesions has been our inability to assess the extent of disease, its malignant potential and its behavior over time.

The biggest challenge for the future is not new systemic approaches of chemoprevention but rather the *development of methods to actively monitor pre-cancerous disease progression. This will result in significant improvements in a patient's state-of-mind and reduce the cost of therapy in the long-term since the requirement for major surgery during the initial course of therapy will be significantly reduced and open the duct for a more scientific approach to the prevention of invasive breast cancer in all women at risk.*

## References


1. Wellings SR, Jensen HM, Marcum RG. An atlas of subgross pathology of the human breast with special reference to possible precancerous lesions. J Natl Cancer Inst. 1975;55(2):231–73.
2. Ewing J. Neoplastic diseases; a treatise on tumors. Philadelphia and London: W. B. Saunders company; 1940. 2p. l., 9–1054p.
3. Holland R, et al. Histologic multifocality of Tis, T1-2 breast carcinomas. Implications for clinical trials of breast-conserving surgery. Cancer. 1985; 56(5):979–90.
4. Mai KT, et al. Pattern of distribution of intraductal and infiltrating ductal carcinoma: a three-dimensional study using serial coronal giant sections of the breast. Hum Pathol. 2000;31(4):464–74.
5. Teboul M, Halliwell M. Atlas of ultrasound and ductal echography of the breast: the introduction of anatomic intelligence into breast imaging. Oxford, United Kingdom: Blackwell Science; 1995.
6. Tot T. DCIS, cytokeratins, and the theory of the sick lobe. Virchows Arch. 2005;447(1):1–8.
7. Lakhani SR, et al. Atypical ductal hyperplasia of the breast: clonal proliferation with loss of heterozygosity on chromosomes 16q and 17p. J Clin Pathol. 1995;48(7):611–5.
8. Lakhani SR, et al. Loss of heterozygosity in lobular carcinoma in situ of the breast. Clin Mol Pathol. 1995;48(2):M74–8.

9. Deng G, et al. Loss of heterozygosity in normal tissue adjacent to breast carcinomas. Science. 1996;274(5295):2057–9.
10. Larson PS, et al. Genetically abnormal clones in histologically normal breast tissue. Am J Pathol. 1998;152(6):1591–8.
11. Cavalli LR, et al. Loss of heterozygosity in normal breast epithelial tissue and benign breast lesions in BRCA1/2 carriers with breast cancer. Cancer Genet Cytogenet. 2004;149(1):38–43.
12. Clarke CL, et al. Mapping loss of heterozygosity in normal human breast cells from BRCA1/2 carriers. Br J Cancer. 2006;95(4):515–9.
13. Kurose K, et al. Genetic model of multi-step breast carcinogenesis involving the epithelium and stroma: clues to tumour-microenvironment interactions. Hum Mol Genet. 2001;10(18):1907–13.
14. Tsai YC, et al. Contiguous patches of normal human mammary epithelium derived from a single stem cell: implications for breast carcinogenesis. Cancer Res. 1996;56(2):402–4.
15. Hildreth NG, Shore RE, Dvoretsky PM. The risk of breast cancer after irradiation of the thymus in infancy. N Engl J Med. 1989;321(19):1281–4.
16. Lundell M, et al. Breast cancer risk after radiotherapy in infancy: a pooled analysis of two Swedish cohorts of 17,202 infants. Radiat Res. 1999;151(5):626–32.
17. Modan B, et al. Increased risk of breast cancer after low-dose irradiation. Lancet. 1989;1(8639):629–31.
18. Myrden JA, Hiltz JE. Breast cancer following multiple fluoroscopies during artificial pneumothorax treatment of pulmonary tuberculosis. Can Med Assoc J. 1969;100(22):1032–4.
19. Miller AB, et al. Mortality from breast cancer after irradiation during fluoroscopic examinations in patients being treated for tuberculosis. N Engl J Med. 1989;321(19):1285–9.
20. Tokunaga M, et al. Incidence of female breast cancer among atomic bomb survivors, 1950–1985. Radiat Res. 1994;138(2):209–23.
21. Diallo R, et al. Monoclonality in normal epithelium and in hyperplastic and neoplastic lesions of the breast. J Pathol. 2001;193(1):27–32.
22. Goldstein NS, Kestin LL, Vicini FA. Monomorphic epithelial proliferations of the breast: a possible precursor lesion associated with ipsilateral breast failure after breast conserving therapy in patients with negative lumpectomy margins. Int J Radiat Oncol Biol Phys. 2011;79(3):818–22.
23. Cooper A. The anatomy and diseases of the breast. Philadelphia: Lea and Blanchard; 1845. p. 74–119.
24. Love SM, Barsky SH. Anatomy of the nipple and breast ducts revisited. Cancer. 2004;101(9):1947–57.
25. Ramsay DT, et al. Anatomy of the lactating human breast redefined with ultrasound imaging. J Anat. 2005;206(6):525–34.
26. Going JJ, Moffat DF. Escaping from Flatland: clinical and biological aspects of human mammary duct anatomy in three dimensions. J Pathol. 2004;203(1):538–44.
27. Moffat DF, Going JJ. Three dimensional anatomy of complete duct systems in human breast: pathological and developmental implications. J Clin Pathol. 1996;49(1):48–52.
28. Ohtake T, et al. Computer-assisted complete three-dimensional reconstruction of the mammary ductal/lobular systems: implications of ductal anastomoses for breast-conserving surgery. Cancer. 2001;91(12):2263–72.
29. Taneri F, et al. Microanatomy of milk ducts in the nipple. Eur Surg Res. 2006;38(6):545–9.
30. Rusby JE, et al. Breast duct anatomy in the human nipple: three-dimensional patterns and clinical implications. Breast Cancer Res Treat. 2007;106(2):171–9.
31. Dietz JR, et al. Directed duct excision by using mammary ductoscopy in patients with pathologic nipple discharge. Surgery. 2002;132(4):582–7; discussion 587–8.
32. Going JJ, Mohun TJ. Human breast duct anatomy, the 'sick lobe' hypothesis and intraductal approaches to breast cancer. Breast Cancer Res Treat. 2006;97(3):285–91.
33. Phillips HA, Howard GC, Miller WR. Nipple aspirate fluid in relation to breast cancer. Breast. 1999;8(4):169–74.
34. King BL, Tsai SC, Gryga ME, et al. Detection of chromosomal instability in paired breast surgery and ductal lavage specimens by interphase fluorescence in situ hybridization. Clin Cancer Res. 2003;9:1509–1516.
35. Mitchell G, et al. Nipple aspiration and ductal lavage in women with a germline BRCA1 or BRCA2 mutation. Breast Cancer Res. 2005;7(6):R1122.
36. Sanchez LM, et al. Identification of the major protein components in breast secretions from women with benign and malignant breast diseases. Cancer Res. 1992;52(1):95–100.
37. Leborgne RA. The breast in Roentgen diagnosis. Montevideo, Uruguay: Impresora Uruguaya SA—Juncal 1511; 1953. p. 14–17.
38. Sartorius OW, et al. Cytologic evaluation of breast fluid in the detection of breast disease. J Natl Cancer Inst. 1977;59(4):1073–80.
39. Dooley WC, et al. Ductal lavage for detection of cellular atypia in women at high risk for breast cancer. J Natl Cancer Inst. 2001;93(21):1624–32.
40. Brogi E, et al. Ductal lavage in patients undergoing mastectomy for mammary carcinoma. Cancer. 2003;98(10):2170–6.
41. Khan SA, et al. Ductal lavage findings in women with known breast cancer undergoing mastectomy. J Natl Cancer Inst. 2004;96(20):1510–7.
42. Kurian AW. Ductal lavage of fluid-yielding and non-fluid-yielding ducts in BRCA1 and BRCA2 mutation carriers and other women at high inherited breast cancer risk. Cancer Epidemiol Biomarkers Prev. 2005;14(5):1082–9.
43. Bhandare D. Endocrine biomarkers in ductal lavage samples from women at high risk for breast cancer.

Cancer Epidemiol Biomarkers Prev. 2005;14(11): 2620–7.

44. Maddux A, et al. Patient and duct selection for nipple duct lavage. Am J Surg. 2004;188(4):390–4.
45. Wood ME, et al. Ductal lavage of cancerous and unaffected breasts: procedure success rate and cancer detection. Acta Cytol. 2009;53(4):410–5.
46. Khan SA, et al. Ductal lavage findings in women with mammographic microcalcifications undergoing biopsy. Ann Surg Oncol. 2005;12(9):689–96.
47. Tondre J, et al. Technical enhancements to breast ductal lavage. Ann Surg Oncol. 2008;15(10): 2734–8.
48. Bender Ö, et al. Scarless endoscopic papillomectomy of the breast. Onkologie. 2009;32(3):94–8.
49. Kapenhas-Valdes E, et al. Mammary ductoscopy for evaluation of nipple discharge. Ann Surg Oncol. 2008;15(10):2720–7.
50. Dooley W. Ductoscopy technique—using ductoscopy anatomically direct breast conservation surgery. 6th International Symposium on the Intraductal Approach to Breast Cancer. Santa Monica, CA. BMC Proc. 2009;3(Suppl 5):S16.
51. Dupont WD, Page DL. Risk factors for breast cancer in women with proliferative breast disease. N Engl J Med. 1985;312(3):146–51.
52. Dupont WD, et al. Breast cancer risk associated with proliferative breast disease and atypical hyperplasia. Cancer. 1993;71(4):1258–65.
53. Wrensch MR, et al. Breast cancer incidence in women with abnormal cytology in nipple aspirates of breast fluid. Am J Epidemiol. 1992;135(2): 130–41.
54. Wrensch MR, et al. Breast cancer risk in women with abnormal cytology in nipple aspirates of breast fluid. J Natl Cancer Inst. 2001;93(23):1791–8.
55. Fabian CJ, et al. Short-term breast cancer prediction by random periareolar fine-needle aspiration cytology and the Gail risk model. J Natl Cancer Inst. 2000;92(15):1217–27.
56. Cyr AE, et al. Correlation of ductal lavage cytology with ductoscopy-directed duct excision histology in women at high risk for developing breast cancer: a prospective, single-institution trial. Ann Surg Oncol. 2011;18(11):3192–7.
57. Page DL, et al. Atypical hyperplastic lesions of the female breast. A long-term follow-up study. Cancer. 1985;55(11):2698–708.
58. Johnson-Maddux A, et al. Reproducibility of cytologic atypia in repeat nipple duct lavage. Cancer. 2005;103(6):1129–36.
59. Krishnamurthy S, et al. Feasibility and utility of using chromosomal aneusomy to further define the cytologic categories in nipple aspirate fluid specimens: a preliminary study. Cancer. 2004;102(5): 322–7.
60. Adduci KM, et al. Fluorescence in situ hybridization of ductal lavage samples identifies malignant phenotypes from cytologically normal cells in women with breast cancer. Cancer. 2007;111(3):185–91.
61. Zhang W, et al. Biomarker analysis on breast ductal lavage cells in women with and without breast cancer. Int J Cancer. 2006;119(2):359–64.
62. Krassenstein R, et al. Detection of breast cancer in nipple aspirate fluid by CpG island hypermethylation. Clin Cancer Res. 2004;10(1 Pt 1):28–32.
63. Fackler MJ, et al. Quantitative multiplex methylation-specific PCR analysis doubles detection of tumor cells in breast ductal fluid. Clin Cancer Res. 2006;12(11 Pt 1):3306–10.
64. King BL, Love SM. The intraductal approach to the breast: raison d'être. Breast Cancer Res. 2006;8(2): 206.
65. Sauter E, et al. Biologic markers of breast cancer in nipple aspirate fluid and nipple discharge are associated with clinical findings. Cancer Detect Prev. 2007;31(1):50–8.
66. Qin W, et al. Proteins and carbohydrates in nipple aspirate fluid predict the presence of atypia and cancer in women requiring diagnostic breast biopsy. BMC Cancer. 2012;12(1):52.
67. Deutscher SL, et al. Carbohydrate antigens in nipple aspirate fluid predict the presence of atypia and cancer in women requiring diagnostic breast biopsy. BMC Cancer. 2010;10(1):519.
68. Chatterton RT, et al. Patterns of sex steroid hormones in nipple aspirate fluid during the menstrual cycle and after menopause in relation to serum concentrations. Cancer Epidemiol Biomarkers Prev. 2010; 19(1):275–9.
69. Sauter ER, et al. Proteomic analysis of nipple aspirate fluid using SELDI-TOF-MS. Int J Cancer. 2005;114(5):791–6.
70. Pavlou MP, et al. Nipple aspirate fluid proteome of healthy females and patients with breast cancer. Clin Chem. 2010;56(5):848–55.
71. Okugawa H, et al. Effect of perductal paclitaxel exposure on the development of MNU-induced mammary carcinoma in female S-D rats. Breast Cancer Res Treat. 2005;91(1):29–34.
72. Murata S. Ductal access for prevention and therapy of mammary tumors. Cancer Res. 2006;66(2):638–45.
73. Love SM, et al. Local drug delivery to the breast: a phase 1 study of breast cytotoxic agent administration prior to mastectomy. BMC Proc. 2009;3 Suppl 5:S29.
74. Rao J, et al. Histopathological responses to a short term intraductal cytotoxic agent treatment: results of a feasibility study. BMC Proc. 2009;3 Suppl 5:S30.
75. Mahoney M, Mills D, Love S. Intraductal therapy of DCIS with liposomal doxorubicin: a preoperative trial in rural California. BMC Proc. 2009;3 Suppl 5:S31.
76. Bittner JJ. Some possible effects of nursing on the mammary gland tumor incidence in mice. Science. 1936;84(2172):162.
77. Etkind P, et al. Mouse mammary tumor virus-like ENV gene sequences in human breast tumors and in a lymphoma of a breast cancer patient. Clin Cancer Res. 2000;6(4):1273–8.

78. Wang Y, et al. Expression of mouse mammary tumor virus-like ENV gene sequences in human breast cancer. Clin Cancer Res. 1998;4(10):2565–8.
79. Wang Y, Holland JF, Bleiweiss IJ. Detection of mammary tumor virus ENV gene-like sequences in human breast cancer. Cancer Res. 1995;55(22): 5173–9.
80. Ford CE, Faedo M, Rawlinson WD. Mouse mammary tumor virus-like RNA transcripts and DNA are found in affected cells of human breast cancer. Clin Cancer Res. 2004;10(21):7284–9.
81. Akil N, et al. High-risk human papillomavirus infections in breast cancer in Syrian women and their association with Id-1 expression: a tissue microarray study. Br J Cancer. 2008;99(3):404–7.
82. Heng B, et al. Human papilloma virus is associated with breast cancer. Br J Cancer. 2009;101(8): 1345–50.
83. Kroupis C, et al. Presence of high-risk human papillomavirus sequences in breast cancer tissues and association with histopathological characteristics. Clin Biochem. 2006;39(7):727–31.
84. Gopalkrishna V, et al. Absence of human papillomavirus DNA in breast cancer as revealed by polymerase chain reaction. Breast Cancer Res Treat. 1996;39(2):197–202.
85. Lindel K, et al. Breast cancer and human papillomavirus (HPV) infection: no evidence of a viral etiology in a group of Swiss women. Breast. 2007;16(2):172–7.
86. Bonnet M, et al. Detection of Epstein-Barr virus in invasive breast cancers. J Natl Cancer Inst. 1999;91(16):1376–81.
87. Luqmani Y, Shousha S. Presence of epstein-barr-virus in breast-carcinoma. Int J Oncol. 1995;6(4):899–903.
88. McCall SA, et al. Epstein-Barr virus detection in ductal carcinoma of the breast. J Natl Cancer Inst. 2001;93(2):148–50.
89. Lespagnard L, et al. Absence of Epstein-Barr virus in medullary carcinoma of the breast as demonstrated by immunophenotyping, in situ hybridization and polymerase chain reaction. Am J Clin Pathol. 1995;103(4):449–52.
90. Glaser SL, et al. Absence of Epstein-Barr virus EBER-1 transcripts in an epidemiologically diverse group of breast cancers. Int J Cancer. 1998;75(4): 555–8.
91. Mittendorf EA, Peoples GE, Singletary SE. Breast cancer vaccines: promise for the future or pipe dream? Cancer. 2007;110(8):1677–86.
92. Disis ML. The ultimate in cancer chemoprevention: cancer vaccines. Cancer Prev Res (Phila). 2010;3(4):406–9.
93. Clive KS, et al. The GP2 peptide: a HER2/neu-based breast cancer vaccine. J Surg Oncol. 2012;105(5): 452–8.
94. Disis ML, Salazar LG, Knutson KL. Peptide-based vaccines in breast cancer. Breast Dis. 2004;20: 3–11.
95. Peoples GE, et al. Clinical trial results of a HER2/neu (E75) vaccine to prevent recurrence in high-risk breast cancer patients. J Clin Oncol. 2005;23(30): 7536–45.
96. Mittendorf EA, et al. Clinical trial results of the HER-2/neu (E75) vaccine to prevent breast cancer recurrence in high-risk patients: from US Military Cancer Institute Clinical Trials Group Study I-01 and I-02. Cancer. 2012;118(10):2594–602.
97. Jaini R, et al. An autoimmune-mediated strategy for prophylactic breast cancer vaccination. Nat Med. 2010;16(7):799–803.
98. Yuan S, et al. MUC1-based recombinant Bacillus Calmette-Guerin vaccines as candidates for breast cancer immunotherapy. Expert Opin Biol Ther. 2010;10(7):1037–48.
99. Czerniecki BJ, Roses RE, Koski GK. Development of vaccines for high-risk ductal carcinoma in situ of the breast. Cancer Res. 2007;67(14):6531–4.
100. Sharma A, et al. HER-2 pulsed dendritic cell vaccine can eliminate HER-2 expression and impact ductal carcinoma in situ. Cancer. 2012;118:4354–62.

# Index




N.M. Hansen (ed.), *Management of the Patient at High Risk for Breast Cancer*,
DOI 10.1007/978-1-4614-5891-3, © Springer Science+Business Media New York 2013

MIX
Papier aus verantwortungsvollen Quellen
Paper from responsible sources
FSC® C105338

If you have any concerns about our products,
you can contact us on
**ProductSafety@springernature.com**

In case Publisher is established outside the EU,
the EU authorized representative is:
**Springer Nature Customer Service Center GmbH**
**Europaplatz 3, 69115 Heidelberg, Germany**

Printed by Libri Plureos GmbH
in Hamburg, Germany